Comprehensive Multiple-Choice Questions in Pathology

Vinay Kumar Kohli • Chitra Kohli
Akanksha Singh

Comprehensive Multiple-Choice Questions in Pathology

A Study Guide

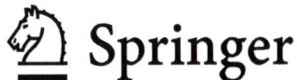 Springer

Vinay Kumar Kohli
MCI Diagnostic Center, LLC
Dallas, TX, USA

Chitra Kohli
Dallas, TX, USA

Akanksha Singh
Department of Pathology
King George's Medical University
Lucknow, India

ISBN 978-3-031-08766-0   ISBN 978-3-031-08767-7   (eBook)
https://doi.org/10.1007/978-3-031-08767-7

This Springer imprint is published by the registered company Springer Nature Switzerland AG
The registered company address is: Gewerbestrasse 11, 6330 Cham, Switzerland

To our mothers, who taught us read and write.
—Vinay Kohli
—Chitra Kohli

Preface

To succeed in pathology academic and competitive examinations, which need a strong base of pathology content and to become an excellent physician, requires one to know and master the basic concepts of pathology. The skills needed to deal with different aspects of pathology, one of the most challenging subjects in medical schools, can be achieved by reading a very concise, to-the-point, and up-to-date text, which covers all topics in a nice summarized and systematic manner. This book contains high-yield questions with short answers, gross and microscopic pictures to cover all aspects to help students achieve high scores. We hope this book will meet the expectations of medical students, postgraduate students of pathology, and candidates appearing for different entrance and licensing examinations. This book will provide all the essential material in brief and clearly expressed and will save a lot of precious time of the medical students. The book contains around 650 questions with detailed answers, which will give students the opportunity to delve further into the topic.

This book is being supported from day one by Mr. Sayeed Khan with his two decades of experience in publication of medical books and by the technical expertise of Mr. Javed Ahmad.

Dallas, TX, USA   Vinay Kumar Kohli
Dallas, TX, USA   Chitra Kohli

Contents

Cellular Pathology, Inflammation, and Repair

1

Multiple Choice Questions

1. Programmed cell death is also called as:
   A. Degeneration
   B. Calcification
   C. Apoptosis
   D. Necrosis
   E. Atrophy
2. Which of the following medical condition is because of inherited defect in DNA repair?
   A. Acanthosis nigricans
   B. Xeroderma pigmentosum
   C. Basal cell nevus syndrome
   D. Bloom syndrome
   E. Werner syndrome
3. Which of the following is a pathologic cause of hyperplasia?
   A. Endometrial hyperplasia
   B. Compensatory hyperplasia after partial hepatectomy
   C. Hormonal stimulation seen in breast development at puberty
   D. Antigenic stimulation seen in lymphoid hyperplasia
   E. Cardiac muscle in hypertension
4. In pathology, what is the name given when there is a reversible change of one cell type to another?
   A. Hyperplasia
   B. Hypertrophy
   C. Metaplasia
   D. Dysplasia
   E. Atrophy
5. Which of the following is the best statement for lipofuscin?
   A. Perinuclear yellow-brown pigment
   B. Black-brown pigment
   C. Golden yellow-brown granular pigment
   D. Protein
   E. Lipid

6. Location of calcifications in interstitial tissues of the stomach, kidneys, lungs, and blood vessels is called as:
   A. Metastatic calcification.
   B. Dystrophic calcification
   C. Hyaline change
   D. Cutaneous mycetoma
   E. Molluscum contagiosum
7. Psammoma bodies belong to which type of pathologic form of calcification?
   A. Dystrophic calcification
   B. Metastatic calcification
   C. Calcifications in interstitial tissues of the stomach
   D. Calcifications in the kidney
   E. Calcifications in the blood vessels
8. A 49-year-old woman has hypertension untreated for years. Which of the following cellular alteration will be seen in the myocardium of this patient?
   A. Apoptosis
   B. Atrophy
   C. Hyperplasia
   D. Metaplasia
   E. Hypertrophy
9. In pathology, what is the name given to abnormal proliferation of cells that is characterized by changes in cell size, shape, and loss of cellular organization?
   A. Hyperplasia
   B. Hypertrophy
   C. Metaplasia
   D. Dysplasia
   E. Atrophy
10. Which type of necrosis is most characteristic of ischemia involving the heart or kidney?
    A. Coagulative
    B. Liquefactive
    C. Caseous
    D. Fibrinoid
    E. Enzymatic

© The Author(s), under exclusive license to Springer Nature Switzerland AG 2022
V. K. Kohli et al., *Comprehensive Multiple-Choice Questions in Pathology*, https://doi.org/10.1007/978-3-031-08767-7_1

11. Apoptosis is an active process regulated by genes and involves RNA and protein synthesis. Which of the following is a central organ in apoptosis?
    A. Ribosomes
    B. Golgi body
    C. Mitochondria
    D. Nucleus
    E. Lysosomes

12. Irreversible, uncontrolled cell death that occurs when antigen-antibody complexes are deposited in the walls of blood vessels along with fibrin is called as:
    A. Gangrenous necrosis
    B. Fat necrosis
    C. Fibrinoid necrosis
    D. Caseous necrosis
    E. Liquefaction necrosis

13. Which of the following organ shows liquefaction necrosis?
    A. Heart
    B. Brain
    C. Gall bladder
    D. Liver
    E. Kidney

14. Degeneration and condensation of nuclear chromatin is defined as:
    A. Karyorrhexis
    B. Karyolysis
    C. Nuclear fusion
    D. Nuclear fission
    E. Pyknosis

15. In tumor metastasis, cancer cells spread from the place where they first formed to another part of the body. What is essential for tumor metastasis?
    A. Apoptosis
    B. Inhibition of tyrosine kinase activity
    C. Angiogenesis
    D. Tumorigenesis
    E. Ischemia

16. A 10-year-old male child suffering from thalassemia comes to the pediatrician office for follow up checkup. On physical examination the skin of the patient has a bronze color. Which of the following findings will be seen in liver biopsy of this male child?
    A. Apoptotic hepatocytes
    B. Hepatocyte swelling
    C. Hepatocyte regeneration
    D. Hemosiderin in hepatocytes
    E. Cholestasis

17. Decrease in cell size and functional ability is defined as:
    A. Atrophy
    B. Apoptosis
    C. Hypertrophy
    D. Hyperplasia
    E. Metaplasia

18. Walerian degeneration is seen in:
    A. Part of nerve attached to cell body in a nerve that is cut peripherally
    B. Cell body that is not attached to the nerve that is cut
    C. Part of nerve not attached to cell body
    D. Cell body that is attached to the nerve that is cut
    E. It is not a type of nerve injury

19. Granuloma is characterized by-
    A. Focal accumulation of activated macrophages
    B. Collection of neutrophils
    C. Newly formed vessels
    D. Collection of eosinophils
    E. Collection of basophils

20. Marked mitochondrial dysfunction, mitochondrial swelling and large densities within the mitochondrial matrix are seen in which type of cell injury?
    A. Cell death
    B. Irreversible cell injury
    C. Reversible cell injury
    D. Necrosis
    E. Apoptosis

21. To which of the following family of chemical mediators of inflammation, lipoxins belong?
    A. Chemokines
    B. Arachidonic acid metabolites
    C. Kinin system
    D. Cytokines
    E. Vasoactive amines

22. Enzyme responsible for respiratory burst is?
    A. Peroxidase
    B. Catalase
    C. NADPH oxidase
    D. Dehydrogenase
    E. Lysozyme

23. Procalcitonin is considered as a marker for?
    A. Sepsis
    B. Medullary carcinoma of thyroid
    C. Vitamin D resistant rickets
    D. Parathyroid adenoma
    E. Hyperthyroidism

24. A 92-year-old man presents to his health care provider with a history of mild dementia, osteoarthritis, emphysema, cataract, and hypertension. What is the most likely diagnosis?
    A. Hypovitaminosis E
    B. Werner syndrome
    C. Natural aging
    D. Progeria (Hutchinson-Gilford syndrome)
    E. Alzheimer's disease

25. What cellular adaptation has occurred in this tissue shown below?

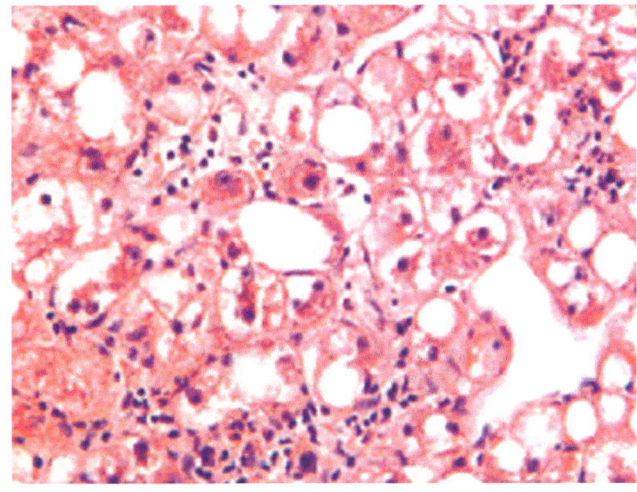

    A. Metaplasia
    B. Hyperplasia
    C. Fatty change
    D. Hypertrophy
    E. Atrophy

26. Which of the following disorder is more likely to be associated with an exudate rather than a transudate?
    A. Congestive heart failure
    B. Inflammation
    C. Nephrotic syndrome
    D. Chronic liver disease
    E. Diabetes mellitus

27. In acute inflammation hemodynamic changes like massive vasodilation are mediated by which of the following chemicals?
    A. Histamine
    B. Bradykinin
    C. Prostaglandins
    D. Histamine, bradykinin, and prostaglandins
    E. Histamine and bradykinin

28. Inflammation is associated with which of the following cytokines?
    A. Cytokines (IL-1)
    B. Cytokines (IL-6)
    C. Tumor necrosis factor-alpha
    D. IL-1, IL-6, and tumor necrosis factor-alpha
    E. Prostacyclin (PGI$_2$)

29. Cytokines IL-8 is produced by which cell?
    A. Neutrophil
    B. Macrophage
    C. Lymphocyte
    D. Eosinophil
    E. Basophil

30. Kupffer cells are found in which system?
    A. Connective tissue
    B. Lung
    C. Liver
    D. Bone
    E. Brain

31. Which of the mitochondrial enzyme that activates caspases and indirectly brings about cell death through intrinsic pathway apoptosis?
    A. Cytochrome c
    B. Monoamine oxidase
    C. Fatty acid CoA ligase
    D. Cytochrome c-reductase
    E. Rotenone-insensitive

32. Virulent organism producing severe tissue damage and extensive cell death is defined as:
    A. Exudative inflammation
    B. Necrotizing inflammation
    C. Granulomatous inflammation
    D. Interstitial inflammation
    E. Cytopathic inflammation

33. Which of the following is a major chemotactic factor for lung macrophages?
    A. CXCL17
    B. N-formylmethionine
    C. Leukotriene B4
    D. Complement system produce C5a
    E. α-Chemokines

34. Which of the following cell plays an important role in parasitic infections?
    A. Neutrophil
    B. Macrophage
    C. Lymphocyte
    D. Eosinophil
    E. Basophil

35. What is the effect of bradykinin?
    A. Pain
    B. Bronchodilation
    C. Vasoconstriction
    D. Decrease vascular permeability
    E. Platelet aggregation

36. What are the mediators of fever?
    A. Cytokines IL-1
    B. Leukotriene B4
    C. Leukotriene C4
    D. Prostacyclin
    E. Thromboxane A2

37. Which of the following cytokine is involved in the pathogenesis of Castleman disease?
    A. IL-2
    B. IL-4
    C. IL-6

D. IL-10

E. IL-5

38. Which of the following important mediators in asthma?

A. Cytokines IL-4, IL-5, and IL-13

B. Interleukin-7 (IL-7)

C. Interleukin-1 (IL-1)

D. Interleukin-6 (IL-6)

E. Interleukin-8 (IL-8)

Answers and Explanations

1. Answer: C. Apoptosis

   Apoptosis is a complex type of programmed cell death. Apoptosis is an active gene regulated process, involving RNA and protein synthesis. It often only affects single cells or small cell groups. Morphologically, cells shrink in size and have dense eosinophilic cytoplasm. There is a condensation of nuclear chromatin followed by fragmentation. There is a cell breakdown into fragments (apoptotic bodies). The conservation of plasma membrane integrity is a key feature of this physiological death process. Apoptosis lack an inflammatory reaction by inducing certain cytokines and producing regulatory T cells. The Bcl-2 oncoprotein inhibits apoptosis and p53 stimulates apoptosis. Embryogenesis and menstrual cycle are physiological manifestations of apoptosis. Sources of pathological apoptosis include viral hepatitis (councilman bodies), graft versus host disease (GvHD), and cystic fibrosis.

2. Answer: B. Xeroderma pigmentosum

   Xeroderma pigmentosum (XP) is a rare disorder that has an increased sensitivity to ultraviolet radiation (UVR). There is an early onset of changes in skin and mucous membrane cancers associated with UVR. Many patients may experience progressive neurodegeneration. Patients with xeroderma pigmentosum are unable to repair the damage DNA. There is an increased risk for skin cancers (SCC, melanoma, and BCC). It is inherited as an autosomal recessive disorder.

3. Answer: A. Endometrial hyperplasia

   Hyperplasia is an increase in the number of cells in a tissue or organ. Physiological causes of hyperplasia are compensatory (after partial hepatectomy), hormonal stimulation (puberty breast development), and antigenic stimulation (lymphoid hyperplasia). Endometrial hyperplasia, benign prostate hyperplasia are pathological causes of hyperplasia. Endometrial hyperplasia usually occurs due to prolonged unopposed action of estrogen on endometrial tissue. Hyperplasia is mediated by cytokines and growth factors. There is an increased expression of growth promoting genes.

4. Answer: C. Metaplasia

   Metaplasia is a reversible change which replaces one type of adult cell with another. It usually occurs in response to irritation. Barrett esophagus exhibits an abnormal (metaplastic) change (normal stratified squamous epithelium to columnar epithelium). Another example of metaplasia is bronchial squamous metaplasia induced by smoking. It also happens when two distinct epithelial tissues cross (e.g., uterine cervix squamocolumnar junction).

5. Answer: A. Perinuclear yellow-brown pigment

   Lipofuscin is a yellow-brown aging pigment. It is commonly seen in the liver and heart. Lipofuscin accumulates in age accumulating hepatocytes, and is also seen in young patients with severe malnutrition, showing an appearance described as "brown atrophy." It is seen in postmitotic cells, such as neurons. For the age of cells including neurons, the fate of postmitotic cells to produce lipofuscin (aging pigment), and is considered a reliable biomarker.

6. Answer: A. Metastatic calcification

   The metastatic calcification is calcium phosphate accumulation due to hypercalcemia in normal tissue. Hyperparathyroidism, chronic renal failure, parathyroid adenomas, paraneoplastic syndrome, vitamin D intoxication, and metastatic cancer to the bone are the most common causes.

7. Answer: A. Dystrophic calcification

   Dystrophic calcification is calcium phosphate deposition in either dying or necrotic tissues. Fat necrosis, psammoma bodies, Monckeberg medial calcific sclerosis, and atherosclerotic plaques are common examples of dystrophic calcification. Psammoma bodies are commonly found as laminated calcifications in meningiomas and papillary carcinomas of the thyroid.

8. Answer: E. Hypertrophy

   Hypertrophy refers to an increase in cell size that leads to an increase in organ size. The hypertrophied organ lacks any new cells, only bigger ones. Physiological causes of hypertrophy are weightlifters striated muscles. Left ventricular hypertrophy (LVH) in hypertension is an example of pathological hypertrophy. Hypertrophy is mediated by cytokines and growth factors.

9. Answer: D. Dysplasia

   Dysplasia is an irregular cell proliferation characterized by changes in cell size, shape, and loss of cell organization. Dysplasia commonly is neoplastic. Common example is cervical dysplasia.

10. Answer: A. Coagulative

    Coagulative necrosis is the most common form of necrosis caused by ischemia or infarction. Light microscopy shows cellular preservation with the loss of the nucleus. It is commonly seen in heart, liver, and kidney.

11. Answer: C. Mitochondria

Mitochondria is a central component of apoptosis (programmed cell death), which is regularly used to rid the body of cells that are no longer useful or properly function.

12. Answer: C. Fibrinoid necrosis

Fibrinoid necrosis is necrotic tissue. Light microscopy shows fibrin accumulation within the blood vessels. It is a cell death pattern due to endothelial damage and plasma protein exudation. Fibrinoid necrosis is usually seen in malignant hypertension.

13. Answer: B. Brain

Hydrolytic enzymes cause cell destruction leading to liquefactive necrosis. This is seen in the brain after ischemic damage. The release of digestive enzymes and neutrophil constituents is the reason for liquefaction in infections. Microscopically, there are multiple neutrophils and inflammatory cells.

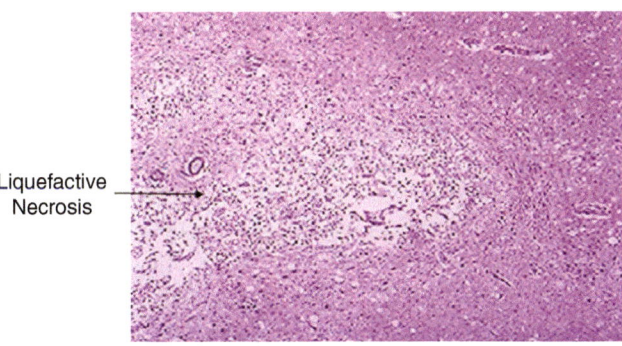

Liquefactive Necrosis

14. Answer: E. Pyknosis

Pyknosis is an irreversible condensation of chromatin and the nucleus. The common causes are apoptotic and necrotic cells. The nucleus undergoes condensation in apoptotic, resulting in fragmentation into large clumps of chromatin. Finally, these clumps of chromatin are stuffed into apoptotic bodies. Nuclei condense into smaller clumps of chromatin in necrotic cells that are usually dissolved later.

15. Answer: C. Angiogenesis

Angiogenesis is a process not only for the preservation of primary tumor ecosystems, but also for the development of new secondary tumor ecosystems at metastasized areas as well as for the invasion and propagation of tumor cells. A strong angiogenic factor is the vascular endothelial growth factor (VEGF). In many tumors, VEGF is upregulated and its tumor angiogenesis role is well known.

16. Answer: D. Hemosiderin in hepatocytes

In hemosiderosis, hemosiderin is usually present in dermal macrophages and fibroblasts. Hepatocytes deposit hemosiderin. In liver, there is heavy periportal depositions of parenchymal iron and Kupffer cells are spared.

17. Answer: A. Atrophy

Atrophy is a decrease in cell size and functional ability. It results due to reduction in blood supply, poor nutrition, and decrease in normal hormonal stimulation. This causes shrinkage of the affected organ. Common examples of atrophy are immobilization, ischemia (atherosclerosis). Light microscopy shows small shrunken cells.

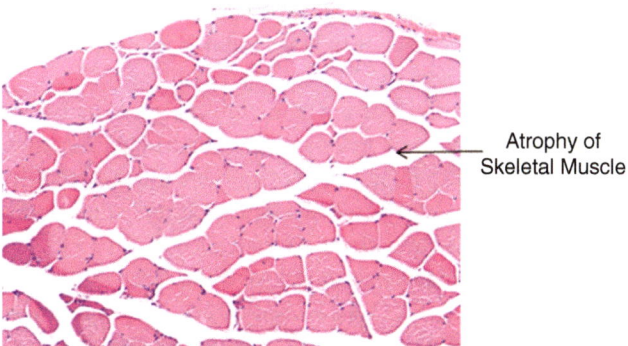

Atrophy of Skeletal Muscle

18. Answer: C. Part of nerve not attached to cell body

A stepwise degeneration process called Wallerian degeneration is the standard response to peripheral nerve injury. It is seen when a nerve fiber is cut which results in the degeneration of part of the axon distal to the injury. Wallerian degeneration is seen in part of nerve not attached to cell body.

19. Answer: A. Focal accumulation of activated macrophages

Granuloma is a mass of granulation tissue produced typically in response to infection, inflammation or foreign substances. These macrophages are important in the development of granuloma cell mediated inflammation. Granuloma is characterized by focal accumulation of activated macrophages.

20. Answer: B. Irreversible cell injury

Irreversible cell damage is a significant membrane damage caused by influx of calcium. There is also an efflux of intracellular enzymes and proteins into circulation. Within the mitochondrial matrix there are marked mitochondrial dysfunction, mitochondrial swelling, and large densities. Common examples of irreversible cell injury are seen in the nucleus. Changes might be pyknosis (degeneration and nuclear chromatin condensation), karyorrhexis (nuclear fragmentation), and karyolysis (nucleus dissolution).

21. Answer: B. Arachidonic acid metabolites

Lipoxins are endogenous, pro-resolving, anti-inflammatory molecules that play a vital part in reducing chronic inflammation. Arachidonic acid, a fatty acid, is enzymatically derived by lipoxins. The metabolites of arachidonic acid contains three hydroxyl residues and four double bonds. Intracellular messengers are called arachidonic acid and its metabolites are prostaglandins and leukotrienes. Arachidonic acid, which results in the synthesis of prostaglandins and leukotrienes, is metabolized by cyclooxygenase (COX) and 5-lipoxygenase.

22. Answer: C. NADPH oxidase

Intracellular killing is oxygen dependent killing. A NADPH oxidase multi-protein complex creates a phagocyte respiratory burst. NADPH oxidase consists of p91-phox and p22-phox membrane bound subunits.

23. Answer: A. Sepsis

The systemic reaction to microbial organisms is sepsis. An appropriate treatment and prognostic evaluation includes a differential diagnosis of diseases, whether by bacteria or other microbial species. Current clinical laboratory procedures are either undefined or need a longer turnaround time for the diagnosis of bacterial infections. Procalcitonin (PCT) is a biomarker that is more accurate for recognizing sepsis patients. It can be used for diagnosing bacterial infections other than proinflammatory markers (for example cytokines).

24. Answer: C. Natural aging

It is suspected that cytokine dysregulation plays a central role in remodeling the immune system at an older age. This is a proof that systemic inflammation is unable to control the prevention of aging. This reconstruction of the model of an expression of cytokine with a steady propensity to an inflammatory phenotype is called the inflammatory aging. Symptoms described in the question are indicative of natural aging.

25. Answer: C. Fatty change

Steatosis or the fatty change is abnormal accumulation of fat (lipids) within a cell or organ. Steatosis frequently affects the liver, which is the primary organ of lipid metabolism, leading to a disorder that is commonly referred to as fatty liver disease.

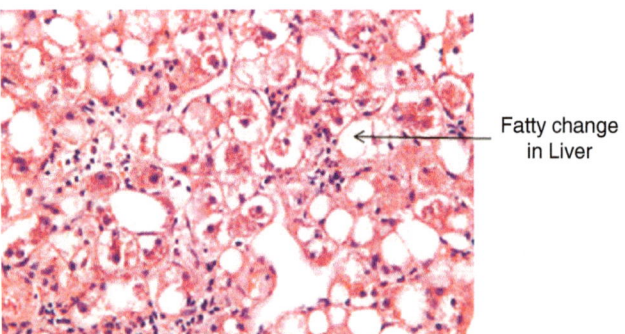

Fatty change in Liver

26. Answer: B. Inflammation

The edema caused by inflammation due to increased permeability of the capillary system. Exudates are called protein rich, high specific gravity, low glucose, cell laden edema fluid. Specific gravity is more than 1.020. Common types of exudates are purulent, fibrinous, and hemorrhagic. Exudates Inflammation belongs to the defense mechanism of the body. Inflammation typically has two types (acute and chronic).

27. Answer: D Histamine, bradykinin, and prostaglandins

Inflammatory mediators such as histamine, bradykinin, and prostaglandins are vasodilators. They also cause an increase in vascular permeability. This causes relaxation of the muscle in the blood vessel walls. This reduces blood flow resistance, increases blood flow, and decreases blood pressure.

28. Answer: D IL-1, IL-6, and tumor necrosis factor-alpha

Imbalance in inflammatory cytokine production such as interleukin-6 (IL-6), TNF-α, interleukin-1 (IL-1), interleukin-10 (IL-10), type I & II interferon contribute to immune dysfunction. They also mediate the inflammation of the tissues and organ damage.

29. Answer: B. Macrophage

In macrophages, cytokines like TNF, IL-1, IL-6, IL-8, and IL-12 are secreted when they are exposed to inflamed stimuli. The primary sources of the cytokines are monocytes and macrophages. Activated lymphocytes, endothelial, and fibroblast cells produce them.

30. Answer: C. Liver

Liver consists of different cell types, including hepatocytes (parenchymal cells). Liver also consists of macrophages (Kupffer cells) and sinusoidal endothelial cells. Kupffer cells reside in the liver sinusoids.

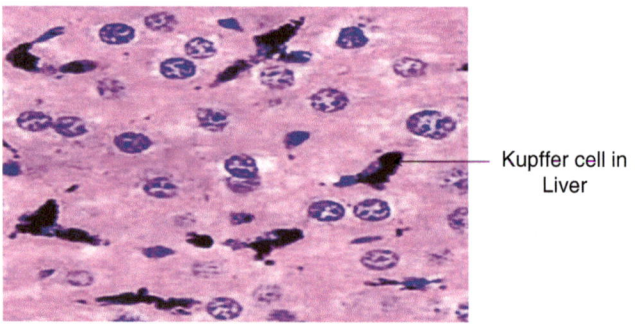

Kupffer cell in Liver

31. Answer: A Cytochrome c

The programmed cell death (PCD) is called apoptosis. There are two main apoptotic pathways: extrinsic one and endogenous one. Intrinsic apoptotic pathway converges with the release of proteins from mitochondria into the cytosol. One such proteins released is called cytochrome c (Cc).

32. Answer: B. Necrotizing inflammation

An inflammatory area in which tissue is dead is called necrotizing granuloma. The conditions caused by necrotizing granulomas are tuberculosis and granulomatosis with polyangiitis. Granulomatous inflammation is a histological tissue reaction which occurs after cell injuries. Common causes of necrotizing inflammation are necrotizing granulomas, non-necrotizing granulomas, and suppurative granulomas. Necrotizing granuloma is seen in mycobacterium tuberculosis. It usually consists of central necrotic regions, epithelioid histiocytes, and multinucleated giant cells. Non-necrotizing granulomas are seen in sarcoidosis.

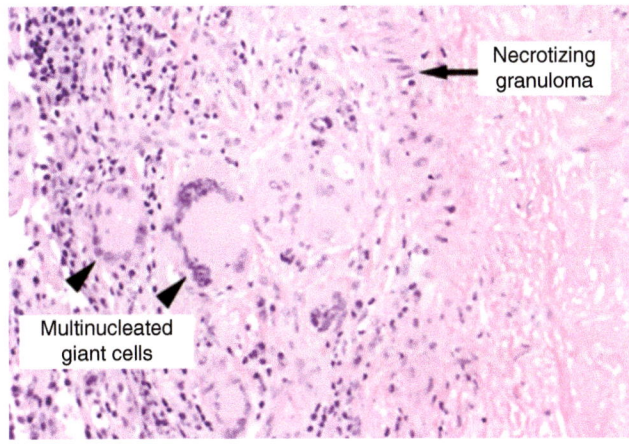

33. Answer: A. CXCL17

Chemokines are a superfamily of chemical cytokines that control the movement of cells in a homeostatic and inflammatory condition. CXCL17 is an important lung macrophage chemotactic factor.

34. Answer: D: Eosinophil

Eosinophils are bilobed cells with large eosinophilic granules. They defend against parasitic infections. Eosinophils may also participate in critical protection tasks against bacterial and viral pathogens including HIV.

35. Answer: A. Pain

Mediators of pain are bradykinin and prostaglandins (E2). Bradykinin increases the vascular permeability. Vasodilation and bronchoconstriction are also caused by bradykinin.

36. Answer: A. Cytokines IL-1

There are several pyrogenic cytokines. Common pyrogenic cytokines are IL-1, IL-6, and TNF. The pyrogenic cytokine interferon (IFN)-alpha is also one of the pyrogenic cytokines.

37. Answer: C. IL-6

IL-6 is a cytokine with a wide range of biological functions including support of hematopoiesis, regulation of immune responses, and generation of acute phase reactions. IL-6 and VEGF are the main cytokines including systemic complications in Castleman disease.

38. Answer: A. Cytokines IL-4, IL-5, and IL-13

TH2 cytokines IL-4, IL-5, and IL-13 are important mediators in asthma.

Bibliography

1. Maximilian Buja L. The cell theory and cellular pathology: discovery, refinements and applications fundamental to advances in biology and medicine. Exp Mol Pathol. 2021;121(12):104660.
2. Elkon K, et al. Apoptosis and autoimmune disease. 2019.
3. Lawrence F Eichenfield. Xeroderma pigmentosum. 2019.
4. Sobczuk K, Sobczuk A. New classification system of endometrial hyperplasia WHO 2014 and its clinical implications. Prz Menopauzalny. 2017;16(3):107–11.
5. Giroux V, Rustgi AK. Metaplasia: tissue injury adaptation and a precursor to the dysplasia–cancer sequence. Nat Rev Cancer. 2017;17(10):594–604.
6. Johnson J, Falck S. Everything you need to know about dysplasia. 2018.
7. Seehafer SS, Pearce DA. Lipofuscin: the "wear and tear" pigment. 2016.
8. Dincay D, et al. Mucosal gastric calcinosis in a hypocalcaemic patient. Prz Gastroenterol. 2017;12(1):70–1.
9. Chan ED, et al. Calcification and ossification of the lungs. 2019.
10. Das DK. Psammoma body: a product of dystrophic calcification or of a biologically active process that aims at limiting the growth and spread of tumor? Diagn Cytopathol. 2009;37(7):534–41.
11. Aronow WS. Hypertension and left ventricular hypertrophy. Ann Transl Med. 2017;5(15):310.
12. Ahmad M. Coagulative necrosis: pathology, causes and regeneration in coagulative necrosis. 2018.
13. Rogers K. Mitochondrion. 2019.
14. Bisognano JD. Malignant hypertension. 2017.
15. Adigun R, Basit H, Murray J. Necrosis, cell (liquefactive, coagulative, caseous, fat, fibrinoid, and gangrenous). 2019.
16. Edlich F. BCL-2 proteins and apoptosis: Recent insights and unknowns. Biochem Biophys Res Commun. 2018;500(1):26–34.
17. Adigun R, et al. Necrosis, cell (liquefactive, coagulative, caseous, fat, fibrinoid, and gangrenous). 2019.
18. Hou L, et al. Necrotic pyknosis is a morphologically and biochemically distinct event from apoptotic pyknosis. J Cell Sci. 2016;129(16).3084–90.
19. Zuazo-Gaztelu I, Casanovas O. Unraveling the role of angiogenesis in cancer ecosystems. Front Oncol. 2018;8:248.
20. Arora K. Liver and intrahepatic bile ducts - nontumor metabolic diseases. Hemochromatosis. 2019.

Genetic Disorders

Multiple Choice Questions

1. A 13-year-old female patient presents with clinical features of failure to develop secondary sex characteristics, short stature, primary amenorrhea, infertility, cystic hygroma, and web neck. What is the diagnosis?
   A. Turner syndrome
   B. Klinefelter syndrome
   C. Edward syndrome
   D. Cri du Chat syndrome
   E. Patau syndrome

2. What is the karyotype of Klinefelter syndrome?
   A. 45 XO
   B. 47 XXY
   C. 46 XX
   D. 47 XX
   E. 47 XY

3. Chromosomal aberrations are due to a change in the normal chromosome number or a change in the structure of a chromosome. What is the genetic abnormality in Cri du Chat syndrome?
   A. 45 XO
   B. 47 XXY
   C. Deletion of chromosome 5p
   D. 47 XX
   E. 47 XY

4. What are the clinical findings of Edward syndrome?
   A. Mental retardation, low set ears, micrognathia, overlapping of the fingers, and rocker-bottom feet
   B. Mental retardation, cleft lip and palate, cardiac defects, and polydactyly
   C. Mental retardation, characteristic high pitched cat-like cry, congenital heart disease, and microcephaly
   D. Testicular atrophy, female distribution of hair, and gynecomastia
   E. Short stature, primary amenorrhea, infertility, cystic hygroma, and webbing of the neck

5. Which of the following is the most frequent form of familial mental retardation, mainly in males, with large ears and macro-orchidism?
   A. Fragile X syndrome
   B. Sotos syndrome
   C. Asperger syndrome
   D. Prader-Willi syndrome
   E. Rett syndrome

6. Which of the following statements is correct regarding Niemann-Pick disease?
   A. Enzyme defect is a deficiency of sphingomyelinase
   B. Enzyme defect is a deficiency of glucocerebrosidase
   C. Enzyme defect is a deficiency of hexosaminidase A
   D. Enzyme defect is a deficiency of glucose-6-phosphatase
   E. Enzyme defect is a deficiency of lysosomal glucosidase (acid maltase)

7. Which of the following is an autosomal recessive mucopolysaccharide storage disease which leads to typical facial dysmorphism with short stature, dementia, corneal clouding, and hepatosplenomegaly?
   A. Hurler syndrome
   B. Hunter syndrome
   C. Sanfilippo syndrome
   D. Maroteaux-Lamy syndrome
   E. Sly syndrome

8. Which of the following syndromes present as a recessive syndrome of primordial growth deficiency, telangiectatic erythema, and tendency to develop malignant tumors?
   A. Turner syndrome
   B. Klinefelter syndrome
   C. Edward syndrome
   D. Cri du Chat syndrome
   E. Bloom syndrome

9. Which of the following condition presents with classic generalized skeletal dysplasia with disproportionate

short stature, large head, coarse facial features, and X-ray findings of thoracolumbar kyphosis and lumbosacral lordosis?

    A. Thanatophoric dysplasia
    B. Achondroplasia
    C. Hypochondroplasia
    D. Pseudoachondroplasia
    E. Metatropic dwarfism

10. Which of the following is a common finding in spontaneously aborted fetuses?
    A. Inversion
    B. Deletion
    C. Polyploidy
    D. Nondisjunction
    E. Trinucleotide repeat mutations

11. Which of the following is a hereditary metabolic disorder with short stature and rachitic bone changes?
    A. Familial hypophosphatemic rickets
    B. Vitamin D deficiency rickets
    C. Metaphyseal chondrodysplasia syndrome
    D. Cartilage-hair hypoplasia
    E. Pseudohypoparathyroidism

12. Which of the following is a syndrome of oculocutaneous albinism, frequent bacterial infections, and large lysosomal granules in the granulocytes?
    A. Cutaneous T cell lymphoma
    B. Oculocutaneous albinism
    C. Chediak-Higashi syndrome
    D. Pyoderma gangrenosum
    E. Hemophagocytic lymphohistiocytosis (HLH)

13. What are the clinical findings of Patau syndrome?
    A. Mental retardation, low set ears, micrognathia, overlapping fixed fingers, and Rocker-bottom feet.
    B. Mental retardation, cleft lip and palate, cardiac defects, and polydactyly
    C. Mental retardation, characteristic high pitched cat-like cry, congenital heart disease, and microcephaly
    D. Testicular atrophy, female distribution of hair, and gynecomastia
    E. Short stature, primary amenorrhea, infertility, cystic hygroma, and webbing of the neck

14. An autosomal dominance is one of the many ways that a trait or disorder can be passed down through families. An autosomal dominant condition is?
    A. Albinism
    B. Huntington's disease
    C. Hurler's syndrome
    D. Hunter's syndrome
    E. Tay-Sachs disease.

15. Which of the following statements is correct regarding Gaucher disease?
    A. Enzyme defect is a deficiency of sphingomyelinase
    B. Enzyme defect is a deficiency of glucocerebrosidase
    C. Enzyme defect is a deficiency of hexosaminidase A
    D. Enzyme defect is a deficiency of glucose-6-phosphatase
    E. Enzyme defect is a deficiency of lysosomal glucosidase (acid maltase)

16. Which of the following medical condition is caused by deficiency of the enzyme hexosaminidase?
    A. Tay-Sachs disease
    B. Hurler syndrome
    C. Fabry disease
    D. Pompe disease
    E. Von Gierke disease

17. Which of the following is a characteristic of hereditary disorder of multiple cafe au lait spots, skin tumors, skeletal and neurological signs?
    A. Multiple lentigines syndrome
    B. McCune-Albright syndrome
    C. Acoustic neuroma
    D. Neurofibromatosis type 2
    E. Neurofibromatosis type 1

18. Marfan syndrome is an autosomal dominant connective tissue disorder. Which of the following mutation is seen in Marfan syndrome?
    A. Fibrillin-1
    B. Fibrillin-2
    C. P mutation in chromosome 12q
    D. DCP mutation in chromosome 15
    E. P mutation in chromosome 11 p

19. Which of the following is a characteristic syndrome of macular hemangiomas, especially of the face, signs of cerebral foci, and mental retardation common?
    A. Sturge-Weber syndrome
    B. Klippel-Trenaunay-Weber syndrome
    C. Beckwith-Wiedemann syndrome
    D. Siderosis
    E. Dyke-Davidoff-Masson syndrome

20. Duchenne muscular dystrophy (DMD) is a rare muscle disorder. Duchenne muscular dystrophy is inherited as:
    A. Mitochondrial DNA
    B. Autosomal dominant
    C. X-linked recessive
    D. X-linked dominant
    E. Multifactorial

21. A 35-year-old woman has Von Hippel-Lindau disease. The gene implicated in the renal tumor associated with Von Hippel-Lindau disease is located on chromosome:
    A. 3p
    B. 5q
    C. 11p
    D. 13q
    E. 17q

22. A 5-year-old child presents with a history of viral and fungal infections and has calcium of 5.6 mg/dL. The most likely diagnosis is:
    A. Fragile X syndrome
    B. X-linked agammaglobulinemia
    C. DiGeorge's syndrome
    D. Ehlers-Danlos syndrome (EDS)
    E. Tay-Sachs disease

23. Which of the following medical condition is an X-linked recessive disorder?
    A. Familial hypercholesterolemia
    B. Von Hippel-Lindau disease
    C. Marfan's syndrome
    D. Wiskott-Aldrich syndrome
    E. Albinism

24. Cystic fibrosis (CF) is a multisystem disease affecting the lungs, digestive system, sweat glands, and reproductive tract. Which chromosome encodes the cystic fibrosis transmembrane conductance regulator (CFTR) protein?
    A. 21
    B. 3
    C. 18
    D. 7
    E. X

25. Clinical triad of chronic sinusitis, bronchiectasis, and situs inversus is found in which of the following condition?
    A. Necrotizing pneumonias
    B. Cystic fibrosis
    C. Wegener's granulomatosis
    D. Kartagener's syndrome
    E. Asthma

26. Which of the following is a characteristic of hereditary disease with neurological (progressive cerebellar ataxia), telangiectasia, and immune deficiency causing frequent respiratory tract infections?
    A. Friedreich disease
    B. Metachromatic leukodystrophy
    C. Ataxia telangiectasia
    D. Krabbe disease
    E. Gaucher disease

27. Which of the following inheritance pattern is most likely to be present in Peutz-Jeghers syndrome?
    A. Autosomal dominant
    B. Autosomal recessive
    C. X-linked recessive
    D. X-linked dominant
    E. Multifactorial

28. Which of the following syndrome is due to deletion of paternal chromosomes 15?
    A. Angelman syndrome
    B. Fragile X syndrome
    C. Marfan syndrome
    D. Ehlers-Danlos syndrome
    E. Prader–Willi syndrome

29. Which of the following is the most common chromosomal disorder because of trisomy 21?
    A. Edward syndrome
    B. Patau syndrome
    C. Cri du Chat syndrome
    D. Down syndrome
    E. Klinefelter syndrome

Answers and Explanations

1. Answer: A. Turner syndrome

   Turner syndrome is a malformation syndrome due to the lack of a second X chromosome (45, XO). It is a common cause of primary ovarian insufficiency. It is characterized by short stature, failure of puberty to occur, webbed neck, cubitus valgus, lymphoedema of the dorsal surfaces of the hands and feet, expressionless face. There is gonadal dysgenesis with rudimentary "streak ovaries," shortening of the fourth and fifth metatarsals. There may be renal anomalies (horseshoe kidney, unilateral renal agenesis), cardiac defects (usually coarctation of aorta). Early treatment to promote growth is required by an experienced pediatric endocrinologist.

2. Answer: B. 47 XXY

   Klinefelter syndrome is a hypogonadism syndrome in males with an additional X chromosome (XXY syndrome). Main signs in childhood are tall stature with unusually long lower extremities, slightly below average intelligence with a delayed onset of puberty, gynecomastia. In adolescent and adulthood, there are eunuchoid proportions with tall stature. There is normally developed penis with small testes, and infertility (azoospermia) noticeable after puberty. Secondary sexual characteristics are poorly developed with female distribution of pubic hair. Most patients are diagnosed after the 14th year of life. Plasma and urine gonadotropins are elevated. X-chromatin is positive on screening (buccal smear). There is an increased risk of psychiatric and autism spectrum disorders.

3. Answer: C. Deletion of chromosome 5p

   Cri du Chat syndrome is a syndrome comprising facial dysmorphism, primordial growth deficiency, low birth weight, psychomotor delay, and affected babies have cat-like high pitched cry in early infancy. Main signs are round flat face, hypertelorism, downslanting palpebral fissures, low broad nasal bridge, micrognathia, and low set ears. A missing piece of chromosome 5 is a cause of this disorder.

4. Answer: A. Mental retardation, low set ears, micrognathia, overlapping fixed fingers, and Rocker-bottom feet

Trisomy 18 (Edward Syndrome) consists of primordial growth deficiency, typical facial dysmorphism, and profound psychomotor retardation. Characteristic facies are distinguished by protruding forehead, upward-slanting palpebral fissures, micrognathia, microstomia, short philtrum and not infrequently cleft lip or palate. Other signs and symptoms include flexion contractures of the fingers with overlapping of the fingers, hypoplastic nails, clenched fists, "rock-bottom feet." There is a short sternum with widely faced nipples. There may be defects in the heart (ventricular septal defect and patent ductus arteriosus).

5. Answer: A. Fragile X Syndrome

Fragile X Syndrome is a form of familial mental retardation of varied severity, mainly in males, with large ears, macro-orchidism, and fragile X chromosome. There is increased weight and head circumference above the 97th percentile at birth. Delayed psychomotor development occurs with muscular hypotonia, thin legs, walking after 18 months, delayed speech. This is an X-linked disorder with anticipation (increasing severity in successive generations). In adolescence, tall stature, flat feet, hyperextensible joints occur along with prolapse of the aortic and mitral valves.

6. Answer: A. Enzyme defect is a deficiency of sphingomyelinase

An autosomal recessive sphingolipidoses with different clinical forms, Niemann-Pick disease (NPD) is characterized by a protruding abdomen due to hepatosplenomegaly. Neurological complications of variable severity, cherry red spot in the macula, thin extremities, and growth deficiency are also found in NPD. Type A is an acute form with neurological complications. Type B is chronic form with or without neurological complications. Regression of speech and intellect, ataxia, grand mal seizures are seen as neurologic complications.

7. Answer: A. Hurler Syndrome

Hurler syndrome is an autosomal recessive mucopolysaccharide storage disease, which leads to the development of typical facial dysmorphism. Characteristic facies have low, flat nasal bridge, broad tip of nose, large nares, hypertelorism, exophthalmos, corneal clouding, thick lips. There is short neck with joint contractures, claw hands. Protruding abdomen and hernias may be present. The mucopolysaccharide type 1-H is not degraded because of the absence of alpha-iduronidase, but are stored in various organs resulting in functional and morphological anomalies of these organs. Gene locus is present on 4p16.3.

8. Answer: E. Bloom syndrome

Bloom syndrome is a recessive hereditary syndrome of primordial growth deficiency and telangiectatic erythema. Main signs are long narrow face with a prominent nose, micrognathia, and microcephaly. Telangiectasia erythema is more marked after exposure to the sun, more commonly in a butterfly distribution on the face. There is a tendency in the younger age group to develop malignant tumors, especially leukemia, lymphoma, and later adenocarcinomas.

9. Answer: B. Achondroplasia

Achondroplasia is a generalized skeletal dysplasia with disproportionate short stature, large head, typical dysmorphism. There is ulnar deviation of the hands, splayed fingers (trident hand). Head is too large for the body with coarse facial features. X-ray findings show thoracolumbar kyphosis and lumbosacral lordosis. It is an autosomal dominant disorder and gene locus is on the short arm of chromosome 4(4p16.3).

10. Answer: C. Polyploidy

In polyploidy, there are more than two paired homologous sets of chromosomes. It is a common finding in spontaneous abortion. Polyploidy is usually lethal irrespective of the sexual phenotype of the embryo.

11. Answer: A. Familial hypophosphatemic rickets

Familial hypophosphatemic rickets is also called vitamin-D resistant rickets. It is a metabolic disorder with short stature and rachitic bone changes. There is a short stature with pronounced bow legs. In childhood, other rachitic bone changes (rachitic rosary, enlargement of the wrists and ankles) are also seen. There may be a dental change with delayed eruptions and dental abscess. In adulthood, abnormal curvature of the spine, osteomalacia, calcification around ligaments, and joint capsules are present. Radiologically, changes as in vitamin-D deficiency rickets are seen but pelvic and spinal regions are spared. Laboratory findings show hypophosphatemia, hyperphosphaturia, increased serum alkaline phosphatase, normal calcium, and parathormone. It is an X-linked dominant disorder, which is triggered by a genetic defect on the short arm of the X chromosome. Combined disorder of phosphate reabsorption and of regulation of 1, 25-(OH) secretion in the proximal renal tubules is present.

12. Answer: C. Chediak-Higashi syndrome

Chediak-Higashi syndrome is a syndrome of oculocutaneous albinism, frequent bacterial infections. Fair skin, fair hair with silvery sheen, light-colored iris, photophobia, and nystagmus are present. There are recurrent bacterial infections, especially of the upper and lower respiratory tract and skin. Giant azure-blue granules in the granulocytes are present. Anemia is found in 80% of all affected individuals. It has an autosomal recessive inheritance. There is an impaired function of the neutrophils in the cell membrane due to giant granules, impaired chemotaxis, and intracellular bacterial killing.

13. Answer: B. Mental retardation, cleft lip and palate, cardiac defects, and polydactyly

    Patau syndrome (trisomy 13) is the result of an extra copy of chromosome 13. Main signs are microcephaly, slanting forehead, hypo or hypertelorism, mongoloid slant of the palpebral fissures, microphthalmia or anophthalmia, cleft lip, palate, and micrognathia. Holoprosencephaly, postaxial polydactyly, mainly of upper extremities are the other main signs. There may be capillary hemangiomas, cryptorchidism, cardiac defects of various types (ventricular septal defect and patent ductus arteriosus).

14. Answer: B. Huntington's disease

    Huntington's disease, an autosomal dominant disorder, is caused by an expansion of the cytosine—adenine—guanine (CAG) trinucleotide in the huntingtin gene (HTT gene), also called the HD gene, that encodes the huntingtin protein, which results in an expanded polyglutamine tract. Huntington's disease (HD) is a neurodegenerative disorder and is characterized by choreiform movements, psychiatric problems, and dementia.

15. Answer: B. Enzyme defect is a deficiency of glucocerebrosidase

    Gaucher disease is a chronic lysosomal storage disease with hepatosplenomegaly, dyshematopoiesis (splenogenic marrow depression, thrombocytopenia, leukopenia, and anemia), and characteristic orthopedic complications. Mental development and nervous system is normal. There is a periodic bone and joint pain, especially in the long bones. Pseudo-osteomyelitic or pseudo arthritic pathologic fractures are usually found in the femur (on radiograph showing an "Erlenmeyer flask deformity"). Demonstration of Gaucher cells in bone marrow aspirates or a cerebroside-beta-glucosidase defect in leukocyte is diagnostic. It is an autosomal recessive disorder due to a defect in glucosylceramidase beta gene (GBA1) coding for enzyme glucocerebrosidase.

16. Answer: A. Tay-Sachs disease

    Tay-Sachs disease is an autosomal recessive GM2 gangliosidosis caused by β hexosaminidase A (HexA) enzyme deficiency. There is a rapid psychomotor deterioration, hypotonia to generalized paralysis and eventual spasticity, progressive deafness, blindness, seizures. Cherry-red spot is present in the macular region in over 95 % of patients.

17. Answer: E. Neurofibromatosis type 1

    Neurofibromatosis type 1 (Von Recklinghausen) is a characteristic hereditary disorder of multiple cafe au lait spots, especially on the trunk. Multiple fibromas or neurofibromas and subcutaneous growth are present. Frequent neurological or ocular disorders are caused by nerve compression. Skeletal anomalies (congenital pseudarthrosis of the tibia, club foot, dislocation of the hip) may be present. NF-type 1 is an autosomal dominant disorder with 100 % penetrance but variable expression. Gene locus is present on 17q11.2.

18. Answer: A. Fibrillin-1

    Marfan syndrome is a hereditary disorder with disproportionate tall stature mainly due to excessively long extremities, resulting in eunuchoid body proportions, and arachnodactyly. There is muscular hypoplasia and hypotonia due to marked deficit of fatty tissue. Main signs are long, narrow face with high palate, and narrowly spaced teeth. Signs of connective tissue weakness include hernias, hyperextensible joints. Dislocation of the lenses is seen in about 75% of the patients. Dislocation of joints, kyphoscoliosis, pes planus, pectus carinatum or excavatum may be present. There may be general dilation of aorta (aortic valve incompetence), dissecting aneurysms. Marfan syndrome is an autosomal dominant disorder. There is a Fibrillin-1 defect. Gene locus is present on 15q21.1.

19. Answer: A. Sturge-Weber syndrome

    Sturge-Weber syndrome (Cerebro Cutaneous Angiomatosis Syndrome) is a characteristic syndrome of macular hemangiomas, especially of the face. Port-wine color, nevus flammeus of the face and head is present preferentially in the trigeminal area, mostly unilateral. Patients may present with focal or generalized cerebral seizures. Spastic hemiparesis is present contralateral to the side of the angioma. Inherited factors are probably of causal significance. This could be the manifestation of a lethal lesion in the mosaic.

20. Answer: C. X-linked recessive

    Duchenne muscular dystrophy is a characteristic hereditary syndrome in males, with onset in childhood of "ascending" muscle atrophy beginning in the pelvis and thigh regions. Main signs are rapid fatigue when climbing stairs, difficulty up from the floor, eventually "climbing up himself" (Gower sign). There is hyperlordosis with protruding abdomen. Pseudohypertrophy (fatty infiltration) especially of the calves, and also of thigh and buttock musculature is present. Ascending degeneration of the musculature starts at the pelvic girdle and thighs. Mental retardation is seen in approximately 30% of the children. Marked increased serum creatine kinase activity is present in the initial stages of the process. The gene product, dystrophin is deficient in Duchenne patients. Absence of dystrophin can be shown immunohistologically. Manifestation is between 3 and 5 years of age. It is an X-linked recessive disorder with 65% of patients show deletion mutations.

21. Answer: A. 3p

    Clear cell carcinoma which typically have a deletion of chromosome 3p, arise from the proximal tubule. In addition to occurring in sporadic disease, clear cell carcinomas are specifically associated with Von Hippel-Lindau disease.

22. Answer: C. DiGeorge's syndrome

    Majority of the cases of DiGeorge syndrome (DGS) are due to a 22q11.2 deletion. Conotruncal cardiac anomalies, hypoplastic thymus, hypocalcemia are the classic triad of features of DGS on presentation.

    Immunodeficiency is common and can range from recurrent sinopulmonary infections (partial DGS) to severe combined immunodeficiency (SCID; complete DGS). The severity of the immunodeficiency is associated to the degree of thymic hypoplasia.

23. Answer: D. Wiskott-Aldrich syndrome

    Wiskott-Aldrich syndrome is an X-linked recessive disorder with the triad of signs; eczema, thrombocytopenia with bleeding tendencies and recurrent infections. The WAS has been localized to the proximal short arm of the chromosome (Xp11.22). There is a clinical onset frequently with eczema due to T cell defect in the first sixth months of life. There are recurrent pneumococcal infections.

24. Answer: D. 7

    CF is a result of mutations in a single large gene on chromosome 7 that encodes the cystic fibrosis transmembrane conductance regulator (CFTR) protein. Disease-causing mutations in both copies of the CFTR gene results in clinical disease. Mutations of the CFTR gene have been divided into five different classes. Mutations in classes I to III cause more severe disease than those in classes IV and V.

25. Answer: D. Kartagener's syndrome

    Kartagener's syndrome, an autosomal recessive inherited disorder, is a subset of primary ciliary dyskinesia, and is characterized by the clinical triad of chronic sinusitis, bronchiectasis, and situs inversus. The main pathophysiologic problem is abnormal ciliary structure or function leading to impaired ciliary motility.

26. Answer: C. Ataxia telangiectasia

    Ataxia telangiectasia (Progressive Cerebellar Ataxia with Telangiectasia) is a characteristic hereditary syndrome with neurological, cutaneous, and immune deficiency signs. Main signs are progressive cerebellar ataxia and telangiectasia. Telangiectasia occurs in the areas of the bulbar conjunctiva that are exposed to light and later on the lids in a butterfly distribution on and alongside of the nose. Immune deficiency causes frequent signs of respiratory tract infections. It is an autosomal recessive disorder. Patients have an increased risk of developing lymphoreticular malignancies.

27. Answer: A. Autosomal dominant

    Peutz-Jeghers Syndrome (PJS) is an autosomal disorder of conspicuous pigmentation, predominantly of the face and oral mucosa, associated with hamartomatous polyposis of the gastrointestinal tract. Main signs are dark, brown or bluish gray-black pigmented spots on the skin of the face, on the oral mucosa, extremities including the nail beds. PJS is an autosomal dominant disorder with almost 100% penetrance.

28. Answer: E. Prader–Willi syndrome

    Prader–Willi syndrome is a syndrome comprising of mental retardation, short stature, obesity, and hypogonadism, following initial marked muscular hypotonia in infancy. In 95 % of patients, it is due to loss of paternal alleles from the region 15q11-13. Common features are short stature, increasing obesity with hyperphagia, severe psychomotor retardation, hypogenitalism, scrotal hypoplasia, and frequent cryptorchidism. Prader–Willi syndrome is the most common syndromic form of obesity. Hypogonadism is present in both sexes.

29. Answer: D. Down syndrome

    Down syndrome (Trisomy 21 syndrome) is a malformation syndrome comprising of mental retardation and characteristic physical appearance. It is frequently associated with increased maternal age. Trisomy of chromosome 21, accounts in over 95% of the patients. Infrequently, in about 3%, it is attached to another chromosome (translocation). In 2% trisomy 21 mosaicism (47+21/46) is present. Main signs are "flat face" with a mongoloid slant of the palpebral fissures, epicanthus, low nasal bridge, a small nose, and dysplastic ears. Short-appearing, neck with loose skin is more apparent in the young child. Muscular hypotonia and generalized hypermobility of the joints with laxity of the ligaments is also seen. Mental retardation is moderate to severe. 80% of all down patients develop microcephaly from the sixth month of life.

Bibliography

1. Angural A, Spolia A, Mahajan A, Verma V, Sharma A, Kumar P, Dhar MK, Pandita KK, Rai E, Sharma S. Understanding rare genetic diseases in low resource regions like Jammu and Kashmir – India. Front Genet. 2020;11:415.

2. Das KK, Srivastava AK. Nerve conduits as replacements of autografts in peripheral nerve surgery: still a work in progress. 2019.

3. Spechler SJ. Barrett's esophagus: epidemiology, clinical manifestations, and diagnosis. 2019.

4. Timmermans WMC, van Laar JAM, van Hagen PM, van Zelm MC. Immunopathogenesis of granulomas in chronic autoinflammatory diseases. Clin Transl Immunol. 2016;5(12):e118.

5. Balan IS, et al. Cellular alterations in human traumatic brain injury: changes in mitochondrial morphology reflect regional levels of injury severity. J Neurotrauma. 2013;30(5):367–81.

6. King MW. Prostaglandins, thromboxanes, leukotrienes, and lipoxins. 2019.
7. Thomas T. The phagocyte respiratory burst: historical perspectives and recent advances. Immunol Lett. 2017;192:88–96.
8. Vijayan AL, et al. Procalcitonin: a promising diagnostic marker for sepsis and antibiotic therapy. J Intensive Care. 2017;5:51.
9. Rea IM, et al. Age and age-related diseases: role of inflammation triggers and cytokines. Front Immunol. 2018;9:586.
10. Tanaka N, et al. Current status, problems, and perspectives of non-alcoholic fatty liver disease research. World J Gastroenterol. 2019;25(2):163–77.
11. Pahwa R, Jialal I. Chronic inflammation. 2019.
12. Branco ACCC, et al. Role of histamine in modulating the immune response and inflammation. Mediat Inflamm. 2018;2018:9524075.
13. Umare V, et al. Effect of proinflammatory cytokines (IL-6, TNF-α, and IL-1β) on clinical manifestations in Indian SLE patients. Mediat Inflamm. 2014;2014:385297.
14. Duque GA, Descoteaux A. Macrophage cytokines: involvement in immunity and infectious diseases. Front Immunol. 2014;5:491.
15. Kermanizadeh A, et al. The importance of inter-individual Kupffer cell variability in the governance of hepatic toxicity in a 3D primary human liver microtissue model. Sci Rep. 2019;9:7295.
16. Elena-Real CA, et al. Cytochrome c speeds up caspase cascade activation by blocking 14-3-3ε-dependent Apaf-1 inhibition. Cell Death Dis. 2018;9:365.
17. Shah KK, Pritt BS, Alexander MP. J Clin Tuberc Other Mycobact Dis. 2017;7:1–12.
18. Burkhardt AM, et al. CXCL17 is a major chemotactic factor for lung macrophages. J Immunol. 2014;193(3):1468–74.
19. Ramirez GA, et al. Eosinophils from physiology to disease: a comprehensive review. Biomed Res Int. 2018;2018:9095275.
20. Kowal K, et al. Overview of in vitro allergy tests. 2019.
21. Zuraw B, et al. An overview of angioedema: pathogenesis and causes. 2019.
22. Porat R, et al. Pathophysiology and treatment of fever in adults. 2019.

Immune System Disorders

Multiple Choice Questions

1. Which is the most common inherited immunodeficiency?
   A. Bruton's X-linked agammaglobulinemia
   B. Common variable immunodeficiency
   C. Severe combined immunodeficiency
   D. Selective IgA deficiency
   E. C1 inhibitor deficiency

2. Which immunoglobulin crosses the placenta?
   A. IgM.
   B. IgG
   C. IgA
   D. IgE
   E. IgD

3. In the lymph node, dendritic cells would be found in the:
   A. Subcapsular sinus
   B. Primary follicle
   C. Germinal center
   D. Outer cortex
   E. Medulla

4. Immunological memory is a unique property of the immune system. Which of the following are the immunological memory cells?
   A. T lymphocytes and NK cells
   B. B lymphocytes and dendritic cells
   C. T and B lymphocytes
   D. Macrophages and B lymphocytes
   E. B lymphocytes and lymphokine-activated killer (LAK) cells

5. Certain drugs may trigger an autoimmune response. Drug induced lupus antibodies are:
   A. Anti-Ro antibodies
   B. Anti-histone antibodies
   C. Anti-U1-ribonucleoprotein antibodies
   D. Anti-Sm antibodies
   E. Anti-Jo-1 antibodies

6. Hypersensitivity reactions are immune responses. Which of the following hypersensitivity immune response is responsible for Myasthenia Gravis?
   A. Type II hypersensitivity
   B. Type I hypersensitivity
   C. Type IV hypersensitivity
   D. Type III hypersensitivity
   E. None of the above

7. Interleukin is defined as any class of glycoproteins produced by leukocytes for regulating immune responses. Which interleukin is required for differentiation of eosinophils?
   A. IL-2
   B. IL-3
   C. IL-4
   D. IL-5
   E. IL-10

8. Which of the following Interleukin is being used as immunotherapy for renal cell carcinoma and metastatic melanoma?
   A. Interleukin-1
   B. Interleukin-2
   C. Interleukin-4
   D. Interleukin-5
   E. Interleukin-10

9. A 1-year-old boy has repeated upper respiratory infections. Stool examination shows giardia lamblia cysts. Which of the following laboratory finding is likely to be useful in this boy?
   A. Deficiencies of C5-C9
   B. Low or absent immunoglobulins
   C. Selective IgA deficiency
   D. Antibodies to human immunodeficiency virus
   E. Low CD4 count

10. Which of the following is produced by human cells in response to viral infection?
    A. Tumor necrosis factors

B. Interferons

C. Interleukin-2

D. Interleukin-5

E. Interleukin-10

11. Which of the following causes increased susceptibility to giardia lamblia?

    A. Common variable immunodeficiency

    B. DiGeorge syndrome

    C. Severe combined immunodeficiency

    D. Wiskott-Aldrich syndrome

    E. Chronic granulomatous disease

12. A child is getting infections of candida, cytomegalovirus (CMV) and pneumocystis jirovecii (carinii). What is the best etiology of these infections?

    A. Common variable immunodeficiency

    B. DiGeorge's syndrome

    C. Severe combined immunodeficiency

    D. Wiskott-Aldrich syndrome

    E. Bruton's X-linked agammaglobulinemia

13. A latent HIV reservoir is a group of immune cells in the body that are infected with HIV but are not actively producing new HIV. Which of the following cells are the reservoirs for the HIV virus?

    A. B lymphocytes

    B. T lymphocytes

    C. Eosinophils

    D. Follicular dendritic cells

    E. Neutrophils

14. Which of the following are examples of Type IV hypersensitivity?

    A. Atopic eczema and contact dermatitis

    B. Tuberculosis and graft-versus-host disease

    C. Leprosy and myasthenia gravis

    D. Poison Ivy and Arthus reaction

    E. Chronic granulomatous disease and chronic allograft rejection.

15. Langerhans cell histiocytosis (LCH) is a rare disease. Which of the following is a marker for Langerhans cells?

    A. CD30

    B. CD1a

    C. CD10

    D. CD34

    E. CD31

16. Amyloidosis is the general term used to refer to the extracellular tissue deposition of fibrils. Amyloid is stained by?

    A. PAS

    B. Congo red

    C. Hematoxylin and eosin

    D. Methenamine silver

    E. Silver nitrate

17. The mechanism by which an antigen triggers an adaptive immune response involves several steps. Which of the following cells do not act as antigen presenting cells?

    A. B lymphocytes

    B. Macrophages

    C. Osteoclasts

    D. Dendritic cells

    E. Basophils

18. Which is the most common specific antibody deficiency?

    A. IgA

    B. IgD

    C. IgE

    D. IgG

    E. IgM

19. A 2-year-old boy presents with fever and a history of recurrent bacterial infections. Physical examination shows lymphadenitis, hepatospleno-megaly, and pneumonia. Which of the following underlying condition best explain these findings?

    A. Cystic fibrosis

    B. Glucose-6-phosphate dehydrogenase (G6PD) deficiency

    C. Leukocyte adhesion deficiency, type 1

    D. DiGeorge syndrome

    E. Chronic granulomatous disease

20. Which of the following diseases is associated with HLA-B27 antigen?

    A. Rheumatoid arthritis

    B. Ankylosing spondylitis

    C. Felty syndrome

    D. Systemic lupus erythematosus (SLE)

    E. Hashimoto thyroiditis

21. Children with selective IgA deficiency are at increased risk for which of the following gastrointestinal condition?

    A. Tufting enteropathy

    B. Celiac disease

    C. Juvenile polyposis

    D. Necrotizing enterocolitis

    E. Autoimmune enteropathy

22. Which of the following type of hypersensitivity is mediated by T cells?

    A. Type I

    B. Type II

    C. Type III

    D. Type IV

23. What is the best marker for enumerating total peripheral blood T cells?

    A. CD4

    B. CD8

C. CD11b

D. CD14

E. CD3

24. The high endothelial venules (HEV) are the sites at which:

A. Memory B cells enter the lymph node

B. Plasma cells leave the lymph node.

C. Foreign antigen enters the lymph node

D. Mature B cells leave the lymph node

E. Secretory antibody leaves the lymph node

25. Which complement factor levels are assayed for defects in the alternate pathway of activation?

A. C1q

B. C3

C. C4

D. C5

E. C9

26. What chromosome is home to the major histocompatibility complex?

A. 3

B. 6

C. 11

D. 13

E. 17

27. Which of the following antibody activates complement through the alternate pathway?

A. IgG

B. IgM

C. IgA

D. IgD

E. IgE

28. What type of immunoglobulin receptor do mast cells express?

A. Fc alpha

B. Fc beta

C. Fc gamma

D. Fc delta

E. Fc epsilon

29. Which chromosome bears the genes for the heavy chains?

A. 2

B. 22

C. 14

D. 16

E. Depends on which heavy chain

30. Which of the following is an underlying cause of Henoch-Schonlein purpura?

A. Type III hypersensitivity reaction

B. Type II hypersensitivity reaction

C. Type IV hypersensitivity reaction

D. Type I hypersensitivity reaction

E. Disseminated bacterial infection

Answers and Explanations

1. Answer: D. Selective IgA deficiency

There is a high prevalence of IgA deficiency. Patients are usually asymptomatic or present with recurrent sinopulmonary and gastrointestinal infections. IgA deficiency patients can cause anaphylactic reactions when exposed to IgA-containing products. Patients with this deficiency should get washed blood products (red blood cells, platelets) to remove IgA against which they could react.

2. Answer: B. IgG

Five immunoglobulin classes (isotypes) are found in serum and only IgG (immunoglobulin G) crosses the human placenta. Immunoglobulin G has four subclasses (IgG1, 2, 3, and 4). All subclasses of immunoglobulin G cross placenta.

3. Answer: C. Germinal center

Germinal center contains proliferating B cells and follicular dendritic cells. It is round or oval zone with pale staining cells, surrounded by darker cells.

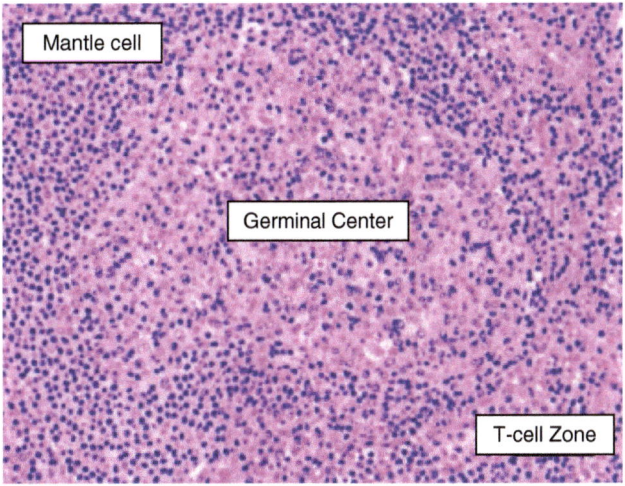

4. Answer: C. T and B lymphocytes

T and B lymphocytes and natural killer (NK) cells are immunological memory cells. They produce an effective response if second encounter occurs with the same antigen.

5. Answer: B. Anti-histone antibodies

Drugs (procainamide, hydralazine) associated lupus produce anti-histone antibodies. In drug-induced lupus, anti-dsDNA antibodies are not found.

6. Answer: A. Type II Hypersensitivity

Myasthenia gravis (MG) is a type II hypersensitivity immune response. The disease produces anti-acetylcholine (ACh) antibodies which block neuromuscular transmission. There is a muscle weakness with drooping eyelids. It may be associated with thymoma (10%).

7. Answer: D. IL-5

Interleukin-5 is produced by T helper type 2 (Th2) cells. It activates B cells. Eosinophils are recruited by Interleukin-5.

8. Answer: B. Interleukin-2

Interleukin-2 (IL-2) is produced by activated T helper cells. It augments T cells, large granular lymphocyte (LGL), and B cells activity. Interleukin-2 (IL-2) is one of the key cytokines used for the therapy of metastatic melanoma and renal cell carcinoma.

9. Answer: B. Low or absent immunoglobulins

X-linked agammaglobulinemia (XLA) of Bruton presents approximately at 2–6 months of age after maternal antibody wanes. It is caused by a defect in B cell maturation. There are extremely low or absent immunoglobulin levels (IgG < 200 mg/dl). CD 19 positive B cells are absent in peripheral blood. Patients present with recurrent respiratory infections due to streptococcus pneumoniae and haemophilus influenzae and gastrointestinal infections by giardia lamblia. In lymph nodes, lymphoid follicles and germinal centers are not formed because of the absence of B cells.

10. Answer: B. Interferons

Type 1 interferons include IFNα and IFNβ. IFNα is produced by leukocytes, inhibits viral replication. It is used to treat Hepatitis C. IFNβ is produced by fibroblast and also inhibits viral replication. Interferon beta (IFNβ) used to treat multiple sclerosis (MS). Type II interferons (IFNs) include IFN-γ (gamma). IFN-γ is produced by T helper cells and increases cell-mediated immunity (CMI).

11. Answer: A. Common variable immunodeficiency

Common variable Immunodeficiency (CVID) may present at any age, often seen in adults. There is impaired B cell differentiation with defective immunoglobulin production. Mutation of genes for inducible costimulator (ICOS) occurs only in a small amount of patients. There are heterogeneous manifestations, including gastrointestinal symptoms and recurrent infections. Common gastrointestinal symptoms are diarrhea, malabsorption, and infections by helicobacter pylori and giardia lamblia.

12. Answer: C. Severe combined immunodeficiency

Severe combined immunodeficiency (SCID) is caused by the IL-2 receptor gamma chain mutation or adenosine deaminase deficiency (20q13, autosomal recessive). Usual presentation is shortly after birth to 6 months of age. T lymphocytes, B lymphocytes, and large granular lymphocytes (LGL) are low or absent. The absence of both cellular and humoral immunity leads to susceptibility to infections. Infections with bacterial, fungal, viral, and protozoal infections are frequently fatal.

13. Answer: D. Follicular dendritic cells

Follicular dendritic cells in the lymphoid tissue are a major reservoir for human immunodeficiency virus.

14. Answer: B. Tuberculosis and graft-versus-host disease

Delayed type hypersensitivity (DTH) is mediated by CD4 cells. It is also known as Type IV hypersensitivity or cell mediated hypersensitivity. DTH occurs 48–72 h after exposure to an antigen. Classic examples are PPD skin test and poison ivy. Graft-versus-host disease (GVHD) and transplant rejection are also type 4 hypersensitivity reactions.

15. Answer: B. CD1a

Langerhans cell histiocytosis (LCH) is common in children from 1–3 years of age, but may be seen in all age groups. CD1a is a common histiocytic marker for Langerhans cells in LCH.

16. Answer: B. Congo red

In amyloidosis, protein fibrils accumulate in various organs. Light chain (AL) amyloid is commonly seen in systemic amyloidosis. Congo red stain is used to demonstrate amyloid deposits in tissues as green birefringence under polarized light.

Congo red stain in renal biopsy (Green birefringence)

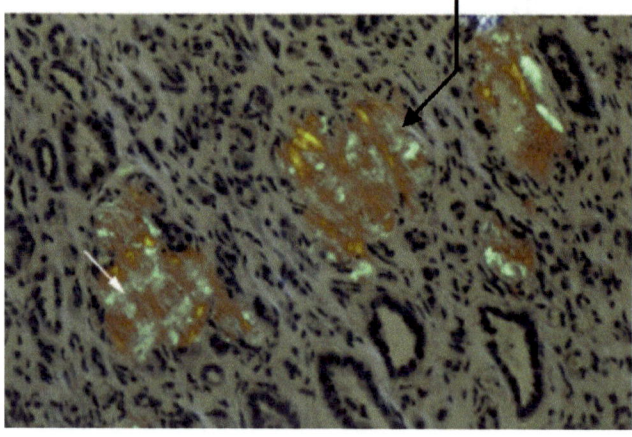

17. Answer: C. Osteoclasts

Antigen elicits and combines with an immune response. Dendritic cells, macrophages, and B lymphocytes are common antigen-presenting cells (APCs). In addition to these APCs, basophils are also considered as antigen-presenting cells. APCs transport antigens from tissues to lymphoid organs and also provide activating signals to T lymphocytes.

18. Answer: A. IgA

There are five immunoglobulin classes of antibody molecules in the serum. They are IgG, IgM, IgA, IgE, and IgD. IgA deficiency is the most common.

19. Answer: E. Chronic granulomatous disease

Chronic granulomatous disease (CGD) usually presents by 2 years of age with lymphadenitis, hepatosplenomegaly, and pneumonia. Diagnosis is made by nitroblue tetrazolium reduction assay or newer, flow cytometric assays. CGD is genetically inherited as an X-linked disorder in most of the cases. There are also autosomal recessive forms.

20. Answer: B. Ankylosing spondylitis

Patients of ankylosing spondylitis (AS) have a higher incidence of HLA-B27. Ankylosing spondylitis causes chronic inflammation of the sacroiliac joints. Majority of patients are young and middle aged males. Patients present with low back pain and stiffness.

21. Answer: B. Celiac disease

Patients with selective IgA deficiency are at increased risk for celiac disease. Diagnosis may be hampered because serum levels (for antigliadin/or antiendomysial antibodies) are often normal. Patients are also at risk for infections, malabsorption, and unusual chronic inflammatory diseases.

22. Answer: D. Type IV

Immunologic reactions are divided into four categories according to the Gell and Coombs system. Antibody-mediated immunologic reactions are types I, II, and III. Type IV immunologic reaction is mediated by T cells.

23. Answer: E. CD3

CD3 (cluster of differentiation 3) is a marker for circulating mature T cells. On routine flow cytometry, CD3 marker is used to identify total T cells including CD4 and CD8 cells.

24. Answer: A. Memory B cells enter the lymph node

Mature B cells exit the spleen and migrate to lymph nodes. The paracortex of the lymph node contains high endothelial venules (HEVs), where circulating lymphocytes leave the bloodstream to enter the lymph node. Postcapillary HEVs are lined by cuboidal endothelial cells.

25. Answer: B. C3

Low level C3 activation is required to kick off the alternate pathway in response to liposaccharide. C3 is a sensitive marker for defects in the alternate pathway.

26. Answer: B. 6

MHC Classes I, II, and III are all located on the short arm of chromosome 6. Class I can be found on all nucleated cells. Class II protein is found on antigen-presenting cells. Class III is a special class composed of diverse complement components of genes such as Bf, C2, and C4 and encodes a hodge-podge of important and varied proteins, such as hydroxylase and TNF-alpha.

27. Answer: C. IgA

There are only three types of immunoglobulin capable of activating complement: IgG, IgA, and IgM. Only IgA activates complement through the alternative pathway.

28. Answer: E. Fc epsilon

Mast cells are capable of binding IgE through Fc epsilon receptors.

29. Answer: C. 14

The gene for mu, gamma, alpha, delta, and epsilon are located on the same chromosome 14. This is important for the mechanism of class type switching.

30. Answer: A. Type III Hypersensitivity reaction

Henoch-Schonlein purpura (HSP) is IgA immune complex mediated type III hypersensitivity reaction. HSP is a systemic vasculitis commonly seen in children between ages 3 and 10. It follows the upper respiratory tract infections. Common clinical manifestations are palpable purpura, arthralgias, abdominal pain. Diagnosis is confirmed by IgA deposits in blood vessels.

Bibliography

1. Angum F, Khan T, Kaler J, Siddiqui L, Hussain A. The prevalence of autoimmune disorders in women. Cureus. 2020;12(5):e118.
2. Chen X, et al. FcγR-binding is an important functional attribute for immune checkpoint antibodies in cancer immunotherapy. Front Immunol. 2019;10:292.
3. Palmeira P, et al. IgG Placental transfer in healthy and pathological pregnancies. Clin Dev Immunol. 2012;2012:985646.
4. Sangueza-Acosta M, Sandoval-Romero E. Epstein-Barr virus and skin. An Bras Dermatol. 2018;93(6):786–99.
5. Ratajczak W, et al. Immunological memory cells. Cent Eur J Immunol. 2018;43(2):194–203.
6. Merola JF, et al. Drug-induced lupus. 2019.
7. Jowkar A. Myasthenia gravis. 2018.
8. Liu M, et al. Pathogenesis of asthma. 2019.
9. Pichler WJ, Adkinson NF, Feldweg AM. An approach to the patient with drug allergy. 2019.
10. Hernandez-Trujillo VP. Agammaglobulinemia. 2019.
11. Cunningham-Rundles C, et al. Clinical manifestations, epidemiology, and diagnosis of common variable immunodeficiency in adults. 2019.
12. Hogan MB, et al. Common variable immunodeficiency in children. 2019.
13. Heimall J, et al. Severe combined immunodeficiency (SCID): an overview. 2019.
14. Kelly SG. HIV reservoirs in lymph nodes and spleen. 2015.
15. Malarvizhi S, Gugan R. Black's medical-surgical nursing. 2019.
16. Radzikowska E. Pulmonary Langerhans' cell histiocytosis in adults. Adv Respir Med. 2017;85(5):277–89.
17. Vaxman I, Gertz M. Recent advances in the diagnosis, risk stratification, and management of systemic light-chain amyloidosis. Acta Haematol. 2019;141(2):93–106.
18. Call ME, et al. Antigen-presenting cells. 2019.
19. Fett N, et al. Evaluation of adults with cutaneous lesions of vasculitis. 2019.
20. Rajkumar SV, et al. Clinical presentation, laboratory manifestations, and diagnosis of immunoglobulin light chain (AL) amyloidosis. 2019.
21. Yu DT, et al. Pathogenesis of spondyloarthritis. 2019.
22. Bloch DB, et al. The anti-Ro/SSA and anti-La/SSB antigen-antibody systems. 2019.
23. Pichler WJ, et al. Drug allergy: pathogenesis. 2019.

Neoplastic Disorders

4

Multiple Choice Questions

1. Which gene is found in Mantle cell lymphoma (MCL)?
   - A. CDK4
   - B. Ki-ras
   - C. Cyclin D1 gene
   - D. L-myc
   - E. N-myc

2. A 35-year-old HIV positive male patient presents with nontender, firm, rubbery lymph nodes in the left side of the neck. Histologically, large Hodgkin–Reed-Sternberg cells with multiple nuclei and prominent nucleoli are present. What is the diagnosis?
   - A. Nodular sclerosis cHL
   - B. Lymphocyte depleted cHL
   - C. Lymphocyte rich cHL
   - D. Non-Hodgkin lymphoma
   - E. Mixed cellularity cHL

3. Which of the oncogene is present in squamous cell carcinoma in the lung?
   - A. ErbB1
   - B. ErbB2
   - C. ErbB3
   - D. Ki-ras
   - E. Cyclin D

4. Which of the following carcinoma shows increased expression of ERBB2 (HER2) gene?
   - A. Carcinoma of the stomach
   - B. Melanoma
   - C. Astrocytoma
   - D. Infiltrating ductal and intraductal carcinoma of the breast
   - E. Ovarian carcinoma

© The Author(s), under exclusive license to Springer Nature Switzerland AG 2022
V. K. Kohli et al., *Comprehensive Multiple-Choice Questions in Pathology*, https://doi.org/10.1007/978-3-031-08767-7_4

5. Microscopic images from lymph node of a 35-year-old male patient are shown below. What is the diagnosis?

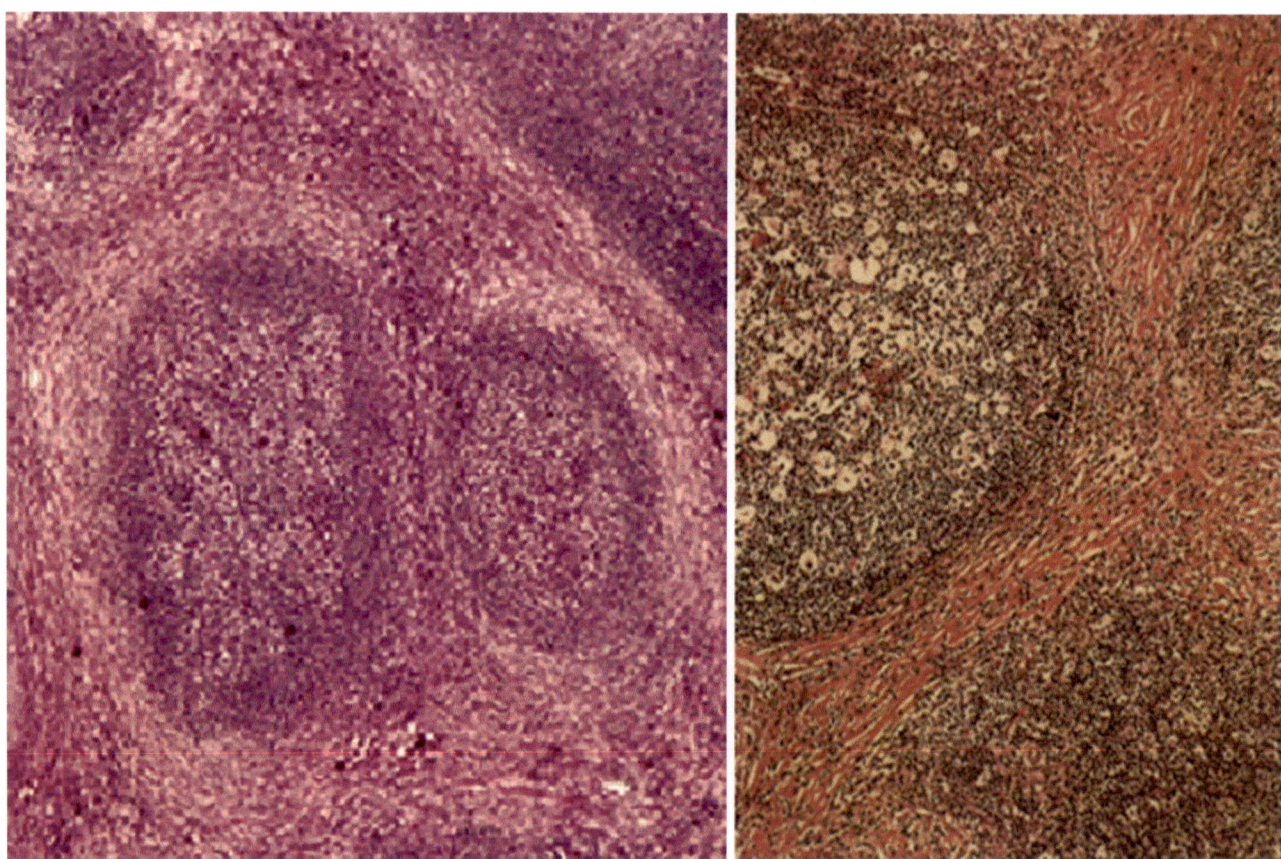

A. Mixed cellularity Hodgkin lymphoma
B. Nodular sclerosis Hodgkin lymphoma
C. Lymphocyte rich classical Hodgkin lymphoma
D. Lymphocyte depleted Hodgkin lymphoma
E. Non-Hodgkin lymphoma

6. Which of the following oncogene is found in the carcinoma of the lung, pancreas, and colon?
A. Ki-ras
B. L-myc
C. N-myc
D. CDK4
E. RET

7. Mediastinal tumors are rare neoplasms. The most common tumor of the mediastinum is:
A. Lymphoma
B. Mediastinal germ cell tumor
C. Thymoma
D. Mediastinal lymphangioma
E. Mediastinal parathyroid adenomas

8. Naphthylamine is a chemical carcinogen responsible for which of the following carcinoma?
A. Angiosarcoma of liver
B. Squamous cell carcinoma of skin
C. Bronchogenic carcinoma
D. Carcinoma bladder
E. Lymphoma

9. Malignant tumor of mesenchymal tissue is referred to as?
A. Choristoma
B. Carcinoma
C. Hamartoma
D. Teratoma
E. Sarcoma

10. A 20-year-old male presents with anterior mediastinal mass. Biopsy of the mass is performed and H&E stained section shows cells which express CD20+, BSAP+, and EMA+. They show CD15 and CD30 expression. What is the diagnosis?
A. Nodular sclerosis Hodgkin lymphoma.
B. Mixed cellularity Hodgkin lymphoma.
C. Lymphocyte depleted Hodgkin lymphoma.
D. Lymphocyte rich Hodgkin lymphoma.
E. Lymphocyte predominant Hodgkin lymphoma

11. A 10-year-old male presents with a rapidly enlarging maxillary mass. Biopsy is done and the microscopic picture shows starry-sky appearance. What is the diagnosis?

A. Follicular lymphoma
B. Mantle cell lymphoma
C. Hodgkin lymphoma
D. Burkitt lymphoma
E. Lymphoblastic lymphoma

12. A 59-year-old female with HIV/AIDS with history of diffuse large B cell lymphoma presents with left supra-clavicular adenopathy. Laboratory findings shows leukopenia and lymphopenia. An excisional biopsy of the enlarged lymph node is performed and H&E picture shows diffuse effacement of the lymph node by sheets of histiocytes. What is the diagnosis?
A. Mycobacterium tuberculosis infection
B. Cytomegalovirus infection
C. Nocardia infection
D. Actinomyces infection
E. Mycobacterium avium-intracellulare infection

13. Some benign tumors of the liver are typically discovered incidentally at laparotomy, autopsy, or during an imaging test performed for unrelated conditions. Which of the following is the most common benign tumor in the liver?
A. Hepatoma
B. Hemangioma
C. Hepatic adenoma
D. Cholangiosarcoma
E. Focal nodular hyperplasia

14. A 39-year-old man comes to the dentist's office with symptoms of enlargement of left tonsil for the last 6 months. Physical examination shows enlargement of right palatine tonsil. Biopsy is done and microscopic picture shows effacement of germinal centers which are replaced by irregular nodules composed of small lymphocytes. What is the diagnosis?
A. Hodgkin's disease
B. Reactive lymphoid hyperplasia
C. Follicular lymphoma
D. Tonsillar abscess
E. Diffuse lymphoma

15. A 55-year-old male with a history of hyperimmunoglobulinemia presents with enlarged cervical lymph nodes. Biopsy of the lymph node is done and microscopic picture shows polymorphous appearance of a lymph node with diffuse effacement of the architecture. There is increased endothelial venules. What is the diagnosis?
A. Multicentric giant lymph node hyperplasia
B. Angioimmunoblastic T cell lymphoma
C. Lymphoma
D. Classic Hodgkin lymphoma mixed cellularity type
E. Sezary syndrome

16. A 37-year-old male presents with lymph nodes in the right side of the neck. Biopsy of a lymph node is done and microscopic picture shows mixed inflammatory background without sclerosis and Hodgkin–Reed-Sternberg cells. What is the diagnosis?
A. Nodular sclerosis cHL
B. Mixed cellularity cHL
C. Lymphocyte rich cHL
D. Lymphocyte depleted cHL
E. Lymphocyte predominant Hodgkin lymphoma

17. Prostate cancer is the second most common cancer in men worldwide. Which fusion gene is found in prostate cancer?
A. TMPRSS2-ERG
B. MYB-NFIB
C. PAX8-PPARG
D. ETV6-NTRK3
E. TFG-GPR128

18. A 17-year-old male presents with recurrent fever, weight loss, and a large painless lump in his groin for the last 8 months. Laboratory findings show pancytopenia. Imaging studies reveal diffuse lymphadenopathy. Cells shows anaplastic lymphoma kinase positivity. What is the diagnosis?
A. Anaplastic large cell lymphoma
B. Classical Hodgkin lymphoma
C. Diffuse large B cell lymphoma
D. Metastatic carcinoma
E. Malignant histiocytosis

19. A 14-year-old boy presents with submandibular lymphadenopathy for the last 2 months. Lymph nodes are freely mobile and firm. Biopsy shows scattered epithelioid histiocytes scattered in the cortical and paracortical areas. What is the diagnosis?
A. Toxoplasmosis
B. Cat scratch disease
C. Histoplasmosis
D. Lymphoblastic lymphoma
E. Metastatic cancer with unknown primary site

20. An 8-year-old boy brought to the pediatrician office by his mother. Physical examination shows hepatosplenomegaly. Laboratory findings show elevated transaminases. Bone marrow biopsy shows numerous macrophages with a wrinkled tissue paper appearance. What is the diagnosis?
A. Niemann-Pick disease
B. GM1 gangliosidosis
C. Gaucher disease
D. Hand-Schuller-Christian disease
E. Mastocytosis

21. Microscopic picture of a type of Hodgkin lymphoma is shown below. Cells have a strong expression of CD20. What is the diagnosis?

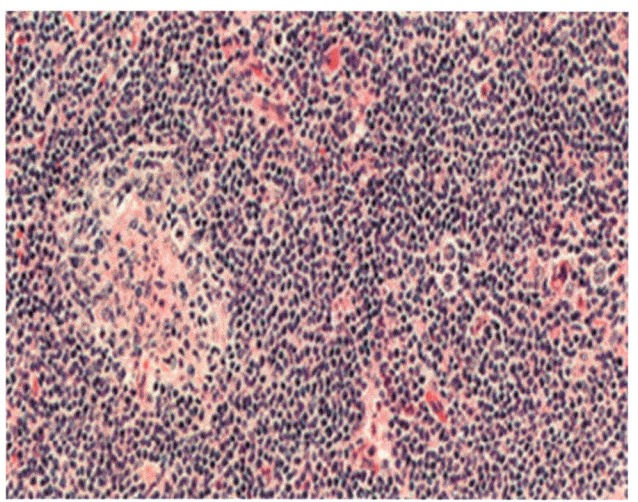

   A. Nodular sclerosis cHL (NSCHL)
   B. Mixed cellularity cHL (MCCHL)
   C. Lymphocyte rich cHL (LRCHL)
   D. Lymphocyte depleted cHL (LDCHL)
   E. Nodular lymphocyte predominant HL (NLPHL)

22. A 57-year-old male present with fever, night sweats, and enlarging lump in his right neck. Imaging studies shows diffuse mediastinal and retroperitoneal lymphadenopathy. Excisional biopsy shows numerous large cells with prominent nucleoli. The tumor shows CD20 positivity. What is the diagnosis?
   A. Follicular lymphoma
   B. Lymphoblastic lymphoma
   C. Diffuse large B cell lymphoma
   D. Mantle cell lymphoma
   E. Mediastinal lymphoma

Answers and Explanations

1. Answer: C. Cyclin D1 gene

   Mantle cell lymphoma (MCL) is B cell lymphoma derived from inner mantle zone cells. This consists of cleaved, distorted small lymphocytes around hyperplastic follicular centers. It is characterized by translocation at t(11:14). Translocation of cyclin D1 leads to the overexpression of cyclin D1. It has poor prognosis. There is frequent involvement of the GI tract causing lymphomatoid polyposis.

2. Answer: B. Lymphocyte depleted cHL

   Lymphocyte depleted cHL (LDCHL) accounts for less than 1% of classic Hodgkin lymphoma (cHL). Histologically, it shows Hodgkin–Reed-Sternberg cells with multiple nuclei and prominent nucleoli. These cells grow within a background which is depleted in lymphocytes. It is found in HIV infected patients. EBV positivity is also seen in the majority of the patients. There is intense staining for CD30.

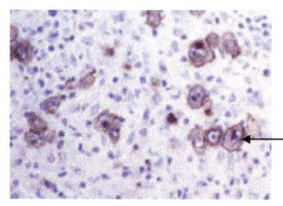

CD30+ in Lymphocyte depleted cHL (Immunohistochemistry)

3. Answer: A. ErbB1

   Epidermal growth factor receptor is a transmembrane glycoprotein that regulate signaling pathways to control cellular proliferation. Some lung cancer develop due to a mutation in an epidermal growth factor (ErbB1) receptor. Tyrosine kinase inhibitors have positive role in lung adenocarcinomas with mutated epidermal growth factor receptor.

4. Answer: D. Infiltrating ductal and intraductal carcinoma of the breast

   Increased expression of ERBB2 (HER2) gene is usually found in infiltrating ductal and intraductal carcinoma of the breast. ERBB2 (HER2) is usually detected immunohistochemically and by fluorescence in situ hybridization (FISH) in the biopsy specimen.

5. Answer: B. Nodular sclerosis Hodgkin lymphoma

   Nodular sclerosis cHL (NSCHL) is characterized by a nodular growth pattern in the lymph node with fibrous bands separating cellular nodules. Diagnostic RS cells may be rare. Typically the majority of Hodgkin–Reed-Sternberg (HRS) cells are lacunar cells. The background is inflammatory and usually consists of eosinophils, neutrophils, macrophages, and areas of necrosis. Tissue fibrosis is commonly found in nodular sclerosis.

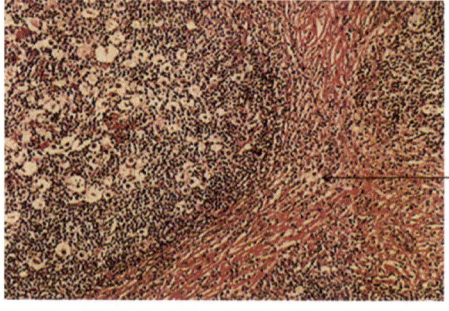

Bands of fibrosis separate nodules

6. Answer: A. Ki-ras

   Mutational activation of KRAS (K-ras or Ki-ras) is commonly found in lung cancer and different types of epithelial cancers. Colon carcinomas and pancreatic adenocarcinomas are also found due to the mutations of KRAS.

7. Answer: C. Thymoma

Tumors of thymus are usually found in the anterior mediastinum. It is commonly found in adults. It can be thymomas and thymic carcinomas. Thymoma is usually incidental finding during imaging studies. Thymoma accounts for 20% of mediastinal neoplasms. Patients usually present with the symptoms of paraneoplastic syndromes such as myasthenia gravis.

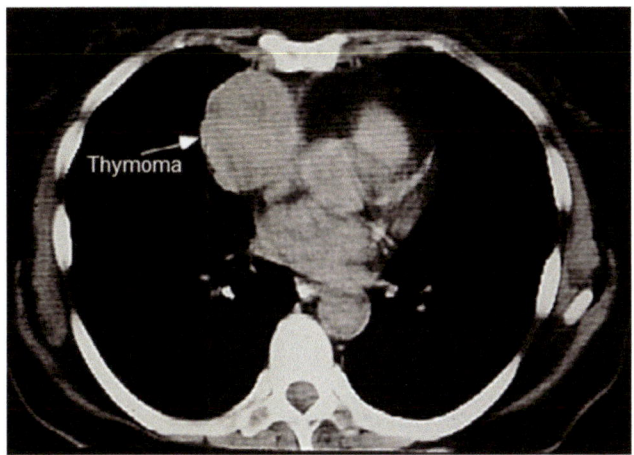

8. Answer: D. Carcinoma bladder

Urinary bladder is caused by chemical carcinogen 2-Naphthylamine. There is an increased incidence of bladder cancer in workers associated with the manufacture and use of 2-naphthylamine. 2-naphthylamine carcinogenicity is commonly due to the genotoxic mechanism of action that involves metabolic activation and induction of mutagenic and clastogenic effects.

9. Answer: E. Sarcoma.

Sarcoma is a malignant tumor arising from mesenchymal tissue. Sarcomas can affect different types of connective tissues. Sarcoma is commonly found in bones, muscles, and cartilages. A common example is bone sarcoma or osteosarcoma. Sarcomas account for around 1% of all adult cancers. It is more common in children and accounts for approximately 15% of pediatric cancers.

10. Answer: E. Lymphocyte predominant Hodgkin lymphoma

Nodular lymphocyte predominant Hodgkin lymphoma (NLPHL) is now recognized as being fundamentally different from other variants of Hodgkin lymphoma, which are collectively referred to as classical Hodgkin lymphoma (cHL). It is believed to arise from a more differentiated B cell than does cHL. As a result, in contrast to cHL (which lacks mature B cell antigens and expresses CD15 and/or CD30), NLPHL is almost always CD20+ and strongly BSAP+ and negative for CD15 and CD30 expression. In addition, it can be positive for EMA (not always present, but strongly supports the diagnosis).

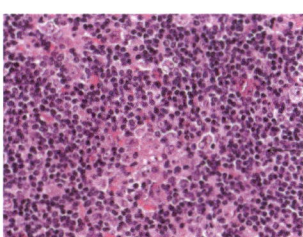

Nodular lymphocyte predominant Hodgkin lymphoma (NLPHL)

11. Answer: D. Burkitt lymphoma

Burkitt lymphoma can be classified as either endemic, sporadic or immunodeficiency associated. They are mostly common in the jaw or abdomen. 95% of the tumors are associated with EBV infection. Immunodeficiency cases generally occur in adults with HIV infection and often involve the cecum or distal ileum. All types are extremely fast growing with numerous mitotic figures. Histologically, there is a distinct starry sky appearance. The tangible body macrophages are the stars sprinkled throughout the sky of deep blue tumor cells. It is characterized by the translocation and deregulation of the MYC gene on chromosome 8.

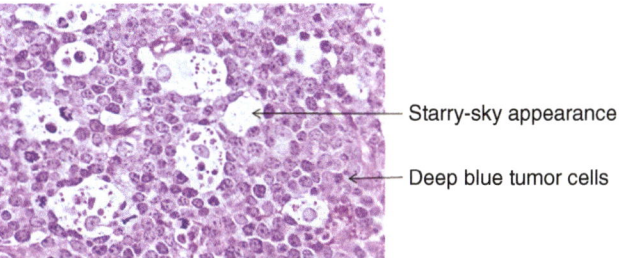

Starry-sky appearance

Deep blue tumor cells

12. Answer: E. Mycobacterium avium-intracellulare infection

Opportunistic infections with HIV/AIDS can occur in large B cell lymphoma. Patients usually prefer with leukopenia and lymphopenia with very low CD4+ T cell count. H&E sections of large B cell lymphoma show diffuse architectural effacement of the lymph node by the sheets of histiocytes. Acid fast stain show numerous intracellular rod shaped acid fast organisms. These findings are typical of mycobacterium avium-intracellulare (MAI) infection.

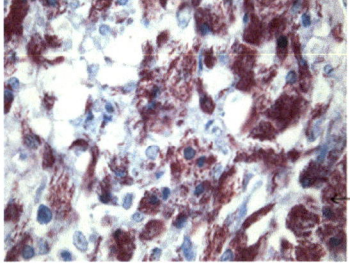

Rod shaped acid-fast organisms-mycobacterium avium-intracellulare (MAI)

13. Answer: B. Hemangioma

The most common benign hepatic mesenchymal tumors are hepatic hemangioma. Hemangiomas are often isolated but in up to 40% of patients multiple lesions may occur both on the right and left lobe in the liver. They range between a few mm to more than 20 cm in size. Majority of them are small (< 5 cm). Bigger than 5 cm are termed as giant hemangiomas. The diagnosis is often made by distinguishing hemangiomas from other lesions.

14. Answer: C. Follicular lymphoma

Follicular lymphoma is a subtype of non-Hodgkin lymphoma. Follicular lymphomas are composed of many large centroblasts. CD43 T cell marker highlights the nodularity or follicular architecture. Negative staining for CD43 is typical for follicular lymphoma. Histologically, the tumor consists of large cells with pleomorphic nuclei and prominent nucleoli.

15. Answer: B. Angioimmunoblastic T cell Lymphoma

Angioimmunoblastic T cell lymphoma is usually an uncommon T cell type of non-Hodgkin lymphoma. It is more common in the elderly males. There is polymorphous lymph node infiltration with diffuse effacement of the architecture. There is a marked increase in follicular dendritic cells and high endothelial venules. Numerous cells are CD2, CD3, and CD5 positive. CD10 co-expression in T cells is characteristic. All these features suggest angioimmunoblastic T cell lymphoma (AILT).

16. Answer: B. Mixed cellularity cHL

Mixed cellularity cHL (MCCHL) accounts for approximately 20–25% of classic Hodgkin lymphoma (cHL). It is a heterogeneous subtype of classic HL. Histologically, it has diffuse or nodular growth pattern. There is no band forming sclerosis. Classic Hodgkin–Reed-Sternberg cells are usually present along with fine interstitial fibrosis. The background usually consists of neutrophils, eosinophils, plasma cells, and macrophages.

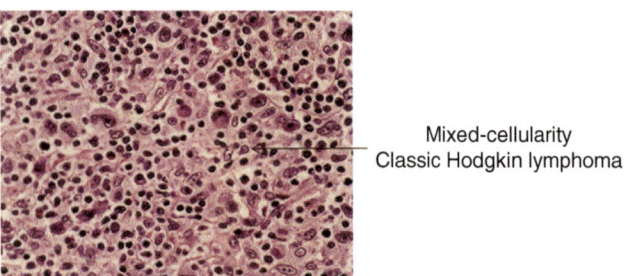

Mixed-cellularity Classic Hodgkin lymphoma

17. Answer: A. TMPRSS2-ERG

Recurrent gene fusion due to chromosomal rearrangement takes place in prostate cancer. The most common recurrent genomic alterations in prostate cancer are the fusion of the TMPRSS2, an androgen-regulated gene, and the ETS transcription family members (ERG, ETV1, ETV4, and ETV5). In almost half of the prostate specific antigen (PSA) screened patients with prostate cancer, TMPRSS2-ERG fusion products are found. Fusion of TMPRSS2-ERG shows a high correlation to disease recurrence for localized prostate cancer after surgery.

18. Answer: A. Anaplastic large cell lymphoma

Patients with anaplastic large cell lymphoma usually present with recurrent fever, weight loss. There may be enlarged painless mass in the lymph nodes areas. Laboratory findings show pancytopenia. Lymphoma is anaplastic lymphoma kinase positive. Histologically, it shows cohesive clusters of large tumor cells with chromatin-poor nuclei and prominent nucleoli. There are also cells with kidney shaped nuclei.

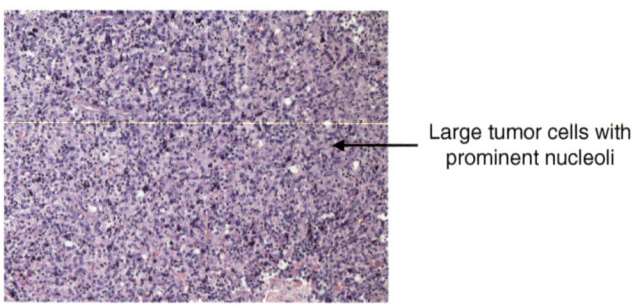

Large tumor cells with prominent nucleoli

19. Answer: A. Toxoplasmosis

In Toxoplasmosis, patients present with lymph nodes enlargement. Lymph nodes are usually mobile and firm. Histologically, there are scattered epithelioid histiocytes scattered haphazardly in the cortical and paracortical areas and encroaching the follicular margins, monocytoid cells, and large germinal centers.

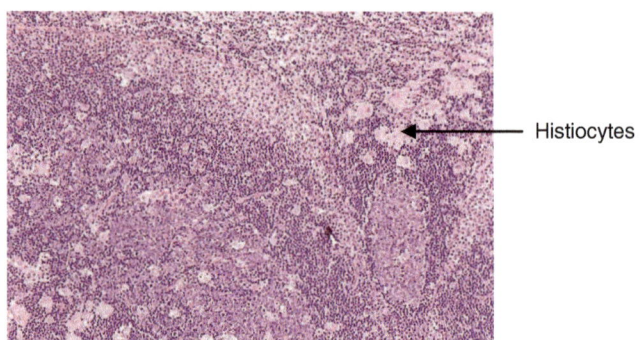

Histiocytes

20. Answer: C. Gaucher disease

Gaucher disease is a type of lipid storage disease. There is a deposition of glucocerebroside in cells of the macrophage-monocyte system. It occurs due to deficiency of glucocerebrosidase. Patient presents with hepatosplenomegaly. Laboratory finding show elevated transaminases. The bone marrow aspirate shows numerous macrophages with a striated tubular pattern described as wrinkled tissue paper in appearance. This is the characteristic of Gaucher disease.

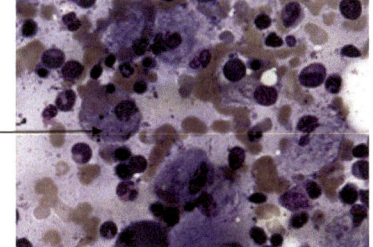

Macrophage with wrinkled tissue paper in appearance

diffuse mediastinal and retroperitoneal lymphadenopathy without organ involvement. Histologically, the tumor is composed of numerous large cells with dispersed chromatin and prominent nucleoli. Positivity of CD20 is important marker for diffuse B cell lymphomas.

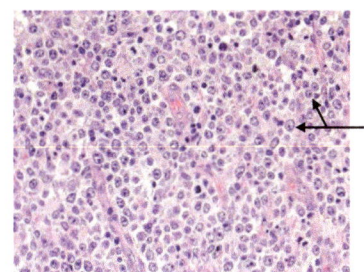

Tumor cells with dispersed chromatin prominent nucleoli

21. Answer: C. Lymphocyte rich cHL (LRCHL)

Lymphocyte rich cHL (LRCHL) is a type of classical Hodgkin Lymphomas (CHL). EBV positivity is found in approximately 40% cases of LRCHL. NSCHL is the predominant subtype followed by MCCHL while lymphocyte rich cHL and lymphocyte dominant CHL are uncommon. Limited stage (Ann Arbor Stage I or II) peripheral lymphadenopathy is usually present in patients with LRCHL. Histologically, common patterns are nodular and diffuse. Small lymphocytes with eccentric and small germinal centers without any eosinophils or neutrophils are seen in LRCHL. Immunohistochemistry for CD20 highlights the nodular pattern with a predominance of B cells.

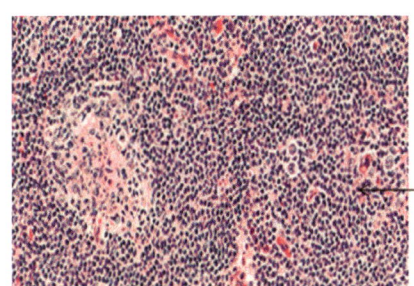

Lymphocyte-rich CHL, nodular variant.

22. Answer: C. Diffuse large B cell lymphoma

Diffuse large B cell lymphoma can affect persons of any age. It is most common in people over 50 years. It is slightly more common in man. Diffuse large B cell lymphoma presents with fever and night sweats. There may be an enlarged lump in the neck. Imaging studies reveal

Bibliography

1. De Falco G, Gibellini D, Piccaluga PP, Murray PG, Mbulaiteye S. Molecular mechanisms of pathogen-driven infectious and neoplastic diseases. Front Cell Dev Biol. 2021;9:696152.
2. Freedman AS, et al. Clinical manifestations, pathologic features, and diagnosis of mantle cell lymphoma. 2019.
3. King TE, Flaherty KR, Hollingsworth H. Asbestos-related pleuropulmonary disease. 2019.
4. Hirsch MS, et al. Anatomy and pathology of testicular tumors. 2019.
5. Aster JC, et al. Pathogenesis of Hodgkin lymphoma. 2019.
6. Meneshian A, et al. Clinical presentation and management of thymoma and thymic carcinoma. 2019.
7. Thomas KW, et al. Overview of the initial evaluation, diagnosis, and staging of patients with suspected lung cancer. 2019.
8. Nagpal M, et al. Tumor markers: a diagnostic tool. Natl J Maxillofac Surg. 2016;7(1):17–20.
9. LaCasce AS, Andrea KN. Treatment of nodular lymphocyte-predominant Hodgkin lymphoma. 2019.
10. Van Etten RA, et al. Cellular and molecular biology of chronic myeloid leukemia. 2019.
11. Curry MP. Hepatic hemangioma. 2019.
12. Aronson MD, et al. Infectious mononucleosis. 2019.
13. Taxy JB, et al. Pathology of head and neck neoplasms. 2019.
14. Griend DV, et al. Molecular biology of prostate cancer. 2019.
15. Win AK, et al. Lynch syndrome (hereditary nonpolyposis colorectal cancer): clinical manifestations and diagnosis. 2019.
16. Kalisz K, et al. An update on Burkitt lymphoma: a review of pathogenesis and multimodality imaging assessment of disease presentation, treatment response, and recurrence. Insights Imaging. 2019;10(1):56.
17. Sax PE, Bartlett JG, Sullivan M. Acute and early HIV infection: clinical manifestations and diagnosis. 2019.

Infectious Diseases

5

Multiple Choice Questions

1. A 39-year-old diabetic patient presents with cough, fever, headache, nasal congestion, facial pain. On examination there is black necrotic eschar in the nasal cavity. Histological examination of the affected tissue shows broad nonseptate hyphae with right-angle branching. What is the diagnosis?
   A. Mucormycosis
   B. Aspergillosis
   C. Actinomyces israelii
   D. Candida albicans
   E. Leishmania major

2. Patient was admitted to the hospital because of bleeding duodenal ulcer. Culture at 37°C grew urease-positive curved bacteria. The most likely causative agent is:
   A. Campylobacter jejuni
   B. Streptococcus faecalis
   C. Enterococcus
   D. Pseudomonas aeruginosa
   E. Helicobacter pylori

3. A patient with uncontrolled diabetes mellitus gets fungal infection. Microscopic examination of the fungus shows that the hyphae are septate and branch at more acute angles. What is the diagnosis?
   A. Mucormycosis
   B. Aspergillosis
   C. Actinomyces israelii
   D. Candida albicans
   E. Blastomycosis

4. A 2-year-old boy presents with symptoms of large volume, watery diarrhea for the last one day. Polymerase chain reaction testing of the stool sample yields a virus with a segmented, double-stranded RNA genome. Which organism is responsible for this presentation?
   A. Rotavirus
   B. Enteric coronaviruses
   C. Norwalk virus
   D. Calicivirus
   E. Entamoeba histolytica

5. A 50-year-old woman is admitted to the hospital with fever, headache, confusion, and ataxia. Similar cases are also reported in a neighboring hospital. Which organism is most likely responsible for this outbreak?
   A. Escherichia coli O157:H7
   B. Streptococcus pneumoniae
   C. Klebsiella pneumoniae
   D. Vibrio cholerae
   E. Listeria monocytogenes

6. Which of the following characteristics is an important virulence factor in Haemophilus influenzae type b?
   A. Exotoxin
   B. Polyribosyl ribitol phosphate
   C. Endotoxin
   D. Adhesins
   E. Yersiniabactin

7. Which of the following pathogens is a leading cause of atypical pneumonia?
   A. Mycoplasma pneumoniae
   B. Streptococcus pneumoniae
   C. Haemophilus influenzae
   D. Chlamydia pneumoniae
   E. Legionella pneumophila

8. Which of the following requires airborne precautions?
   A. Disseminated varicella zoster
   B. Allergic contact dermatitis
   C. Influenza A
   D. Rubella
   E. Ebola

9. A 42-year-old patient presents with fever, sore throat, tachypnea and shortness of breath, and maculopapular rash on the trunk is hospitalized in the emergency. Patients also developed bleeding in the stool, petechiae, ecchymoses, oozing from venipuncture sites and mucosal bleeding. Patient also develops meningoencephalitis. Unfortunately the patient died due to multi-organ failure

V. K. Kohli et al., *Comprehensive Multiple-Choice Questions in Pathology*, https://doi.org/10.1007/978-3-031-08767-7_5

and shock. Which of the following infectious agents is most likely to produce these findings?

- A. Influenza virus
- B. Ebola virus
- C. Lassa virus
- D. Yellow fever virus
- E. Cytomegalovirus

10. A 40-year-old homosexual man presents with anorectal spasms, pain, bloody discharge, and peri-anal sores. Patients also reported a genital ulcer. Which of the following is responsible for this patient conditions?

- A. Human papillomavirus
- B. Trichomoniasis
- C. Chlamydia trachomatis
- D. Neisseria gonorrhoeae
- E. Herpes simplex virus (HSV) infection

11. Which of the following pathogenic bacteria produces swarming growth on blood agar?

- A. Proteus species
- B. Clostridium botulinum
- C. Staphylococcus aureus
- D. Escherichia coli
- E. Klebsiella pneumoniae

12. Most common virus associated with laryngeal papilloma is:

- A. HPV 6
- B. HPV 24
- C. HPV 32
- D. HPV 36
- E. HPV 17

13. A photograph is shown below. What is the diagnosis?

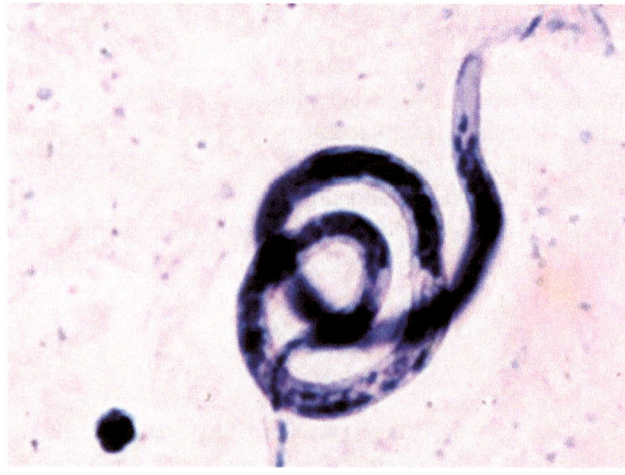

- A. Loa loa
- B. Mansonella species
- C. Brugia malayi
- D. Brugia timori
- E. Wuchereria bancrofti

14. Which of the following organism requires fatty-acid supplementation for growth?

- A. Aspergillus fumigatus
- B. Histoplasma capsulatum
- C. Coccidioides immitis
- D. Malassezia furfur
- E. Candida albicans

15. A 65-year-old man presents with fever, severe headache, and nuchal rigidity. Physical examination in the emergency department shows a Glasgow coma score of 7. Lumbar puncture reveals cloudy cerebrospinal fluid (CSF) with 1200 neutrophils/mm^3, elevated protein, and decreased glucose. Which of the following is the most probable etiologic agent of this condition?

- A. Arbovirus
- B. Herpesvirus
- C. Mycobacterium tuberculosis
- D. Neisseria meningitidis
- E. Streptococcus pneumoniae

16. A 33-year-old woman presents with severe, acute, right upper quadrant abdominal pain. She had several months of bloody diarrhea. CT scan of the liver demonstrates lesions that are interpreted to be abscesses. Which of the following is the most likely cause of her illness?

- A. Ascaris lumbricoides
- B. Entamoeba histolytica
- C. Enterobius vermicularis
- D. Salmonella typhi
- E. Shigellosis

17. A 2-month-old male infant is brought to the emergency room by his mother with symptoms of paroxysms of coughing and choking spells. During the examination the infant was found gasping for breath. Complete blood picture shows 84% lymphocytes. Which of the following organism is responsible for these symptoms?

- A. Streptococcus pneumoniae
- B. Bordetella pertussis
- C. Streptococcus pyogenes
- D. Klebsiella pneumoniae
- E. Mycoplasma pneumoniae

18. Which of the following is transmissible between people?

- A. Epidermophyton
- B. Histoplasma capsulatum
- C. Coccidioides immitis
- D. Trichophyton rubrum
- E. Microsporum

19. There is an incidental finding of a common nematode infection in a colon biopsy of a 52-year-old female daycare worker. Which of the following organism is likely to be present?

- A. Enterobius vermicularis
- B. Ascariasis

C. Giardiasis

D. Entamoeba histolytica

E. Tropheryma whipplei

20. A 62-year-old man presents with symptoms of high grade fever and productive cough for the last 10 days. X-ray of the chest shows areas of consolidation of the left lower lobe. Unfortunately the patient died in the hospital. Autopsy shows bronchopleural fistula and abscess formation with sulfur granules. Which of the following organism is responsible for this patient's condition?

A. Nocardia asteroides

B. Staphylococcus aureus

C. Klebsiella pneumoniae

D. Actinomyces israelii

E. Mycobacterium kansasii

21. A 35-year-old male patient with a diagnosis of acute myelogenous leukemia underwent a stem cell transplant. The patient develops fever and becomes unresponsive after 10 days. Lumbar puncture is done. CSF culture is performed and shows organisms which are catalase negative, LAP positive, PVR positive, and positive for the Lancefield D antigen. Which of the following organism causing this infection?

A. Enterococcus species

B. Escherichia coli

C. Klebsiella pneumoniae

D. Streptococcus pyogenes

E. Staphylococcus aureus

22. A 59-year-old diabetic male patient with a diagnosis of acute myeloid leukemia status post bone marrow transplant presents with right sided facial swelling. Invasive fungus is suspected which is confirmed by fungal culture. Histology shows non septate hyaline hyphae. Which of the following organisms is most likely to produce these findings?

A. Aspergillosis

B. Mucor species

C. Zygomycota

D. Ascomycota

E. Basidiomycota

23. Which of the following parasites is associated with megaloblastic anemia?

A. Necator americanus

B. Ancylostoma duodenale

C. Diphyllobothrium latum

D. Entamoeba histolytica

E. Ascariasis

24. A 19-year-old high school athlete presents with excruciating left ear pain. Physical examination shows diffused inflamed, encrusted, ear canal with weeping lesion. Which of the following organism is most likely to produce these findings?

A. Escherichia coli

B. Aspergillus niger

C. Proteus vulgaris

D. Pseudomonas aeruginosa

E. Klebsiella pneumoniae

25. A 39-year-old woman presents with symptoms of intermittent bloody urine. A diagnosis of infection with an adult worm is suspected. This adult worm resides in the veins of the urine bladder. Which of the following is most likely to cause these clinical findings?

A. Schistosoma haematobium

B. Trematodes (flukes)

C. Diphyllobothriasis

D. Strongyloidiasis

E. Cysticercosis

26. A 14-year-old male with sickle cell anemia presents with shortness of breath that has been getting worse over the past several days. Laboratory finding shows relatively low reticulocyte count (0.5%). Which of the following virus is most likely to produce these findings?

A. Retrovirus

B. Parvovirus B 19

C. Adenovirus

D. Epstein–Barr virus

E. Calicivirus

27. A 28-year-old woman with HIV infection presents with symptoms of fever, sweats, malaise, and sore throat for the last 2 weeks. Physical examination shows swollen tender cervical lymph nodes. Endoscopic examination shows plaques throughout her esophagus. Which of the following is the diagnosis related to the sore throat?

A. Disseminated pneumocystis carimi

B. Candida esophagitis

C. Hairy leukoplakia

D. Cytomegalovirus ulcers of the esophagus

E. Lymphoma of the esophagus

28. A 24-year-old recently married female with symptoms of dysuria. A urine nitrite test is negative. The bacteria is cultured. Biochemical tests are catalase+/coagulase-/novobiocin resistant bacteria. Which of the following infectious agents is most likely to produce these findings?

A. Staphylococcus saprophyticus

B. Escherichia coli

C. Staphylococcus aureus

D. Pseudomonas aeruginosa

E. Proteus vulgaris

29. A 10-year-old child brought to the pediatrician office with the symptoms of fever. Mother states that the fever has been occurring every 2 days. A CBC with peripheral blood smear is ordered. Peripheral blood smear shows a parasite causing the fever. What is the diagnosis?

A. Plasmodium ovale

B. Plasmodium knowlesi

C. Plasmodium malariae

D. Plasmodium vivax

E. Plasmodium falciparum

Answers and Explanations

1. Answer: A. Mucormycosis

   The risk factor for the formation of rhino-orbital-cerebral mucormycosis is diabetic ketoacidosis. Diabetics can also experience cutaneous mucormycosis, most commonly caused by skin trauma. Erythematous indurated plaques or bullae on the wound frequently lead to a necrotic ulcer in the form of eschar. Histologically, pseudohyphae and hyphae are seen along with rectangular arthroconidia, and blastoconidia.

2. Answer: E. Helicobacter pylori

   The spiral shaped, microaerophilic helicobacter pylori (H. pylori) is a gram-negative bacterium with a length of about 3.5 microns and a width of 0.5 micron. The organism has two to seven unipolar sheathed flagella which enhances the mobility of the organism through viscous solutions. Diagnosis of H. pylori is based on biopsy, urease breath test, and stool antigen and serum antibody testing.

3. Answer: B. Aspergillosis

   The most common fungal infections involving maxillary sinuses are aspergillosis and mucormycosis. There are three types of bronchopulmonary aspergillosis infections: invasive aspergillosis, chronic aspergillosis, and allergic aspergillosis. They can be expressed in two ways—noninvasive or invasive. These infections can be treated early without causing significant tissue damage if properly diagnosed. Immunocompromised persons are more susceptible to this infection, especially long-term uncontrolled diabetics. Uncontrolled diabetes mellitus may alter the patient's normal immunological response to infections. Biopsy specimens can be observed with acute angle hyphae (45 degrees) using Gomori methenamine silver or periodic acid-Schiff staining. If left untreated, invasive aspergillosis can have mortality approaching 100%. There is a need for extensive diagnostic testing in cases of suspected invasive aspergillosis but treatment should be started early to minimize morbidity and mortality.

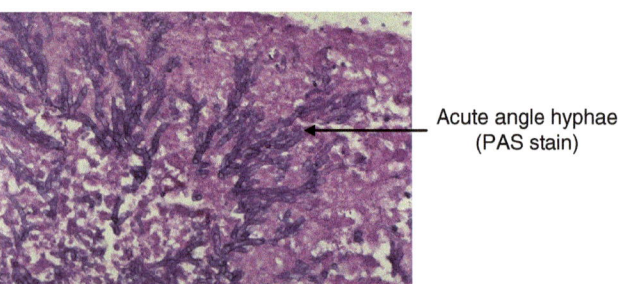

Acute angle hyphae (PAS stain)

4. Answer: A. Rotavirus

   The major cause of serious, dehydrating gastroenteritis in children is a rotavirus infection. It commonly affects less than 5 years old. Acute watery diarrhea is most often due to rotavirus. In older children, it is most often due to *E. coli* (ETEC). Rotavirus infects primarily enterocytes and contributes to diarrhea due to the destruction of absorptive enterocytes. Rotavirus infection control is based on prevention and treatment of dehydration.

5. Answer: E. Listeria monocytogenes

   In immunosuppressed patients, neonates and older adults, pregnant women and sometimes previously healthy individuals are infected by bacterial pathogen, Listeria monocytogenes. Common clinical infestations are an invasion of nervous system including meningitis or meningoencephalitis.

6. Answer: B. Polyribosyl ribitol phosphate

   Haemophilus influenzae is a gram-negative coccobacillus. An essential virulence factor in the Haemophilus influenzae type b is a polyribosyl-ribitol (PRP) capsule. Polyribosyl-ribitol (PRP) is a capsular polysaccharide. This prevents phagocytosis of the type b H influenzae due to the absence of a certain anticapsular antibody.

7. Answer: A. Mycoplasma pneumoniae

   Mycoplasma pneumoniae is a cause of atypical (walking) pneumonia. It lacks a cell wall and is therefore, not visible on the gram stain. It is one of the smallest free-living pathogens. Due to the lack of cell wall, it is not susceptible to antibiotics such as penicillins. Patients usually present with mild infections of the respiratory system. Imaging studies show unilateral, multilobar, or bilateral infiltrates. Outbreaks are frequently seen among military recruits and in prisons. It is associated with cold agglutinin (IgM) autoimmune hemolytic anemia.

8. Answer: A. Disseminated varicella zoster

   Varicella zoster is highly infectious. In patients with disseminated herpes zoster, precautions are to be taken until lesions are dry and crusted. Varicella zoster infection has two distinct diseases. Primary infection results in varicella (chickenpox) which consists of vesicular lesions on face trunk and extremities. Herpes Zoster occurs from the reactivation of latent VZV infection in sensory ganglia. Immunocompromised patients are at increased risk of developing varicella zoster.

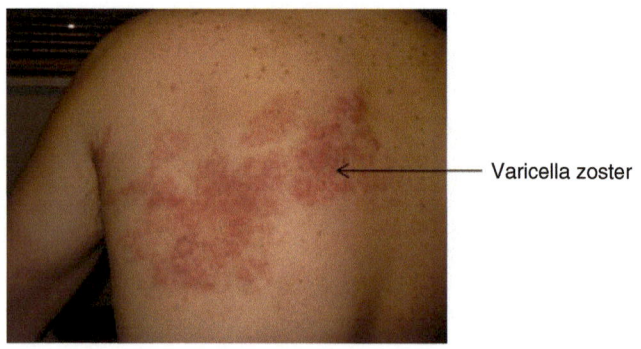

Varicella zoster

9. Answer: B. Ebola virus

Ebola virus is the Filoviridae family consisting of three different genera: Ebola virus, Marburgvirus, and Cuevavirus. Ebola virus is transmitted by contact with fomites, symptomatic individuals, and infected corpse. Viable virus has been isolated up to 7 days after death. There have been numerous infections during mourning and funeral or while the bodies have been removed or transported by burial teams. Therefore, appropriate safety precautions should be taken.

10. Answer: C. Chlamydia trachomatis

Chlamydia trachomatis L1, L2, and L3 serovars causes Lymphogranuloma venereum (LGV). Patients present with ulcerative disease. The ulcers are usually small. After the resolution of ulcers, there are two main presentations of this disease: the classical inguinal syndrome and the anorectal syndrome. Inguinal syndrome causes inguinal lymphadenopathy with the formation of buboes (unilateral painful inguinal lymph nodes). Anorectal symptoms include fever, spasms, anal pain, perianal sores, bloody discharge, constipation, and tenesmus.

11. Answer: A. Proteus species

Proteus species are gram-negative bacilli and belong to Enterobacteriaceae family. Proteus organisms cause infections in humans. Proteus species swarm on blood agar. They form concentric circles (swarming).

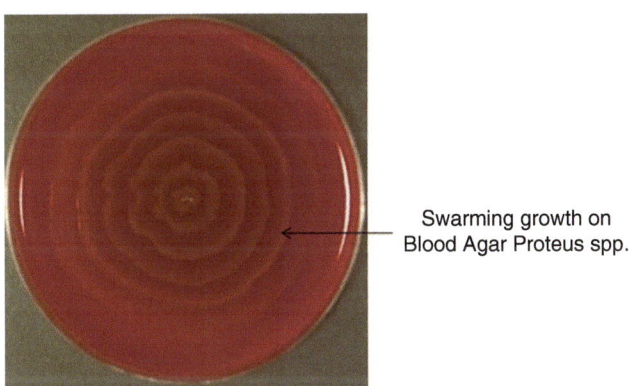

Swarming growth on Blood Agar Proteus spp.

12. Answer: A. HPV 6

Recurrent respiratory papillomatosis (RRP) usually present with the development of small, wart-like growths (papillomas) in the respiratory tract. Papillomas can grow in any part of the respiratory tract. They are mostly found in the larynx and the vocal cords (laryngeal papillomatosis). Human papillomavirus (HPV) commonly causes recurrent respiratory papillomatosis. There are different subtypes of HPV. HPV 6 and HPV 11 account for about 90% cases of RRP.

13. Answer: C. Brugia malayi

Brugia malayi is endemic in Asia. It results in lymphatic filariasis. Brugia malayi can also cause pulmo-

nary tropical eosinophilia. Brugia malayi circulates in the blood stream with nocturnal periodicity. Therefore, blood specimens should be collected between sunset and sunrise. The range of length of B. malayi is 175–230 µm.

14. Answer: D. Malassezia furfur

Malassezia furfur requires fatty-acid supplementation. M. Furfur causes tinea versicolor. Patients usually present with hypopigmented or hyperpigmented macules. Common sites are upper trunk, proximal extremities, neck, or face. It can also cause sepsis in patients who receive parenteral nutrition. The organism is isolated from skin scrapings from the hypopigmented epidermal patches. Classically, the fungal elements from the skin scrapings reveal yellow-green fluorescence under a wood lamp. Microscopically, they are described as spaghetti and meatballs because of the mixture of hyphal elements and yeast forms. Diagnosis is confirmed with a potassium hydroxide (KOH) preparation.

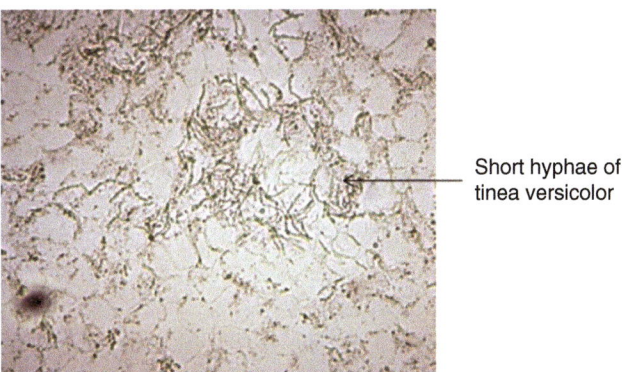

Short hyphae of tinea versicolor

15. Answer: E. Streptococcus pneumoniae

Bacterial meningitis in adults is usually caused by streptococcus pneumoniae. Other pathogens which can cause bacterial meningitis in adults are Neisseria meningitidis and Listeria monocytogenes. It is seen in patients over 50 years old. It may also be seen in patients with deficiencies in cell mediated immunity. Patients usually present with unexplained fever and headache. CSF findings show WBC count of 1000 to 5000/microL. Majority of WBCs are neutrophils (usually greater than 80%). Protein is usually more than 200 mg/dL and glucose is less than 40 mg/dL.

16. Answer: B. Entamoeba histolytica

Entamoeba histolytica is a protozoan parasite. Human infection occurs with ingestion of fecally contaminated food and water. Infected individuals most commonly have non-invasive disease with mild diarrhea and abdominal cramping. Almost 10% of the patients, though, will have an invasive, dysenteric course of disease. Identification of E. histolytica can be made on morphology. Amebae may invade the cryptids of colonic glands and burrow down into the submucosa creating flask-shaped ulcers. They can penetrate the portal venous system and spread to the liver, causing liver abscesses. E. histolytica cysts usually measure 10–15 μm and have four nuclei with centrally-located karyosomes. Diagnosis is made by examination of stool for parasites or stool E. histolytica antigen.

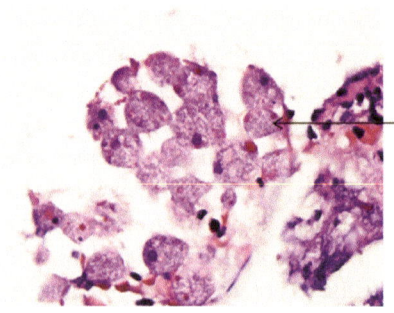

Trophozoite of Entamoeba histolytica

17. Answer: B. Bordetella pertussis

Bordetella pertussis is a common pathogen causing pertussis (whooping cough). It is commonly seen in children less than 10 years old. Patients usually present with prolonged cough, inspiratory whoop, paroxysmal cough. Bordetella pertussis is a fastidious gram-negative coccobacillus. It survives only a few hours in respiratory secretions. It is commonly spread by respiratory droplets. It can also be transmitted by coughing and sneezing. In unvaccinated children, classic pertussis occurs. Classic pertussis consists of three stages: catarrhal stage (lasts 1–2 weeks), a paroxysmal stage (lasts 2–8 weeks) with the symptoms of coughing and inspiratory whoop and a convalescent stage.

18. Answer: D. Trichophyton rubrum

The most common of the superficial fungi is Trichophyton rubrum. Trichophyton rubrum is a dermatophytic fungus. It belongs to the phylum Ascomycota. The upper layers are colonized by an anthropophilic saprotroph. It is the main cause of the fungal infection of the nails and athlete's foot. It may also cause jock itch and ringworm infection.

19. Answer: A. Enterobius vermicularis

Two of the most common nematode infections around the world are Enterobius vermicularis (pinworm) and Trichuris trichiura (whipworm). It affects people of all ages. Common infection is by fecal-oral route. Children in day-care preschool and their attendants are at increased risk for contracting this nematode infection. Patients usually present with intense anal itching which is worse at night. Ileum or cecum are the common sites where adult pinworms are found.

20. Answer: D. Actinomyces israelii

Actinomycosis usually causes chronic granulomatous disease. It is caused by actinomyces israelii. Actinomyces israelii is a gram-positive, filamentous, and an anaerobic bacterium. It commonly affects middle-aged males. Actinomyces are normal inhabitants of the gastrointestinal tract. Pathogenicity is acquired by the invasion of breached tissue leading to the formation of abscesses, draining sinuses, and fistulas. Diagnosis is confirmed by histological identification of actinomycotic sulfur granules or culture of Actinomyces. Pus is a preferred specimen. Sulfur granules are colonies of actinomyces. They consist of granulation tissue surrounding eosinophilic granules.

21. Answer: A. Enterococcus species

Enterococcus species are responsible for the conditions of the patient described in the question. Biochemically, enterococci are Leukocyte alkaline phosphatase (LAP) and pyrrolidonyl arylamidase (PYR) positive and Lancefield D antigen positive. They are also catalase negative and oxidase negative.

22. Answer: B. Mucor species

Mucor species is responsible for the condition of this patient. Rhizopus, absidia, and mucor are considered Zygomycetes and in the laboratory they are distinguished by both the presence and location of the rhizoids, or root-like projections. Mucormycosis infections are usually life-threatening. Diabetic ketoacidosis and neutropenia are the risk factors. Patients usually present with a severe infection of the facial sinuses, which may extend into the brain. Mucormycosis can also cause pulmonary, cutaneous, and gastrointestinal infections.

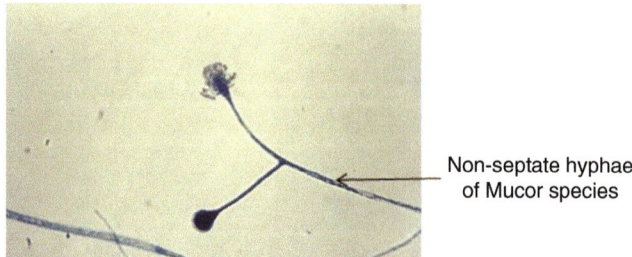

Non-septate hyphae of Mucor species

23. Answer: C. Diphyllobothrium latum

Diphyllobothrium latum is associated with vitamin B12 deficiency which causes megaloblastic anemia. D. Latum is also called the fish tapeworm. It is mainly found in cold freshwater. D. Latum has a unique affinity for vitamin B12. The adult worm attaches to the mucosa of the ileum inhibiting the absorption of vitamin B12. D. latum infection can be transmitted by consumption of a variety of freshwater fish. Individuals who eat various forms of raw fish, such as sushi, sashimi, ceviche, are at risk of infection.

24. Answer: D. Pseudomonas aeruginosa

Otitis externa is caused by pseudomonas aeruginosa. Otitis externa is caused by inflammation due to infection in the external auditory canal. It is commonly seen in swimmers. Common risk factors of otitis externa include swimming, trauma, and occlusive ear devices. Antibiotic therapy cures the majority of cases but diabetic and immunocompromised patients can develop malignant otitis externa. In malignant otitis externa bacteria invade deep into the surrounding tissues and if left untreated has a mortality rate that approaches 50%. P. aeruginosa is a oxidase positive gram-negative rod. It causes a variety of infections such as folliculitis, pneumonia (cystic fibrosis), and urine tract infection.

25. Answer: A. Schistosoma haematobium

Schistosoma haematobium is not an uncommon infection. The adult worms reside in the bladder veins and deposit eggs in the bladder wall. This can cause irritation leading to intermittent hematuria. It also leads to bladder wall thickening, calcifications. Eventually, it can lead to squamous cell carcinoma. The eggs of S. haematobium are about 100 μm and have a terminal spine.

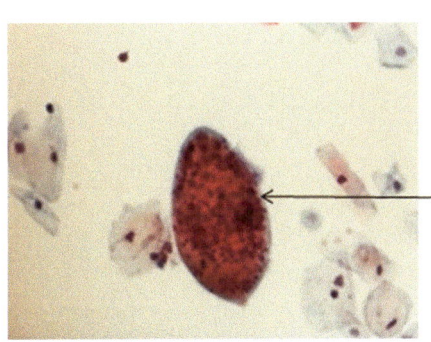

Egg of Schistosoma haematobium

26. Answer: B. Parvovirus B19

Human parvovirus B19 is a virus of erythroparvovirus genus of the parvoviridae family. Aplastic crisis in sickle cell patients is generally caused by infection with parvovirus B19. The virus infects erythroid precursor cells in bone marrow, causing destruction of reticulocytes. Parvovirus is a non-enveloped, single-stranded DNA virus. Parvovirus B 19 infection occurs primarily in children. Patients usually present with erythema infectiosum (fifth disease). Parvovirus B 19 is transmitted via respiratory secretions.

27. Answer: B. Candida esophagitis

Candida albicans causes opportunistic infection in immunocompromised patients. Candida albicans causes candida esophagitis, a common infection of the esophagus. Patients present with dysphagia, odynophagia (pain with swallowing). Candida albicans can also cause oral thrush. Diagnosis of Candida esophagitis is confirmed by endoscopy which shows visible white mucosal plaque-like lesions.

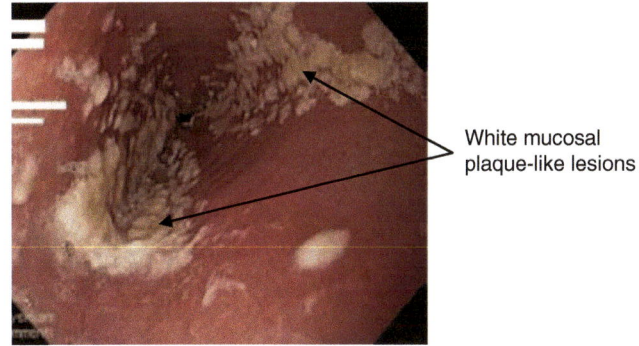

White mucosal plaque-like lesions

28. Answer: A. Staphylococcus saprophyticus

Staphylococcus saprophyticus is a common cause of urinary tract infections in recently married sexually active women. Patients usually present with dysuria. Urine nitrite test is negative. Staphylococcus saprophyticus is a gram positive/catalase+/coagulase-/novobiocin resistant bacteria.

29. Answer: D: Plasmodium vivax

The child is having an infection with Plasmodium vivax. Clinically, the patient presented with fever since 2 days (ternary) typical for Plasmodium vivax. 3-day fevers (quaternary) is commonly seen in Plasmodium malariae. Peripheral blood smear shows amoeboid amorphous trophozoite that occupies red blood cell. This is seen in Plasmodium vivax. Schuffner's dots are usually seen in the trophozoites of Plasmodium vivax.

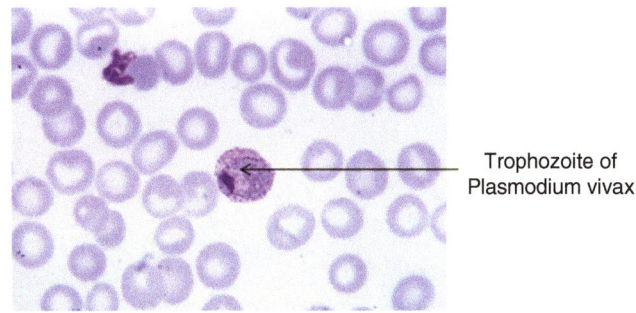

Trophozoite of Plasmodium vivax

Bibliography

1. Galeotti C, Bayry J. Autoimmune and inflammatory diseases following COVID-19. Nat Rev Rheumatol. 2020;16:413–4.
2. Lopez FA, et al. Fever and rash in immunocompromised patients without HIV infection. 2019.
3. Dhakal OP, Dhakal M. Prevalence of Helicobacter pylori infection & pattern of gastrointestinal involvement in patients undergoing upper gastrointestinal endoscopy in Sikkim. Indian J Med Res. 2018;147(5):517–20.

4. Barthunia B, et al. Aspergillosis of maxillary sinus in an uncontrolled diabetic patient: a case report. J Indian Acad Oral Med Radiol. 2017;29(4):337–40.
5. Harris JB, et al. Approach to the child with acute diarrhea in resource-limited countries. 2019.
6. Gelfand MS, et al. Epidemiology and pathogenesis of Listeria monocytogenes infection. 2019.
7. Sexton DJ, et al. Tetanus. 2019.
8. Baum SG, et al. Mycoplasma pneumoniae infection in adults. 2019.
9. Albrecht MA, et al. Epidemiology, clinical manifestations, and diagnosis of herpes zoster. 2019.
10. Lopez FA, et al. Fever and rash in HIV-infected patients. 2019.
11. Tuddenham S, et al. Approach to the patient with genital ulcers. 2019.
12. Palefsky JM, et al. Virology of human papillomavirus infections and the link to cancer. 2019.
13. Derkay C. Recurrent respiratory papillomatosis. 2019.
14. Apicella M, et al. Clinical manifestations of meningococcal infection. 2019.
15. Coates TD, et al. Approach to the child with lymphocytosis or lymphocytopenia. 2019.
16. Tunkel AR, Calderwood SB, Mitty J. Clinical features and diagnosis of acute bacterial meningitis in adults. 2019.
17. Leder K, et al. Intestinal entamoeba histolytica amebiasis. 2019.
18. Cornia P, et al. Pertussis infection in adolescents and adults: treatment and prevention. 2019.
19. Boakes E, et al. Breast infection: a review of diagnosis and management practices. Eur J Breast Health. 2018;14(3):136–43.
20. Groopman JE, Aboulafia DM, Shah S. AIDS-related Kaposi sarcoma: clinical manifestations and diagnosis. 2019.
21. Wong L-M, Song K, et al. Abdominal actinomycosis. 2019.
22. Stover DE, et al. Approach to the HIV-infected patient with pulmonary symptoms. 2019.
23. Chopra S, et al. Clinical manifestations and natural history of chronic hepatitis C virus infection. 2019.
24. Vichinsky EP, et al. Sickle cell trait. 2019.
25. Sax PE, et al. Techniques and interpretation of measurement of the CD4 cell count in HIV-infected patients. 2019.
26. Bernardo J, von Reyn CF, Baron L. Diagnosis of pulmonary tuberculosis in adults. 2019.
27. Vuong MF, Waymack JR. Aspergillosis. 2018.
28. Nassar Y, Eljabbour T, Lee H, Batool A. Possible risk factors for candida esophagitis in immunocompetent individuals. Gastroenterology Res. 2018;11(3):195–9.
29. Jordan JA. Clinical manifestations and diagnosis of parvovirus B19 infection. 2019.
30. Tayal S, et al. A case of syphilitic anal condylomata lata mimicking malignancy. Int J Surg Case Rep. 2015;17:69–71.
31. Kaner RJ, et al. Pulmonary complications after allogeneic hematopoietic cell transplantation. 2019.
32. Marra CM, et al. Neurosyphilis. 2019.
33. Khanal S, Ghimire P, Dhamoon AS. The repertoire of adenovirus in human disease: the innocuous to the deadly. Biomedicine. 2018;6(1):30.
34. Fayyaz J, Mosenifar Z. Histoplasmosis. 2019.

Blood Vessels

6

Multiple Choice Questions

1. Medial calcification is seen in:
   A. Atherosclerosis
   B. Arteriosclerosis
   C. Monckeberg sclerosis
   D. Dissecting aneurysm
   E. Malignant hypertension
2. Neointimal hyperplasia causes vascular graft failure as a result of hypertrophy of:
   A. Smooth muscle cells
   B. Endothelial cells
   C. Collagen fibers
   D. Elastic fibers
   E. Epithelial cells
3. Atheromatous changes of blood vessels affects early in:
   A. Kidney
   B. Heart
   C. Liver
   D. Spleen
   E. Brain
4. Most common cause of aortic aneurysm is:
   A. Syphilis
   B. Marfan's syndrome
   C. Atherosclerosis
   D. Congenital
   E. HIV
5. Most common cause of aortic dissection is:
   A. Hypertension
   B. Diabetes melitus
   C. Trauma
   D. Marfan's syndrome
   E. Myocardial infarction
6. Muscle biopsy in polyarteritis nodosa (PAN) show:
   A. Necrotizing arteritis
   B. Atrophy
   C. Granulomatous lesion
   D. Ring lesion
   E. Fragmentation of the internal elastic lamina

7. Hypersensitivity vasculitis is seen most commonly in:
   A. Post capillary venules
   B. Arterioles
   C. Veins
   D. Capillaries
   E. Elastic arteries
8. Hypersensitivity vasculitis is seen in which complication:
   A. Systemic lupus erythematosus
   B. Polyarteritis nodosa
   C. Henoch-Schonlein purpura
   D. Buerger's disease
   E. Wegener's granulomatosis
9. The tissue of origin of Kaposi sarcoma is:
   A. Lymphoid
   B. Vascular
   C. Neural
   D. Muscular
   E. Bone
10. A 20-year-old female presents with low grade fever, fatigue, and arthralgia. Physical examination shows absence or weak peripheral pulse of radial artery. What is the diagnosis?
    A. Giant cell arteritis
    B. Takayasu arteritis
    C. Bechet syndrome
    D. IgG4-related disease
    E. Fibromuscular dysplasia
11. A 60-year-old male presents with headache visual disturbance jaw claudication, sudden onset of visual changes. Laboratory findings show elevated erythrocyte sedimentation rate. What is the diagnosis?
    A. Giant cell arteritis
    B. Migraine headache
    C. Polymyalgia rheumatica
    D. Postherpetic neuralgia
    E. Transient ischemic attack
12. A middle-aged man presents with bilateral pneumonitis with nodular and cavitary pulmonary infiltrates, chronic

V. K. Kohli et al., *Comprehensive Multiple-Choice Questions in Pathology*, https://doi.org/10.1007/978-3-031-08767-7_6

sinusitis, nasopharyngeal ulcerations, and renal disease. Laboratory findings show cytoplasmic antineutrophil cytoplasmic autoantibodies (c-ANCA). Which of the following diagnosis is most compatible with the findings in this case?
    A. Wegener's granulomatosis
    B. Goodpasture's disease
    C. Buerger's disease
    D. Lupus nephritis
    E. Postinfectious glomerulonephritis

13. A 32-year-old male smoker develops gangrenous toes of the left foot. His serum cholesterol level is 135 mg/dL. What is the diagnosis?
    A. Monckeberg's arteriosclerosis
    B. Severe atherosclerosis
    C. Thromboangiitis obliterans
    D. Giant cell arteritis
    E. Kawasaki's disease

14. A 45-year-old man injures his left knee while skiing and undergoes arthroscopic surgery. He continues to have considerable left knee pain despite receiving analgesic medication. He spends the next few days in bed. On the fifth postoperative day, he develops acute right-sided chest pain. What is the most likely diagnosis?
    A. Pulmonary embolism
    B. Drug reaction
    C. Aspiration pneumonia
    D. Diffuse alveolar damage
    E. Viral pneumonia

15. Which of the following substances is most likely to reduce serum level of cholesterol?
    A. Apolipoprotein
    B. Lipoprotein
    C. Omega-3 fatty acids
    D. C-reactive protein
    E. Exercise

16. Which of the following is true about atherogenesis?
    A. Vascular cell adhesion molecule 1 (VCAM-1)
    B. Activated endothelial cells and leukocytes release growth factors
    C. Calcification and peripheral neovascularization
    D. A and B
    E. All of the above

17. An increase in which of the following is most likely to increase the risk for the development of cardiovascular risk?
    A. Erythrocyte sedimentation rate (ESR)
    B. White blood cell count
    C. C-reactive protein (CRP)
    D. Total protein
    E. Cryoglobulin

18. A 52-year-old woman presents with severe headache. CT scan shows an intracranial hemorrhage. Which of the following complication is most likely to occur as a consequence of her condition?
    A. Antiphospholipid syndrome
    B. Mycotic aneurysm
    C. Atrial myxoma
    D. Systemic lupus erythematosus
    E. Polymyalgia rheumatica

19. An exaggerated vascular response to cold temperatures or emotional stress is seen in which of the following vascular disorder?
    A. Antiphospholipid syndrome
    B. Cryoglobulinemia
    C. Mixed connective tissue disease
    D. Scleroderma
    E. Raynaud's phenomenon

20. Which of the following arteries is most commonly affected in Kawasaki disease?
    A. External carotid artery
    B. Subclavian artery
    C. Coronary artery
    D. Renal artery
    E. Femoral artery

21. Unilateral leg swelling, warmth, erythema Homan's sign are characteristics of which of the following vascular disease?
    A. Lymphangitis
    B. Deep vein thrombosis
    C. Cellulitis
    D. Septic thrombophlebitis
    E. Pulmonary embolism

Answers and Explanations

1. Answer: C. Monckeberg sclerosis

    Mönckeberg sclerosis (Mönckeberg arteriosclerosis) is a type of arteriosclerosis leading to vessel hardening. Calcium deposits are present in the middle muscular layer of the walls of the arteries. It is an example of dystrophic calcification. Monckeberg sclerosis is a benign medial calcification of the elastic lamina not involving the intima leading to vascular stiffening without obstruction. It usually affects medium-sized arteries (radial, ulnar, tibial, uterine, or femoral arteries). Imaging studies show Pipestem appearance. It is generally asymptomatic and benign. It is commonly associated with type II diabetes and chronic kidney disease.

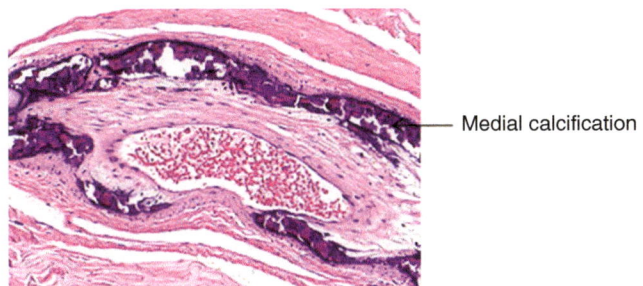
Medial calcification

2. Answer: A. Smooth muscle cells

   Atherosclerosis is a common cause of morbidity and mortality. Many interventions are done to treat atherosclerosis such as balloon angioplasty (with or without stenting), endarterectomy or surgical bypass grafting. Occasionally, interventions fail from restenosis due to neointimal hyperplasia (NIH). Neointimal hyperplasia and vascular thrombosis are some of the common causes of AV graft or fistula failures.

3. Answer: B. Heart

   Atherosclerosis is caused by the deposition of cholesterol plaques in the intima of medium and large arteries. Atherosclerosis commonly affects arteries in the heart, brain, and kidneys. Commonly affected arteries are abdominal aorta, coronary artery and internal carotid artery. The common carotid arteries are often spared. The common risk factors of atherosclerosis include dyslipoproteinemia, hypertension, smoking, diabetes, sedentary lifestyle, and genetic abnormalities.

4. Answer: C. Atherosclerosis

   Abdominal aortic aneurysm (AAA) is the most common form of aneurysm. It affects male smokers over the age of 50 years. The patients usually have atherosclerosis. The common site of AAA is between the renal arteries and aortic bifurcation at the L4 level. It manifests as a palpable pulsating abdominal mass. The patients usually present with sudden severe and constant low back, flank pain. Complications of AAA are rupture, obstruction or compression of other structures. It can also results in release of emboli which can cause stroke and MI. Imaging studies are recommended for the male smokers between 65 and 75 years old.

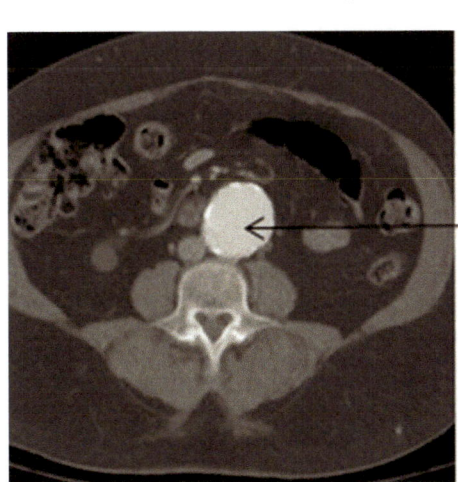
Abdominal aortic aneurysm

5. Answer: A. Hypertension

   Hypertension is a risk factor for several cardiovascular diseases. Hypertension confirmation is obtained by blood pressure exceeding 140/90 mm Hg, confirmed at least on two occasions. Common risk factors include advanced age, obesity, physical inactivity, excess salt, alcohol consumption, smoking, and diabetes. Primary hypertension is the most common type of hypertension, comprising approximately 95% of the cases. Long-term hypertension causes left ventricular hypertrophy, heart failure and is also a risk factor of coronary artery disease. Aortic dissection is commonly seen in patients with hypertension.

6. Answer: A. Necrotizing arteritis

   Polyarteritis nodosa (PAN) is a necrotizing, immune complex-mediated inflammation of small to medium arteries. It frequently causes destruction of the media and internal elastic lamina. It commonly affects middle-aged to older men. Polyarteritis Nodosa is seen in approximately 30% of patients infected with hepatitis B. The blood vessels most commonly affected are vessels of the mesentery, pancreas, and testes, but lesions may also occur in the hepatic, coronary, uterine, cerebral, adrenal, and renal arteries. It does not involve the lung.

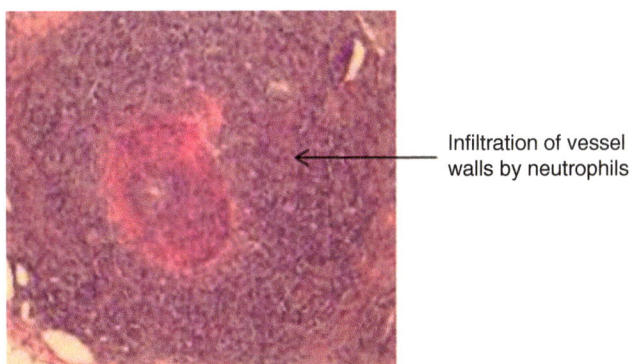
Infiltration of vessel walls by neutrophils

7. Answer: A. Post capillary venules

   The histopathology diagnosis given to the cutaneous small vessel vasculitis, especially a vasculitis of the dermal postcapillary venules is also called leukocytoclastic vasculitis. Most cases are idiopathic. Leukocytoclastic vasculitis present with visible purpura on lower extremities, small vessel involvement, and is extracutaneous in about 30% of cases.

8. Answer: C. Henoch-Schonlein purpura

   Henoch-Schonlein purpura is the most common childhood systemic vasculitis. It is an inflammatory disorder secondary to IgA complex deposition affecting small vessels. It usually occurs after an upper respiratory infection in children. The triad of Henoch-Schonlein purpura is palpable purpura on the buttocks and legs, polyarthralgias, and colicky abdominal pain. Histologically, it involves IgA, C3, and immune complex deposition in arterioles, venules, and capillaries.

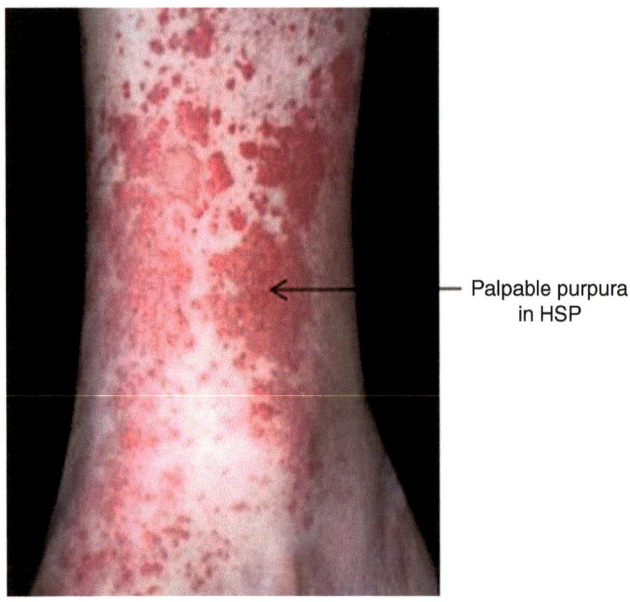

Palpable purpura in HSP

9. **Answer: B. Vascular**

The tissue of the origin of Kaposi sarcoma is vascular. Kaposi sarcoma is a low grade malignant tumor of endothelial cells caused by virus HHV8. It is multicentric vascular tumor. Grossly, there are multiple red-purple patches, plaques, or nodules. They may remain confined to the skin or may disseminate. Light microscopy shows the proliferation of spindle-shaped endothelial cells that line blood and lymphatic vessels. It also shows extravasated RBCs.

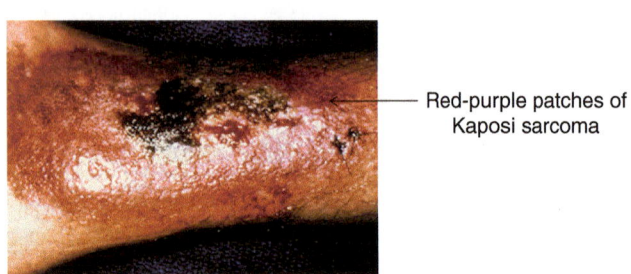

Red-purple patches of Kaposi sarcoma

10. **Answer: B. Takayasu arteritis**

Takayasu arteritis (TAK) commonly affects the aorta and its primary branches. It commonly affects women in approximately 80–90% of cases. Patients usually present with constitutional symptoms (weight loss, fever, and fatigue), arthralgias. Other symptoms include limb claudication. GIT symptoms may include abdominal pain, diarrhea, and hemorrhage. Patients may also present with neurological symptoms (lightheadedness, vertigo, headaches, and convulsions). Physical examination may reveal arterial bruits, unequal blood pressures between extremities and diminished pulses. In severe cases, inflammation of vessels may cause ischemic changes leading to visual disturbances, chest pain or strokes. ESR and CRP are elevated. Imaging studies

including arteriography and magnetic resonance angiography (MRA) are useful for establishing the diagnosis of TAK.

11. **Answer: A. Giant cell arteritis**

Giant cell arteritis is a large vessel vasculitis. It is characterized by granulomatous inflammation of the internal elastic lamina. It may also involve any of the large branches of the carotid. Patients usually present with temporal headaches, tenderness, jaw claudication and visual changes (when the ophthalmic artery is involved). Approximately 50% of patients have symptoms of polymyalgia rheumatica. The disease affects older individuals (rarely less than 50 years old). Laboratory findings show an elevated erythrocyte sedimentation rate (ESR more than 50 mm/h). Definitive diagnosis requires temporal artery biopsy. Light microscopy shows epithelioid histiocytes, multinucleated giant cells, T lymphocytes, and macrophages. Fragmentation of elastic fibers in a vessel wall can be seen by elastic stain. Most dreaded complication of temporal arteries is loss of vision.

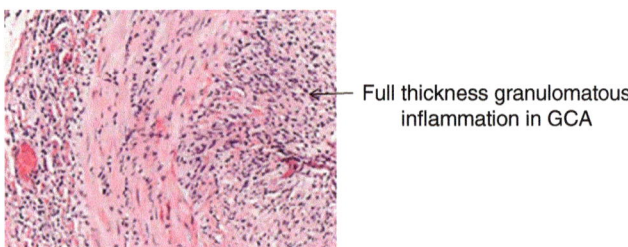

Full thickness granulomatous inflammation in GCA

12. **Answer: A. Wegener's granulomatosis**

Wegener's granulomatosis is a small vessel necrotizing vasculitis. It usually involves the upper and lower respiratory tract with extravascular granulomatous inflammation, glomerulonephritis. Renal involvement is usually asymptomatic until advanced uremia develops. It affects patients of all ages and both sexes. Patients present with constitutional symptoms, chronic sinusitis, epistaxis, mucosal ulceration, and visual changes.

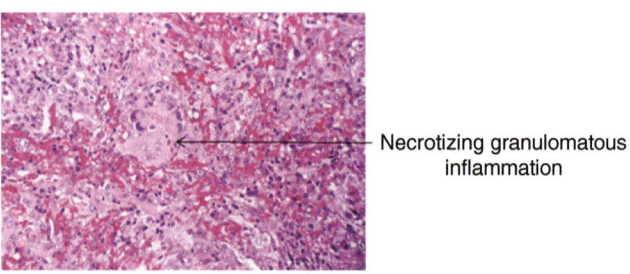

Necrotizing granulomatous inflammation

13. **Answer: C. Thromboangiitis obliterans**

Thromboangiitis obliterans is a full thickness, segmental, thrombosing inflammation of small- to medium-sized arteries, veins, nerves of the distal extremities. It is commonly seen in young men who are heavy smokers. This thromboangiitis obliterans present with a triad of distal arterial occlusion, Raynaud phenomenon, and migrating superficial vein thrombophlebitis. Patients present with pain at rest. Gangrene occurs due to intermittent claudication. In extreme cases, autoamputation of digits may occur. Diagnosis is confirmed by arteriography. Arteriography may show stenotic corkscrew vessels. Tissue biopsy is the definitive diagnosis.

14. Answer: A. Pulmonary embolism

Pulmonary embolism occurs when a blood clot from a systemic vein lodged one or more branches of pulmonary artery. Pulmonary embolism commonly arises from a deep vein thrombosis. It can also result from embolization of fat, air, bacteria, amniotic fluid, and tumor cells. Patients usually present with tachypnea, tachycardia, hypoxemia, sudden onset dyspnea with pleuritic chest pain. Bronchoconstriction can occur due to the release of inflammatory mediators. There is V/Q mismatch and hypoxemia. Hypotension, syncope, and shock can occur due to reduced output of the right ventricle. Pulmonary embolism is often missed clinically and seen in more than 60% of autopsies.

15. Answer: C. Omega-3 fatty acids

Fatty acids omega-3 are commonly found in fish, flaxseeds, and fish oil. Vegetable oils including such as flaxseed, soybean, and canola contain alpha-linolenic acid. Patients with high triglycerides who cannot tolerate statin fenofibrate, omega-3 ethyl esters are used in the treatment. Triglyceride levels are lowered by fibrates, omega-3 fatty acids derived from the marine and statins. Most sources of fish oil make up only 30–50% of omega-3 fatty acids. Omega-3 ethyl esters (for example, Lovaza and Omacor) contain about 85% of omega-3 fatty acids.

16. Answer: B. All of the above

Endothelial cells release VCAM-1. Vascular cell adhesion molecule 1 promotes adhesion and intimal migration of monocytes and T lymphocytes. Activated endothelial cells and leukocytes release growth factors that recruit and promote smooth muscle cell proliferation and extracellular matrix elaboration. Calcification and peripheral neovascularization are frequent features of atheromatous plaques. All these factors are essential for the pathogenesis of atherogenesis.

17. Answer: C. C-reactive protein (CRP)

C-reactive protein is a non-specific marker of inflammation. Elevated C-reactive protein is an important predictor of atherosclerosis in both sexes. In myocardial infarction, ischemic stroke, hypertension, and peripheral artery disease, CRP is an important predictor for an early diagnosis. C-reactive protein being an important bio-

marker of inflammation is a known factor in the development of atherosclerosis.

18. Answer: B. Mycotic aneurysm

Mycotic aneurysms usually occur due to bacterial infection involving the wall of the abdominal aorta. It is commonly seen in intracranial arteries. It can also occur in visceral arteries and upper or lower extremity arteries, usually at arterial bifurcations. An aneurysm can develop due to the destruction of the vessel wall by infection. It can also develop in preexisting aneurysm when secondarily infected. Common organisms causing infected aneurysm are salmonella species and staphylococcus species. Other organisms which can cause mycotic aneurysm due to infection include streptococcus pneumoniae, treponema pallidum, and mycobacterium tuberculosis. Common risk factors for infected aneurysm are trauma, endocarditis and advanced age. Patients usually present with painful, pulsatile, and enlarging mass along with fever and malaise. Imaging studies help in the diagnosis.

19. Answer: E. Raynaud's phenomenon

Raynaud's phenomenon occurs when cold or stress exposure induces the vasoconstriction of digital arteries. This leads to white or blue coloration of fingers/toes. Raynaud's phenomenon occurs in the absence of any underlying cause. It is usually found in women. Secondary Raynaud's phenomenon is usually found in men associated with secondary systemic disorders, such as systemic lupus erythematosus or systemic sclerosis.

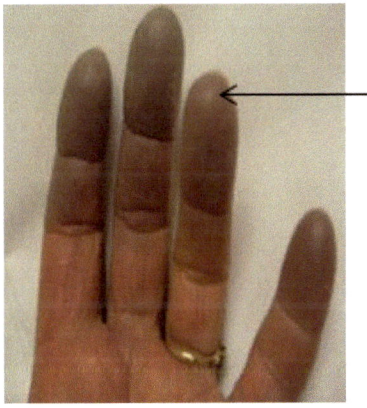

Digital cyanosis (Raynaud's phenomenon)

20. Answer: C. Coronary artery

Kawasaki disease is a mucocutaneous disease. It is characterized by acute necrotizing inflammation of the small, medium and large arteries. It is commonly seen in children younger than 4 years. The most serious sequelae of Kawasaki disease includes coronary vessel involvement leading to aneurysms. Patients usually present with fever (present for at least 5 days), cervical lymphadenitis, and bilateral conjunctival injection. Other symptoms may include red, fissured lips, strawberry tongue. There may be a maculopapular erythematous rash. Diagnosis is made clinically. Coronary angiogram is commonly performed to diagnose coronary artery aneurysm. Currently, Kawasaki disease is a leading cause of acquired cardiac disease in young children.

21. Answer: B. Deep vein thrombosis

In deep vein thrombosis (DVT), blood clots most often occur in calf veins. DVT can also affect popliteal, femoral or iliac veins. Common risk factors include stasis of blood flow, vascular endothelium damage, and hypercoagulability (usually summarized in Virchow triad). Patients may be asymptomatic. They may present with calf or thigh discomfort, unilateral leg swelling, edema, warmth, and erythema. Physical examinations show tenderness on palpation over the veins. Homan's sign (dorsiflexion of the foot producing calf pain) is often used as a test but it is not reliable. Laboratory findings show increase D-dimer (fibrin degradation product). It is sensitive, but not specific test. Lower extremity venous duplex ultrasonography is commonly used to assess blood flow within the vein. The gold standard test is angiography.

Bibliography

1. Hayashi K, Watanabe H, et al. Granulomatosis with polyangiitis with obstructive pneumonia progressing to hypertrophic pachymeningitis. Medicine. 2021;100(3):24028.
2. Lanzer P, et al. Medial vascular calcification revisited: review and perspectives. Eur Heart J. 2014;35(23):1515–25.
3. Zain MA, Jamil RT; Siddiqui WJ. Neointimal hyperplasia. 2019.
4. Bergheanu SC, et al. Pathophysiology and treatment of atherosclerosis. Current view and future perspective on lipoprotein modification treatment. Neth Heart J. 2017;25(4):231–42.
5. Rahimi SA, Rowe VL. Abdominal aortic aneurysm. 2019.
6. Levy D, Jacqueline K. Aortic dissection. 2018.
7. Lee HS, et al. Four cases of polyarteritis nodosa presenting initially as pain and pitting edema in both lower extremities. J Rheum Dis. 2017;24(1):48–54.
8. Blood vessel - polyarteritis nodosa. 2017.
9. Baigrie D, Crane JS. Leukocytoclastic vasculitis (hypersensitivity vasculitis). 2019.
10. Cabral D. Hypersensitivity vasculitis in children. 2019.
11. MacGill M, Murrell D. What is Kaposi sarcoma? 2018.
12. Jacobs-Kosmin D, Diamond HS. What is the relationship between polyarteritis nodosa (PAN) and hepatitis B virus (HBV)? 2017.
13. Wang AL, Raven ML, Surapaneni K, Albert DM. Studies on the histopathology of temporal arteritis. Ocul Oncol Pathol. 2017;3(1):60–5.
14. Nordqvist C, Biggers A. Granulomatosis with polyangiitis (GPA): what you need to know. 2018.
15. Mohareri M, et al. Thromboangiitis obliterans episode: autoimmune flare-up or reinfection? Vasc Health Risk Manag. 2018;14:247–51.
16. Yamamoto T. Management of patients with high-risk pulmonary embolism: a narrative review. 2018.
17. Frogoudaki AA, Gatzoulis MA. Pulmonary arterial hypertension in congenital heart disease. 2018.
18. Fett N, et al. Evaluation of adults with cutaneous lesions of vasculitis. 2019.
19. Crea F, et al. C-reactive protein in cardiovascular disease. 2019.
20. Spelman D, et al. Overview of infected (mycotic) arterial aneurysm. 2019.
21. Wigley FM, et al. Clinical manifestations and diagnosis of the Raynaud phenomenon. 2019.
22. Newburger JW, et al. Cardiovascular sequelae of Kawasaki disease: clinical features and evaluation. 2019.
23. Kearon C, et al. Clinical presentation and diagnosis of the nonpregnant adult with suspected deep vein thrombosis of the lower extremity. 2019.

The Heart

7

Multiple Choice Questions

1. A 46-year-old woman with a history of systemic lupus erythematosus comes to the physician office due to frequent thromboembolic events due to a mitral valve mass. Transesophageal echocardiography demonstrated verrucous vegetations on the mitral valve. What is the diagnosis?
   A. Degenerative valvular disease
   B. Rheumatic valvular disease
   C. Infective endocarditis
   D. Libman–Sacks endocarditis
   E. Non-bacterial thrombotic endocarditis
2. What is the characteristic feature of rheumatic carditis?
   A. Pericarditis
   B. Endocarditis
   C. Myocarditis
   D. Pancarditis
   E. Reflux carditis
3. What is the characteristic diagnostic histological feature of rheumatic heart disease?
   A. Aschoff body
   B. Bread butter pericarditis
   C. Eosinophilic infiltration
   D. Patchy infarction
   E. Deep granuloma annulare
4. The commonest type of pericarditis in acute rheumatic fever is:
   A. Serous pericarditis
   B. Fibrinous pericarditis
   C. Purulent pericarditis
   D. Myxomatous pericarditis
   E. Constrictive pericarditis
5. A 14-year-old male died suddenly while playing basketball. An autopsy is performed, and a gross photograph of the heart opened to reveal the left ventricle, is shown here. What is the diagnosis?

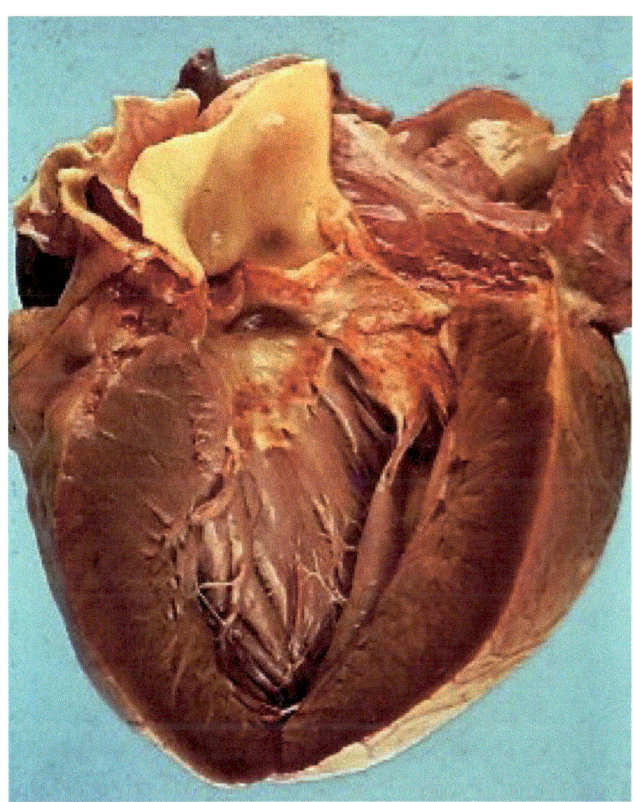

   A. Hypertrophic cardiomyopathy (HCM)
   B. Hypertensive heart disease
   C. Aortic stenosis
   D. Restrictive cardiomyopathy
   E. Fabry disease
6. Gross picture of heart with marked left ventricular hypertrophy is shown below. What is the diagnosis?

V. K. Kohli et al., *Comprehensive Multiple-Choice Questions in Pathology*, https://doi.org/10.1007/978-3-031-08767-7_7

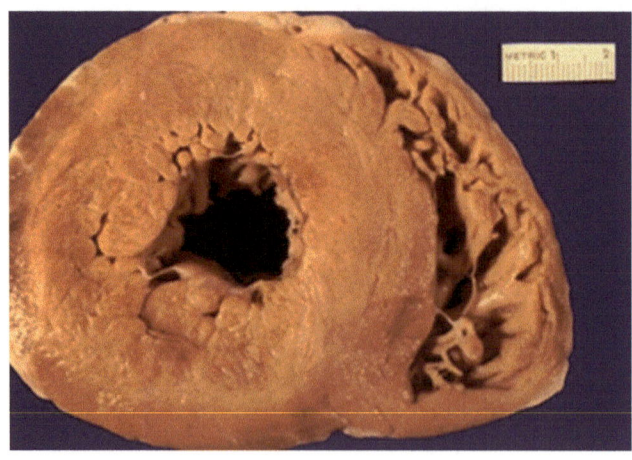

A. Pheochromocytoma
B. Hypertension
C. MEN I (Wermer's syndrome)
D. MEN II (IIa or Sipple's syndrome)
E. MEN III

7. Tetralogy of Fallot is defined as:
   A. Right ventricular hypertrophy
   B. Ventricular septal defect
   C. Pulmonary stenosis
   D. An aorta that overrides the ventricular septal defect
   E. All of the above

8. A surgically resected mitral valve has a "fish-mouth" shape due to commissural fusion. These changes are most likely the result of:
   A. Infective endocarditis
   B. Rheumatic heart disease
   C. Left ventricular enlargement
   D. Myxomatous degeneration
   E. Papillary muscle rupture

9. A 22-year-old man who has multiple cutaneous xanthomas presents to a local emergency room complaining an acute onset of chest pain while jogging. There is a family history of myocardial infarction in his 26-year-old brother and his father at young age. An EKG is done which shows ST elevation in the left precordial leads. Laboratory studies show elevated Troponin I. Patient dies due to ventricular fibrillation. Which of the following risk factors is most likely responsible for this man's cardiac disease?
   A. Niemann–Pick disease
   B. Glycogen storage disease type 1
   C. Gaucher's disease
   D. Familial hypercholesterolemia
   E. Tay–Sachs disease

10. A 59-year-old woman has metastatic breast carcinoma. Which of the following condition is well described phenomenon associated with malignancies?
    A. Calcific valvular disease
    B. Antiphospholipid syndrome

C. Acute infectious endocarditis
D. Atrial myxoma
E. Marantic endocarditis

11. What is the earliest microscopic sequence of changes in the heart after myocardial infarction?
    A. Wavy myocyte fibers
    B. Coagulative necrosis
    C. Neutrophilic infiltrate
    D. Macrophages
    E. Granulation tissue

12. What is the most common cardiovascular manifestation associated with systemic lupus erythematosus?
    A. Myocarditis
    B. Cardiomyopathy
    C. Pericarditis
    D. Pancreatitis
    E. Pulmonary hypertension

13. Rupture of the free wall of the ventricle is most common within how many days postmyocardial infarction?
    A. 48 h post-MI
    B. 24 h post-MI
    C. 3–7 days post-MI
    D. 2 weeks post-MI
    E. 3 weeks post-MI

14. In order to make a morphologic diagnosis of definite myocarditis, which of the following changes are required?
    A. Inflammatory infiltration and myocyte necrosis
    B. Eosinophilic infiltration
    C. Giant cells
    D. Inflammatory infiltration
    E. Inflammatory infiltration and fibrosis

15. Which of the following is associated with cardiac rhabdomyoma?
    A. Hibernoma
    B. Reticulohistiocytoma
    C. Myxoma
    D. Tuberous sclerosis
    E. Hemangiomas

16. Microscopic findings intra-alveolar hemosiderin-laden macrophages are suggestive of:
    A. Acute respiratory distress syndrome
    B. Bacterial pneumonia
    C. Cardiogenic pulmonary edema
    D. Congestive heart failure
    E. Serous pericarditis

17. Which of the following serum marker is used to diagnose myocardial infarction in 3–6 h?
    A. CK-MB
    B. LDH
    C. Alanine aminotransferase (ALT)
    D. Troponin I & T
    E. Aspartate aminotransferase (AST)

18. Which of the following is associated with Marfan's syndrome?

A. Mitral regurgitation

B. Pulmonary regurgitation

C. Mitral valve prolapse

D. Pulmonic stenosis

E. Tricuspid valve atresia

19. Microscopic findings of amorphous extracellular matrix with scattered stellate or globular myxoma cells within abundant mucopolysaccharide ground substances are characteristic of which cardiac tumor?

A. Cardiac myxoma

B. Cardiac rhabdomyoma

C. Lipoma

D. Primary malignant cardiac tumor

E. Carcinoid tumor

20. The congenital heart anomaly that is least likely to cause neonatal cyanosis is:

A. Ventricular septal defect

B. Tricuspid atresia

C. Tetralogy of fallot

D. Transposition of great vessels

E. Truncus arteriosus

21. What is the diagnosis regarding the disease process seen in this heart microscopic section?

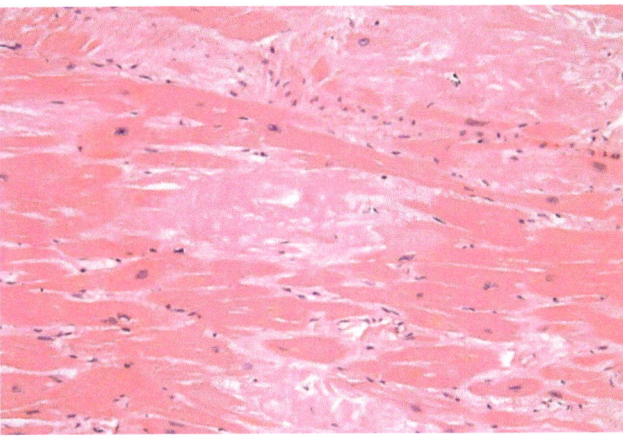

A. Cardiac amyloidosis

B. Hypertensive heart disease

C. Hypertrophic cardiomyopathy

D. Glycogen storage disease

E. Fabry disease

22. A complete atrioventricular (AV) canal defect is comprised of an atrial septal defect, a ventricular septal defect, and a common A/V valve. This congenital cardiac anomaly is associated with which of the following medical conditions?

A. Zellweger syndrome

B. Trisomy 18

C. Down syndrome

D. Congenital hypothyroidism

E. DiGeorge syndrome

23. A 33-year-old male is brought dead to the emergency department. Autopsy shows a ruptured cerebral aneurysm with extensive intracranial hemorrhage. Which of the following disease is associated with this patient's condition?

A. Patent ductus arteriosus

B. Transposition of the great arteries

C. Atrial septal defect

D. Coarctation of the aorta

E. Bicuspid aortic valve

24. A 27-year-old male patient is brought by his friends to the emergency room with severe shortness of breath. The patient dies suddenly. Troponin and CK-MB were elevated. What is the diagnosis?

A. Dilated cardiomyopathy (DCM)

B. Hypertrophic cardiomyopathy

C. Restrictive cardiomyopathy

D. Acute coronary syndrome

E. Cardiac tamponade

25. A 51-year-old male patient with about 2 years of dyspnea on exertion dies in a motor vehicle accident. Autopsy shows 5 cm atrial mass. What is the diagnosis?

A. Angioma

B. Rhabdomyosarcoma

C. Myxoma

D. Liposarcoma

E. Teratoma

Answers and Explanations

1. Answer: D. Libman–Sacks endocarditis

   Libman–Sacks endocarditis (LSE) is seen in patients with lupus erythematosus. Vegetations cover both sides of valve surfaces causing fibrinoid necrosis and inflammation. These verrucous vegetations result in valvular dysfunction and embolization.

2. Answer: D. Pancarditis

   Rheumatic heart disease is an acquired heart disease in children and young adults. Acute rheumatic fever causes pancarditis. Pancarditis affects the valve leaflets, pericardium, epicardium, myocardium, and endocardium. The most common valve lesion is mitral regurgitation.

3. Answer: A. Aschoff body

   Acute rheumatic fever is an immune-multisystem complication following group A streptococcal pharyngitis. The histologic hallmark of acute rheumatic carditis is the Aschoff body. Aschoff bodies are found in myocardium and consist of interstitial perivascular areas of fibrinoid necrosis surrounded by inflammatory infiltrate and Anitschkow cells. Anitschkow cells are histiocytes with a caterpillar pattern of nucleus and abundant cytoplasm. Aschoff body is pathognomonic for acute rheumatic fever. Rheumatic cardiac disease is a late complication of acute fever and occurs approximately after 10–20 years of acute rheumatic fever.

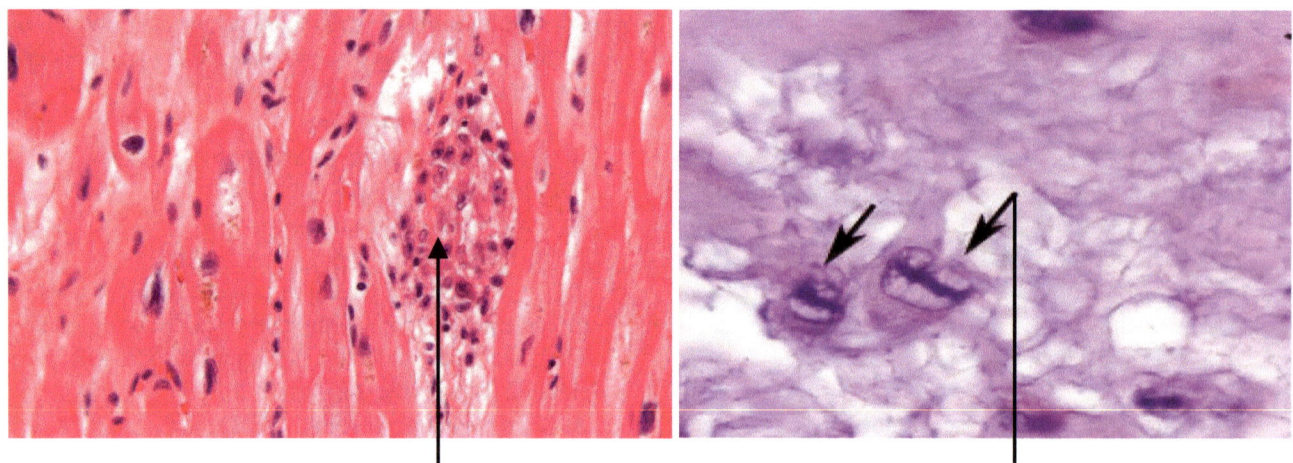

Aschoff body   Anitschkow cells: caterpillar chromatin pattern of nucleus

4. Answer: B. Fibrinous pericarditis

There are four subtypes of pericarditis; serous, fibrinous, suppurative, and hemorrhagic. Fibrinous pericarditis patients present with chest pain and friction rub. Exudate in fibrinous pericarditis is usually fibrin-rich with plasma proteins. It is associated with rheumatic fever, myocardial infarction (Dressler syndrome), and uremia. Fibrinous pericarditis leads to scar formation and diastolic filling defects.

5. Answer: A. Hypertrophic cardiomyopathy (HCM)

Hypertrophic cardiomyopathy can be seen at any age but classically is seen in young healthy patients. HCM may be completely silent in some patients. Patients may present with symptoms of dyspnea or syncope. There may be a family history of HCM. Genetic defect is found in the beta-myosin heavy chain on chromosome 14. Septal hypertrophy is seen in about 90% of cases with a thick mitral valve. Left atrium is large with a small left ventricle. Echocardiography is a useful diagnostic tool. Echocardiography findings include mitral valve prolapse and regurgitation, left ventricular hypertrophy, left atrial enlargement, and small ventricular chamber size. It is inherited as an autosomal dominant. Histologically, myocytes are hypertrophied and disorganized. It is recommended that first-degree relatives of an affected patient be screened for the disease.

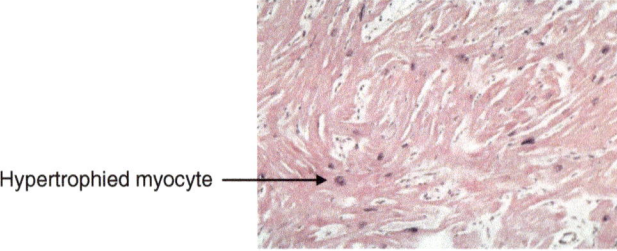

Hypertrophied myocyte →

6. Answer: B. Hypertension

Primary (essential) hypertension is diagnosed with BP > 140/90 mmHg on at least two occasions or a single

reading of 170/110 mmHg. Hypertension is a risk for several cardiovascular diseases. Long-term hypertension causes left ventricular hypertrophy.

7. Answer: E. All of the above

Tetralogy of Fallot is a common congenital cardiac defect. Tetralogy of Fallot leads to right-to-left shunts, causes cyanosis and reduction of PaO_2. There are four abnormalities in tetralogy of Fallot. They are overriding aorta and ventricular septal defect (VSD). Other two of the four abnormalities are pulmonic stenosis, right ventricular hypertrophy.

8. Answer: B. Rheumatic heart disease

Gross evaluation of surgical specimens is crucial in the diagnosis of cardiac valvular disease. Commissural fusion is highly characteristic of rheumatic heart disease. Many patients present with Rheumatic valve disease with stenotic and regurgitant components due to commissural fusion, giving rise to a "fish mouth" appearance imparted by the pathologic process.

9. Answer: D. Familial hypercholesterolemia

Familial hypercholesterolemia results from a mutation in the gene encoding the LDL receptor gene (LDLR) found on chromosome 19. This causes a loss of the main mechanism by which cholesterol is removed from serum and loss of negative feedback normally exerted through LDL on the endogenous production of cholesterol. The net effect is hypercholesterolemia (type II hyperlipidemia). The diagnosis of LDL receptor defects is suspected in patients with tendonous xanthomas and a family history of premature coronary artery disease (CAD). Elevated levels of LDL cholesterol have a direct impact on the risk of CAD.

10. Answer: E. Marantic endocarditis

Non-bacterial thrombotic endocarditis (NBTE) is commonly known as marantic endocarditis. Histologically, these lesions consist of fibrin, platelets and are composed of bland thrombi that are loosely attached to the underlying valve. The vegetations are free of inflammation. The vegetations rarely cause symptoms. Symptoms usually result from embolization to the brain, kidneys, and spleen. NBTE most commonly affects severe debilitated patients and its association with many types of cancer is well established. There is an association with mucinous adenocarcinomas, which is attributed to the procoagulant effects of tumor-derived

Non-bacterial thrombotic endocarditis (NBTE) mucin or tissue factor.

11. Answer: A. Wavy myocyte fibers

Wavy pattern of myocytes is the earliest microscopic changes seen in myocardial infarction (MI).

Sequence of changes in MI.

Time	Gross	Microscopic
0-½ h	None	None
½-4 h	None	Thin wavy myofibers
4-12 h	Occ dark mottling	Loss of striations, shrunken myocytes, loss of nucleus, hypereosinophilic cytoplasm
12-24 h	Dark mottling	Coagulation necrosis, many PMNs
1-3 d	Pallor	Complete necrosis, many PMNs

12. Answer: C. Pericarditis

There are different subtypes of pericarditis. Serous pericarditis is found in systemic lupus erythematosus (SLE). Exudate of serous pericarditis is protein-rich, straw-colored with few inflammatory cells. Many patients present with dyspnea, fatigue, and hypotension. It may be an incidental finding during echocardiography or computed tomography of the chest. There are four subtypes of pericarditis; serous, fibrinous, suppurative, and hemorrhagic. Fibrinous pericarditis patients present with chest pain and friction rub. Exudate in fibrinous pericarditis is usually fibrin-rich with plasma proteins. It is associated with rheumatic fever, myocardial infarction (Dressler syndrome), and uremia. Fibrinous pericarditis leads to scar formation and diastolic filling defects.

13. Answer: C. 3–7 days post-MI

The rupture of the free wall of the ventricle is the most frequent 3–7 days after the onset of myocardial infarction.

14. Answer: A. Inflammatory infiltration and myocyte Necrosis

Myocarditis is an inflammation of the heart muscle. Common causes include infections, toxins, autoimmune diseases, and drug reactions. The most common cause of myocarditis in developed countries is a viral infection. Viral infection could be due to coxsackie B virus, rubella virus, and cytomegalovirus. Worldwide, the most common cause of myocarditis is Chagas disease (caused by *Trypanosoma cruzi*). Patients may present with symptoms of chest pain, congestive heart failure, dyspnea, and peripheral edema. ECG may show T wave inversions and ST segment elevation. To establish a definitive diagnosis of myocarditis, inflammatory infiltration must be present in association with myocyte necrosis.

15. Answer: D. Tuberous sclerosis

Cardiac rhabdomyomas in newborns are frequently in association with the typical signs and symptoms of tuberous sclerosis, including cortical

tubers, renal angiomyolipomas, and pulmonary hamartomas. Rhabdomyoma is the most common primary tumor of the heart in children. Most cardiac rhabdomyomas occur in the ventricular myocardium, and show a solid, tan, homogeneous cut surface. Spontaneous regression is common. However, larger tumors are associated with increased risk of arrhythmias.

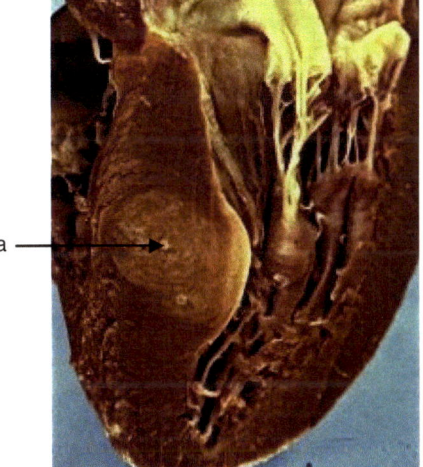

Cardiac rhabdomyoma

16. Answer: D. Congestive heart failure

Left-sided, cardiac dysfunction leads to pulmonary congestion. Patients present with orthopnea, paroxysmal nocturnal dyspnea, and orthopnea. Pulmonary congestion causes dilation of capillaries leading to the accumulation of blood in macrophages of alveolar spaces (hemosiderin-laden macrophages). RBCs breakdown appears as brown granules of hemosiderin and get accumulated in the cytoplasm of macrophages. Histologically, the findings are intra-alveolar hemosiderin laden macrophages, cardiac myocyte hypertrophy, and alveolar edema. Hemosiderin-laden macrophages are called heart-failure cells.

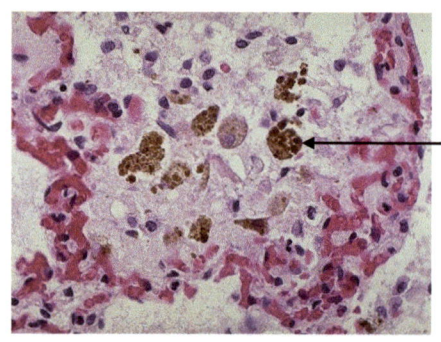

Hemosiderin-Laden macrophages

17. Answer: D. Troponin I & T

Troponin I & T serum markers peak at 12–48 h after myocardial infarction. They remain elevated for 4–10 days. Sensitivity of troponin I & T is near 100% after myocardial infarction if serum sample is taken within 6–12 h. Troponin I & T are specific and sensitive markers of myocardial infarction.

Serum marker	Elevated by	Peak	Returns to normal by
Troponin I & T	3-6 hrs	16 hrs	7-10 days

18. Answer: C. Mitral valve prolapse

In Marfan syndrome, there is involvement of the pulmonary artery or the mitral and tricuspid valves (prolapse of the mitral valve). General dilation of the aorta (aortic valve incompetence), dissecting aneurysm also occurs in Marfan syndrome. Marfan syndrome is an autosomal dominant disorder with Fibrillin-1 defect. Mitral valve prolapse affects 55% of the adult population between ages 20 and 40. Mitral valve becomes floppy or incompetent.

19. Answer: A. Cardiac myxoma

Myxoma is the most common tumor with unknown histogenesis. Majority of myxomas are located in the left atrium (75%). They are mostly sporadic. Some are associated with Carney's complex/triad, familial myxomatous syndrome or TS complex.

20. Answer: A. Ventricular septal defect

Most congenital heart anomalies that cause neonatal cyanosis are due to right-to-left shunting defects that causes deoxygenated blood to enter the systemic circulation. Ventricular septal defects along with atrial septal defects are left-to-right shunt and do not cause neonatal cyanosis.

21. Answer: A. Cardiac amyloidosis

The image shows cardiac myofibrils surrounded by an amorphous eosinophilic extracellular material. Eosinophilic material is positive with Congo Red stain and polarized light, consistent with amyloid. Amyloidosis can be primary, secondary, hereditary, or age related. Primary form is related to plasma cell neoplasms, while secondary is due to inflammatory conditions. Hereditary forms are related to various gene mutations while senile forms can be localized or systemic. Cardiac amyloidosis restrictive features due to poor ventricular compliance. Grossly, the heart is enlarged with a rubbery or waxy myocardium.

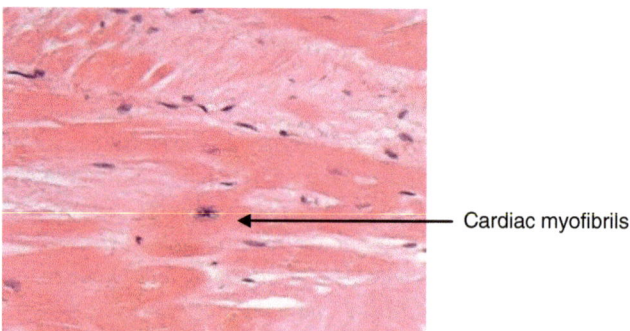

Cardiac myofibrils

22. Answer: C. Down syndrome

Cardiac defects occur in almost one-half the patients (usually septal defects, e.g. arteriovenous canal) in Down syndrome (Trisomy 21 syndrome). It is a malformation syndrome comprising mental retardation and very characteristic physical appearance.

23. Answer: D. Coarctation of the aorta

Berry aneurysms occur in coarctation of the aorta in about 10% of cases. Aneurysm size and risk of rupture increases with age. Cerebral aneurysms are congenital saccular lesions and are seen commonly in the circle of Willis. These lesions develop at congenital sites of weakness at the bifurcation of cerebral arteries. Uncontrolled hypertension promotes the growth of aneurysms which can lead to rupture causing subarachnoid hemorrhage. Patients usually present with the worst headache of life.

24. Answer: A. Dilated cardiomyopathy (DCM)

Dilated cardiomyopathy is the most common type of idiopathic cardiomyopathy. DCM affects younger patients. Patients usually present with symptoms of congestive heart failure or, occasionally, with sudden death. Echocardiography is the most reliable test to diagnose the DCM.

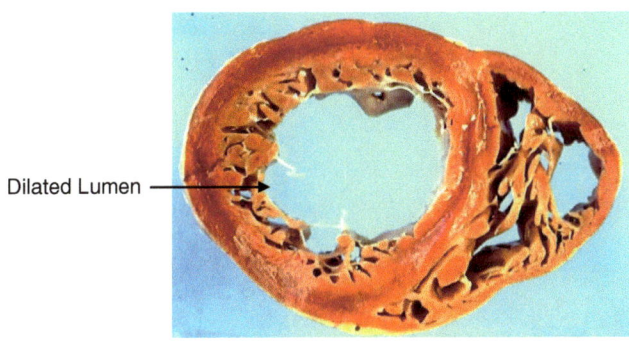

Dilated Lumen

25. Answer: C. Myxoma

Myxoma is the most common tumor of heart. Patients may present with one or more symptoms of myxoma triad which includes embolic phenomena, intracardiac flow obstruction, and constitutional symptoms. Myxomas are benign tumors. Complete resection is the treatment of choice.

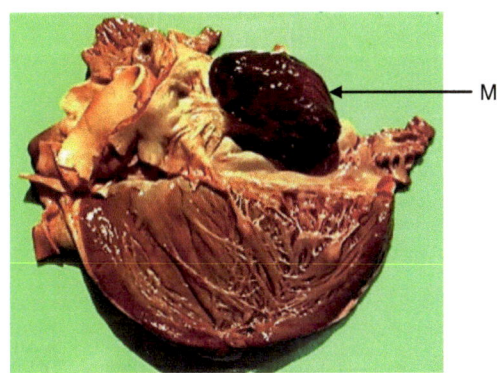

Myxoma of heart

Bibliography

1. Azeem A, Alexander-Nickens ME, Majithia V, Hall M. Is it Libman–Sacks endocarditis? J Am Coll Cardiol. 2016;67(13):1193.
2. Sika-Paotonu D, Beaton A, Raghu A, Steer A, Carapetis J. Acute rheumatic fever and rheumatic heart disease. Oklahoma City: University of Oklahoma Health Sciences Center; 2017.
3. Thomas L, Khetrapal A. Rheumatic heart disease: pathophysiology. Treasure Island: StatPearls; 2019.
4. Nair AR, Samavedam S, Tharakan JM, Karunakaran J. Acute rheumatic valvulitis with palisading: a rare but classic histopathological finding in a surgical specimen. Heart India. 2015;3(4):121–2.
5. Singhal P, Luk A, Rao V, Butany J. Molecular basis of cardiac myxomas. Int J Mol Sci. 2014;15(1).1315–37.
6. Liu T, Xie M, Lv Q, Li Y, Fang L, Zhang L, Deng W, Wang J. Bicuspid aortic valve: an update in morphology, genetics, biomarker, complications, imaging diagnosis and treatment. Front Physiol. 2019;9:1921.
7. Neto FL, Marques LC, Aiello VD. Myxomatous degeneration of the mitral valve. Autopsy Case Rep. 2018;8(4):e2018058.
8. https://www.nature.com/subjects/hypertension.
9. Diaz-Frias J, Guillaume M. Tetralogy of Fallot. Dellas: American Heart Association; 2019.
10. Jun J-I, Kim K-H, Lau LF. The matricellular protein CCN1 mediates neutrophil efferocytosis in cutaneous wound healing. Nat Commun. 2015;6:7386.
11. Mytilinaiou M, Kyrou I, Khan M, Grammatopoulos DK, Randeva HS. Familial hypercholesterolemia: new horizons for diagnosis and effective management. Front Pharmacol. 2018;9:707.
12. (A) Arvold ND, Hsu L, Chen WY, Benzaquen LR, Weiss SE. Marantic endocarditis with cardioembolic strokes mimicking leptomeningeal metastases in breast cancer. J Clin Oncol. 2011;29(29):e743–6. (B) Starobinska E, Robinson EA, Brucks E, Scott S. Marantic endocarditis: incidental infarcts leading to diagnosis of pancreatic cancer. 2018.
13. https://librepathology.org/wiki/Myocardial_infarction.
14. Michaud K, et al. Diagnosis of myocardial infarction at autopsy: AECVP reappraisal in the light of the current clinical classification. Virchows Arch. 2019;476(2):179–94.
15. Imazio M, et al. Pericardial involvement in systemic autoimmune diseases. Heart. 2019;97(22):1882–92.
16. Davies RE, Gilchrist IC. Contemporary management of post-MI myocardial rupture. Washington, DC: American College of Cardiology; 2018.
17. EM MN. β-Myosin heavy chain gene mutations in familial hypertrophic cardiomyopathy: the usual suspect? Circ Res. 2018;90(3):246–7.
18. Castro-Monsalve J, Alvarado-Socarras JL, Mantilla KA, Forero L, Moreno A, Prada CE. Cardiac rhabdomyomas in tuberous sclerosis complex. 2018;192:264.
19. (A) https://www.pathologyoutlines.com/topic/liverCHF.html. (B) Türkmen N, Eren B, Fedakar R, Akgöz S. The significance of hemosiderin deposition in the lungs and organs of the mononucleated macrophage resorption system in infants and children. J Korean Med Sci. 2008;23(6):1020–26.
20. (A) Garg P, Morris P, Fazlanie AL, Vijayan S, Dancso B, Dastidar AG, Plein S, Mueller C, Haaf P. Cardiac biomarkers of acute coronary syndrome: from history to high-sensitivity cardiac troponin. Intern Emerg Med. 2017;12(2):147–155. (B) https://librepathology.org/wiki/Myocardial_infarction.
21. Bhatti R, Dhamoon AS. Fibrinous pericarditis. Treasure Island: StatPearls; 2019.
22. Thacoor A. Mitral valve prolapse and Marfan syndrome. Congenit Heart Dis. 2017;12(4):430–4.
23. Karabinis A, Samanidis G, Khoury M, Stavridis G, Perreas K. Clinical presentation and treatment of cardiac myxoma in 153 patients. Medicine (Baltimore). 2018;97(37):e12397.
24. Arnautovic JZ, Yamasaki H, Rosman HS. Multiple embolic strokes as a result of Libman–Sacks endocarditis associated with lupus and secondary antiphospholipid antibody syndrome: a case report. Eur Heart J Case Rep. 2018;2(3):yty094.
25. (A) Ondrus T, Kanovsky J, Novotny T, Andrsova I, Spinar J, Kala P. Right ventricular myocardial infarction: from pathophysiology to prognosis. Exp Clin Cardiol. 2013;18(1): 27–30. (B) Dima C, Yang EH. Right ventricular infarction. 2017.
26. Ammash NM, Connolly HM, Silversides C, Yeon SB. Clinical manifestations and diagnosis of ventricular septal defect in adults. Waltham: UpToDate; 2018.
27. Atrioventricular canal defect. https://www.mayoclinic.org/diseases-conditions/atrioventricular-canal-defect/symptoms-causes/syc-20361492. Accessed 14 Jul 2018.

Hematopathology of Red Blood Cells and White Blood Cells

8

Multiple Choice Questions

1. Paroxysmal nocturnal hemoglobinuria (PNH) is associated with deficiency of:
   A. MIRL (Membrane inhibitor of reactive lysis)
   B. DAF (Decay accelerating factor)
   C. LFA-1 (Lymphocyte function-associated antigen 1)
   D. GPI (Glycosylphosphatidylinositol) anchored proteins
   E. LFA-3 (Lymphocyte function-associated antigen 3)

2. A 20-year-old female comes to the physician office with symptoms of increased menstrual flow and easy bruising. Laboratory investigations show platelet count of 26,000/mm³. A diagnosis of idiopathic thrombocytopenic purpura (ITP) is made. Which of the following is responsible for low platelet count in ITP?
   A. Antiplatelet antibodies
   B. Defective platelet aggregation
   C. Hypersplenism
   D. Ineffective megakaryopoiesis
   E. Mechanical trauma

3. A 70-year-old male presents with bone pain in the back and renal failure. Bone marrow aspirate shows abnormal blasts. Which finding is expected in the red blood cells of the peripheral blood smear?
   A. Rouleaux formation
   B. Schistocytes
   C. Teardrop-shaped red cells
   D. Dacrocytes
   E. Bite cells

4. Thrombocytosis refers to an increased platelet count. Which of the following is correct statement regarding thrombocytosis?
   A. Platelet count of >200,000/μL (>200 × 10⁹/L)
   B. Platelet count of >250,000/μL (>250 × 10⁹/L)
   C. Platelet count of >350,000/μL (>350 × 10⁹/L)
   D. Platelet count of >325,000/μL (>325 × 10⁹/L)
   E. Platelet count of >450,000/μL (>450 × 10⁹/L)

5. Howell–Jolly bodies are a cytopathological findings of basophilic nuclear remnants (clusters of DNA) in circulating erythrocytes. Howell–Jolly bodies are found in which of the following condition?
   A. Asplenia (surgical or functional)
   B. Iron deficiency anemia
   C. β-Thalassemia minor
   D. Glucose-6-phosphate dehydrogenase deficiency
   E. Megaloblastic anemia

6. A 29-year-old female is scheduled for elective surgery. Screening tests for bleeding disorder are done. Prothrombin time (PT) = 13.7 s, Partial thromboplastin time (PTT) = 100 s, PTT (50:50 MIX) = 29.3 s, PTT (50:50 MIX-1 h) = 28.6 s. Which of the following factor is likely to be deficient?
   A. Factor XII
   B. Factor XI
   C. Factor VIII
   D. Factor IX
   E. Factor X

7. The cytogenetic defect t(15;17) is associated with which of the following leukemia?
   A. Chronic myeloid leukemia
   B. Acute promyelocytic leukemia
   C. Acute lymphoblastic leukemia
   D. Chronic lymphocytic leukemia
   E. Acute monocytic leukemia

8. A 59-year-old female with breast cancer presents with fatigue. Complete blood count shows pancytopenia. Peripheral blood smear shows nucleated red cells, dacrocytes, and immature granulocytes but no blasts. What is the diagnosis?

A. Acute myeloid leukemia
B. Myelodysplastic syndrome
C. Myelophthisic anemia
D. Chronic lymphocytic leukemia
E. Chronic myeloid leukemia.

9. Laboratory findings of anemia, thrombocytopenia, and leukopenia are characteristic of which of the following type of anemia?
   A. Megaloblastic anemia
   B. Iron deficiency anemia
   C. Aplastic anemia
   D. Sickle cell anemia.
   E. β Thalassemia

10. Ineffective erythropoiesis is characteristic of which one of the following conditions?
    A. β Thalassemia major
    B. Iron deficiency anemia.
    C. Aplastic anemia
    D. Sickle cell anemia.
    E. Glucose-6-Phosphate Dehydrogenase (G6PD) Deficiency.

11. Which of the following is a poor prognostic indicator in acute lymphoblastic leukemia (ALL)?
    A. t(4;11)(q21;q23)
    B. t(1;19)(q23;p13)
    C. t(5;14)(q31.1;q32.1)
    D. t(12;21)(p13.2;q22.1)
    E. t(v;11)(q23.3)

12. Macro-ovalocytes and hypersegmented neutrophils are seen in which of the following type of anemia?
    A. Megaloblastic anemia.
    B. Aplastic anemia
    C. Iron deficiency anemia
    D. Hereditary spherocytosis
    E. Autoimmune hemolytic anemia

13. Classical pentad of transient neurologic problems, fever, thrombocytopenia, microangiopathic hemolytic anemia, and acute renal failure are found in which of the following condition?
    A. Idiopathic thrombotic thrombocytopenic purpura
    B. Paroxysmal nocturnal hemoglobinuria
    C. Hemolytic-uremic syndrome
    D. Thrombotic thrombocytopenic purpura
    E. Disseminated intravascular coagulation

14. Bone marrow biopsy of a 72-year-old man is shown below. What is the diagnosis?

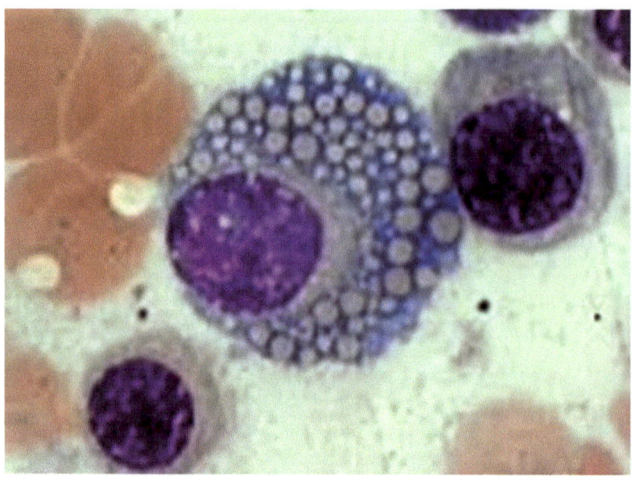

A. Primary (Malignant) lymphoma of bone
B. Metastatic bone disease
C. Multiple myeloma
D. Monoclonal gammopathies of undetermined significance (MGUS)
E. Waldenstrom macroglobulinemia

15. Schistocytes (fragmented red cells) in peripheral blood smear are characteristics of which of the following anemia?
    A. Iron deficiency anemia
    B. Anemia of chronic disease
    C. Aplastic anemia
    D. Sideroblastic anemia
    E. Microangiopathic hemolytic anemia

16. Pappenheimer bodies are composed of:
    A. Copper
    B. Iron
    C. Zinc
    D. Manganese
    E. Silicates

17. Basophilic stippling of red cells is found in which of the following condition?
    A. Lead poisoning
    B. Hemophilia
    C. Paroxysmal nocturnal hemoglobinuria
    D. Hemoglobin C disease
    E. G6PD deficiency

18. Abnormal shaped red blood cells are found in different medical conditions. Bite cells are characteristic of which of the following condition?
    A. G6PD deficiency

B. Thalassemia

C. Hereditary spherocytosis

D. Sideroblastic anemia

E. Anemia of chronic disease

19. An 8-year-old girl is brought to the emergency by her mother with symptoms of nose bleed and hematomas. Laboratory investigations show prolonged bleeding time, normal prothrombin time, and prolonged partial thromboplastin time. What is the diagnosis?

A. Immune thrombocytopenic purpura

B. Von Willebrand disease

C. Hemophilia A

D. Hemophilia B

E. Disseminated intravascular coagulopathy

20. Peripheral blood smear of a male patient is shown below. What is the diagnosis?

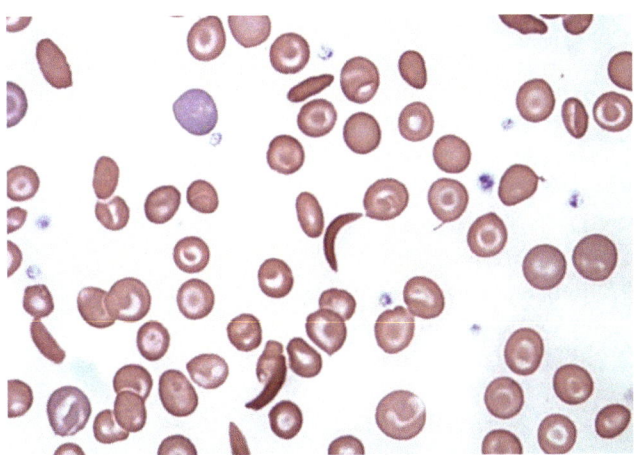

A. Anemia of chronic disease

B. Megaloblastic anemia

C. Sideroblastic anemia

D. Sickle cell anemia

E. Iron deficiency anemia

21. Which of the following vitamins is an essential cofactor for gamma-glutamyl carboxylase, an enzyme that carboxylates coagulation factors II, VII, IX, and X?

A. Vitamin K

B. Vitamin A

C. Vitamin D

D. Vitamin B-12

E. Thiamine (Vitamin B1)

22. Which of the following statements about Von Willebrand factor (vWF) is correct?

A. Von Willebrand factor activity is higher in adults than newborns

B. Patients with blood group O have the highest mean vWF levels

C. Von Willebrand factor activity is equal in adults and newborns

D. Von Willebrand factor activity is higher in newborns than adults

E. Von Willebrand factor is only synthesized by endothelial cells

23. An 80-year-old male patients present with fatigue, malaise, and anemia. Peripheral blood smear shows increased number of normal-appearing lymphocytes. What is the diagnosis?

A. Chronic myelogenous leukemia

B. Polycythemia vera

C. Acute myelogenous leukemia

D. Chronic lymphocytic leukemia

E. Myelofibrosis with myeloid metaplasia

24. Microscopic picture is shown below. What is the diagnosis?

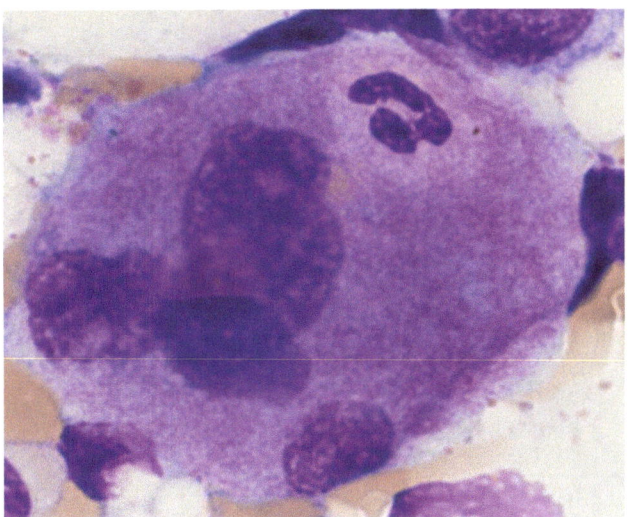

A. Langerhans cell

B. Giant cells

C. Macrophage

D. Megaloblastosis

E. Emperipolesis

25. Which of the following test is the best indicator of response to therapy on patients being treated for thrombotic thrombocytopenic purpura (TTP)?

A. Prothrombin time

B. Fibrinogen levels

C. Platelet count

D. Activated partial thromboplastin time

E. LDH level

26. A 47-year-old male presents with fatigue, dyspnea and easy bruisability. Echocardiogram shows reduced left ventricular ejection. Endomyocardial biopsy is done which shows amyloid deposition. PT and aPTT values are increased. What is the diagnosis?

A. Factor V deficiency

B. Factor II deficiency

C. Factor X deficiency

D. Factor XII deficiency

E. Factor VIII deficiency

27. Which of the following is an indicator of good prognosis for pre-B Childhood ALL?

A. Age of diagnosis

B. Hypodiploidy

C. Hyperdiploidy

D. WBC count

E. (1, 19) translocation

28. Platelets are tiny, disc-shaped pieces of cells that are found in the blood. Platelets are stored at:

A. 20–24 °C

B. 4 °C

C. −20 °C

D. 0 °C

E. 8 °C

29. Which antibody is commonly elevated in Waldenstrom macroglobulinemia?

A. IgG

B. IgA

C. IgM

D. IgD

E. IgE

30. Prothrombin time (PT) is a blood test that measures the time it takes for the liquid portion (plasma) of blood to clot. Prolonged prothrombin time is seen in:

A. Hemophilia A

B. Hemophilia B

C. Thrombocytopenia

D. Factor VII deficiency

E. Factor XIII deficiency

31. Red blood cells are prepared from whole blood by removing the plasma. Shelf life of whole blood is:

A. 35 days

B. 120 days

C. 7 days

D. 85 days

E. 100 days

32. A 15-year-old male presents with fever, sore throat, and enlarged cervical lymph nodes. CBC shows total WBC of 22,000. Peripheral blood smear shows atypical lymphocytes. Monospot test is positive. What is the diagnosis?

A. Infectious mononucleosis

B. Acute mumps

C. Diphtheria

D. Scarlet fever

E. Toxoplasmosis

33. Cabot's ring in RBCs is seen in:

A. Acquired hemolytic anemia

B. Hemochromatosis

C. Thalassemia

D. After splenectomy

E. Iron deficiency anemia

34. Deficiency of which of the following causes hereditary spherocytosis?

A. Actin

B. Glycoprotein

C. Ankyrin

D. Band 4

E. G-6PD deficiency

35. A 37-year-old male presents with severe fatigue, frequent nose bleeds, and gingival masses. The abnormal cells seen in the blood smear show tissue paper nuclei. What is the diagnosis?

A. Acute myelogenous leukemia

B. Acute monocytic leukemia

C. Chronic lymphocytic leukemia

D. Acute lymphocytic leukemia

E. Acute myelomonocytic leukemia

36. Which of the following is a marker of B or T cell acute lymphoblastic leukemia?

A. CD138 positivity

B. CD33 positivity

C. CD52 positivity

D. TdT positivity

E. CD10 positivity

37. Reticulocytes are stained by:

A. Wright stain

B. Brilliant cresyl blue

C. Alcian blue

D. Giemsa stain

E. Trichrome stain

38. Which of the following findings will be found in iron deficiency anemia?

A. Decreased MCV, increased RDW

B. Increased MCV, increased RDW

C. Normal MCV, Increased RDW

D. Decreased MCV, decreased RDW

E. Normal MCV, normal RDW

39. Most sensitive test for disseminated intravascular coagulation (DIC) is:

A. Platelet count

B. D-Dimer

C. Fibrinogen Degradation Products (FDP)

D. PT

E. Bleeding time

40. PAS-positive coarse granules are found in which kind of leukemia?

A. Acute lymphoblastic leukemia

B. Acute myeloblastic leukemia

C. Acute promyelocytic leukemia

D. Chronic lymphocytic leukemia

E. Chronic myeloid leukemia

41. Which of the following cytochemical stains differentiate acute myeloid leukemia (AML) from Acute lymphoblastic leukemia (ALL)?
    A. Acid phosphatase
    B. Nonspecific esterase
    C. Myeloperoxidase
    D. Toluidine blue
    E. Giemsa stain

42. A 9-year-old male child comes to the pediatrician office with symptoms of fatigue, weakness, infections, nose bleed, and gingival bleeding. Laboratory investigations show hemoglobin of 5.5 g/dL. Flow cytometry reveals biphenotypic patterns of antigen expressions. There is strong expression of CD19 and Myeloperoxidase (MPO) + ve. What is the diagnosis?
    A. Acute lymphoblastic leukemia
    B. Acute myeloid leukemia
    C. Undifferentiated leukemia
    D. Mixed phenotype acute leukemia
    E. Chronic myelogenous leukemia

43. A 49-year-old female presents with fever, fatigue, and a dragging sensation in her upper left quadrant. Complete blood count shows low hemoglobin and elevated white blood cells count. Bone marrow aspirates shows immature cells, segmented neutrophils, and basophils. What is the diagnosis?
    A. Acute lymphoblastic leukemia
    B. Acute myeloid leukemia
    C. Myelodysplastic syndrome
    D. Chronic myeloid leukemia
    E. Chronic lymphocytic leukemia

44. Macrocytosis of red blood cells are seen in:
    A. Folate deficiency
    B. Myelodysplasia
    C. Alcoholism
    D. Vitamin B12
    E. All of the above

45. A 72-year-old patient comes to the physician office with complaints of fatigue and low energy. Detailed laboratory and imaging investigations were done. Serum M-protein shows <3 g/dL. Bone marrow shows plasma cells <10 percent. There are no lytic lesions, anemia, hypercalcemia, and renal insufficiency. What is the diagnosis?
    A. Multiple myeloma
    B. Reactive systemic amyloidosis
    C. Non-Hodgkin lymphoma
    D. Monoclonal gammopathy of undetermined significance (MGUS)
    E. Waldenstrom macroglobulinemia

46. Peripheral blood smear of a 54-year-old patient is shown below. What is the diagnosis?

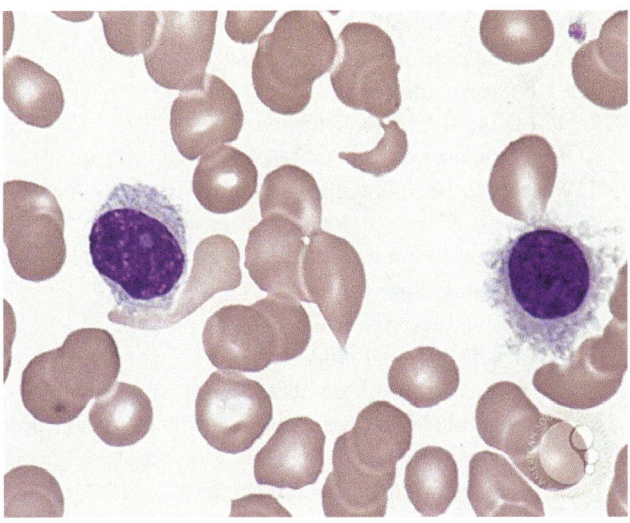

    A. Hairy cell leukemia
    B. Chronic lymphocytic leukemia
    C. Myelodysplastic syndrome
    D. Myelophthisic anemia
    E. Primary myelofibrosis

47. Bence Jones proteins in the urine are found in which of the following condition?
    A. Multiple myeloma
    B. Waldenstrom macroglobulinemia
    C. Mantle cell lymphoma
    D. Acute lymphoblastic lymphoma
    E. Chronic lymphocytic leukemia

48. A 60-year-old man presents with pancytopenia, a markedly enlarged spleen and extramedullary hematopoiesis. He is found to have a JAK-2 mutation. What is the diagnosis?
    A. Myelodysplastic syndrome
    B. Chronic myeloid leukemia
    C. Hairy cell leukemia
    D. Chronic myelofibrosis
    E. Acute myeloid leukemia

49. The combination of erythrocytosis leukocytosis and thrombocytosis along with splenomegaly is highly characteristic of which of the following condition?
    A. Essential thrombocytosis
    B. Chronic myelogenous leukemia
    C. Primary myclofibrosis
    D. Acute lymphoblastic leukemia
    E. Polycythemia vera

50. Cytopenias (anemia, neutropenia, thrombocytopenia) and morphological evidence of significant dysplasia in all the cell lines (erythroid, myeloid, and megakaryocytes) are characteristics of which of the following condition?

A. Myelodysplastic syndrome
B. Acute myelogenous leukemia
C. Polycythemia vera
D. Essential thrombocythemia
E. Chronic myelogenous leukemia

51. Which of the following lab finding would support a diagnosis of anemia of chronic disease (ACD)?
  A. Normal serum iron
  B. Low serum transferrin
  C. Elevated serum ferritin
  D. Elevated hemoglobin A2
  E. Normal erythrocyte sedimentation rate

52. A 39-year-old female patient present with intractable nose bleeds. Complete blood counts show low hemoglobin and elevate in the white blood cells count (122×10^9/L). Some of the abnormal cells show thin linear structures either side of the nucleus. What is the diagnosis?
  A. Acute myeloblastic leukemia without maturation (AML-M1)
  B. Acute monoblastic and monocytic leukemia
  C. Acute myelomonocytic leukemia
  D. Acute lymphoblastic leukemia
  E. Acute megakaryoblastic leukemia (AML-M7)

53. Bone marrow aspirate of a patient shows several blasts stained with PAS. What is the diagnosis?
  A. Acute lymphoblastic leukemia (ALL)
  B. Acute myeloid leukemia (AML)
  C. Acute erythroid leukemia
  D. Myelodysplastic syndrome
  E. Pernicious anemia

Answers and Explanations

1. Answer: D. GPI (Glycosylphosphatidylinositol) anchored proteins

   Paroxysmal nocturnal hemoglobinuria is a rare, acquired clonal hematologic disorder that arises from a mutation in the phosphatidylinositol glycan anchor biosynthesis class A (PIGA) gene. There is decreased glycosylphosphatidylinositol (GPI)-linked proteins, especially decay accelerating factor (DAF). RBCs are subjected to increased sensitivity to lysis due to deficiency of membrane-bound GPI-anchored proteins. Patients present with pancytopenia (anemia, leukopenia, and thrombocytopenia). Symptoms are episodes of hemolysis which usually occur at night. Acidosis in vivo, which occurs in sleep causes activation of complement leading to episodes of hemolysis. There is episodic hemoglobinuria on awakening which can lead to iron deficiency. There is an increased risk of aplastic anemia, leukemia, and venous thrombosis. Flow cytometry is used to detect lack of CD55 decay-accelerating factor (DAF) on blood cells.

2. Answer: A. Antiplatelet antibodies

   Idiopathic thrombocytopenic purpura is an acquired thrombocytopenia caused by antiplatelet antibodies. Thrombocytopenia is present with normal or increased megakaryocytes. Antiplatelet antibodies attach to platelets (anti-GpIIb/IIIa antibodies) and lead to removal by splenic macrophages. Patients present with fatigue, cutaneous petechiae, and bleeding. Severe bleeding occurs when platelet counts are below 20,000/microL. In adults, ITP is a chronic autoimmune condition and occurs more often in females. In children it is an acute, self-limited reaction to viral infection.

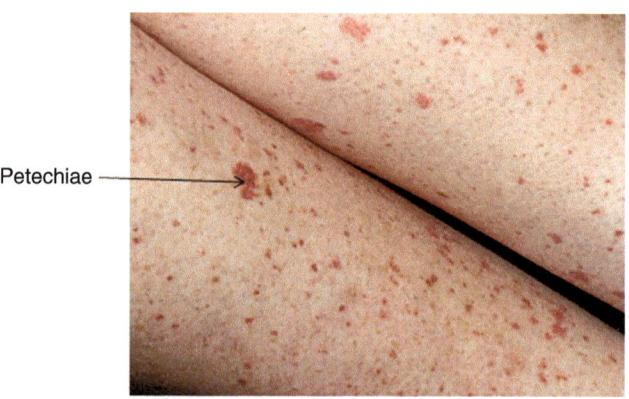

Petechiae

3. Answer: A. Rouleaux formation

   The diagnosis of multiple myeloma is confirmed by the presence of numerous plasma cells in bone marrow. The malignant plasma cells resemble blasts and may contain large globular inclusions. The plasma cells have clock-face chromatin, eccentric nuclei, and perinuclear hofs. Red blood cells in multiple myeloma show rouleaux formation. Rouleaux formation occurs due to excess immunoglobulin serum, which disrupts the normal repellent force between the red cells leading to piling up of red blood cells like stacks of coins.

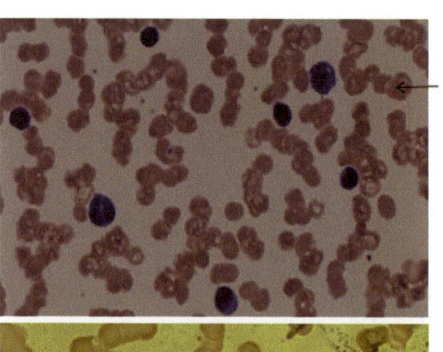

Rouleaux formation

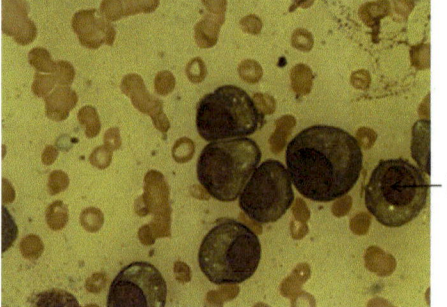

Myeloma cell

4. Answer: E. Platelet count of >450,000/μL (>450 × 10⁹/L)

Essential thrombocythemia is neoplastic proliferation of myeloid stem cells, which lead to increased megakaryocytes in bone marrow. There is an increased number of platelets in the peripheral blood smear. In thrombocytosis, platelets count is more than 450,000/μL (>450 × 10⁹/L). Patients may present with excessive bleeding. Thrombocytosis could be due to reactive processes or autonomous processes. Some causes of reactive processes are iron deficiency/blood loss and post-splenectomy. Autonomous processes may include myeloproliferative neoplasms, hematologic malignancies, and familial thrombocytosis.

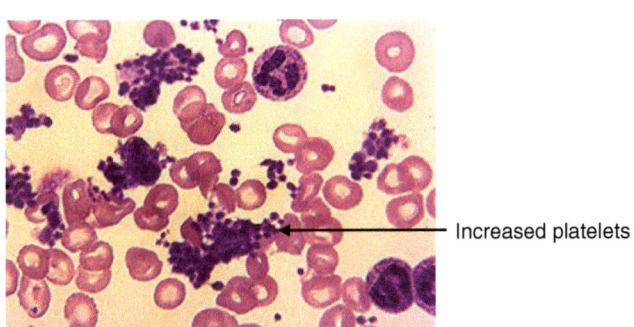
Increased platelets

5. Answer: A. Asplenia (surgical or functional)

Howell–Jolly bodies are remnants of nuclear chromatin. They are founds in patients who had undergone splenectomy. Howell–Jolly bodies may also be seen in sickle cell disease patients who have functional asplenia.

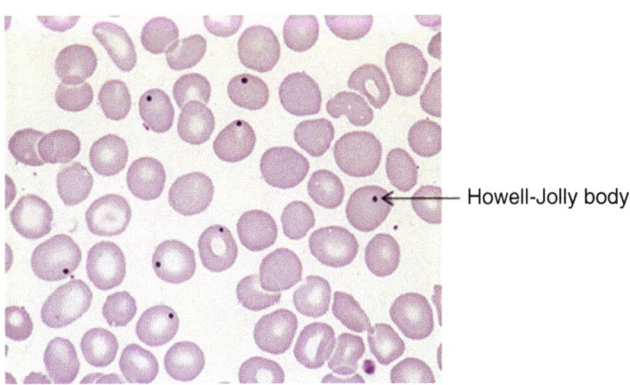
Howell-Jolly body

6. Answer: A. Factor XII

Coagulation factor XII, also called Hageman factor, is a plasma protein. It is the zymogen of a serine protease that begins the contact activation reactions and intrinsic blood coagulation in vitro. Factor XII deficiency causes an isolated increase in partial thromboplastin time (PTT) without any bleeding symptoms. The 50:50 PTT mix corrects, ruling out an inhibitor. Factor VIII, IX, and XI deficiencies also cause an isolated elevation in the PTT,

but the patients usually present with a history of bleeding.

7. Answer: B. Acute promyelocytic leukemia

Acute myeloid leukemia is an acquired genetic mutation in stem cells lead to the proliferation of undifferentiated myeloid blasts. Acute promyelocytic leukemia is a type of acute myeloid leukemia. It results from a translocation due to a rearrangement of genetic material resulting in the formation of chromosome t(15;17) (q24.1;q21.2). Patients usually present with weakness, fatigue, hemorrhage and frequent infections. The diagnosis of APL is confirmed by the identification of the PML-RARA fusion gene.

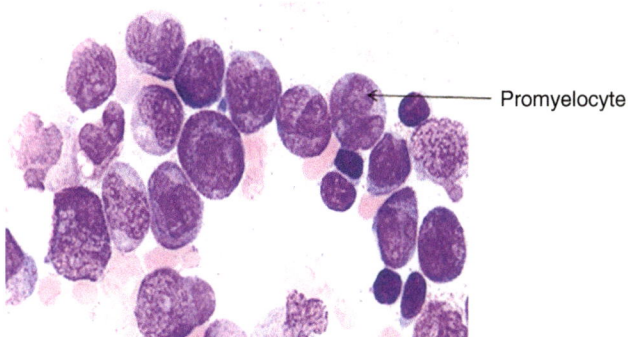
Promyelocyte

8. Answer: C. Myelophthisic anemia

Myelophthisic anemia is a type of marrow failure caused by a destructive marrow lesion that disturbs normal hematopoiesis, such as metastatic disease. Peripheral blood smears of myelophthisic anemia is characterized by nucleated red cells, dacrocytes and immature granulocytes. Myelophthisic anemia occurs because fibrosis and crowding out of the normal bone marrow due to infiltration by abnormal cells such as metastatic cancers or hematologic malignancy.

9. Answer: C. Aplastic anemia

Aplastic anemia is a type of pancytopenia characterized by severe anemia, neutropenia, and thrombocytopenia. It affects men and women equally. Failure or destruction of multipotent myeloid stem cells causes inadequate production of different cell lines. It may be idiopathic (immune-mediated). Other causes of aplastic anemia include radiation, drugs (Chloramphenicol, sulfonamides), viral agents (parvovirus B19, Epstein–Barr virus). Patients present with fatigue, malaise, pallor. Other clinical manifestations include purpura, mucosal bleeding, petechiae, and infection. Laboratory findings show pancytopenia. Bone marrow is hypercellular with decreased megakaryocytes and fatty infiltration.

10. Answer: A. β Thalassemia major

β Thalassemia is mainly due to a point mutation, which form either some β chains (β+). β Thalassemia major lacks HbA and is characterized by alpha-chain aggregation. Aggregation causes decrease in the life span of red blood cells. Apoptotic death of red blood cells precursors occurs resulting in ineffective erythropoiesis. Laboratory findings show elevation in fetal hemoglobin. Patients are usually normal at birth and symptoms develop at about 6 months when fetal hemoglobin starts declining. Hemoglobin electrophoresis shows increasing fetal hemoglobin (90%), an increase in hemoglobin A2 and decrease in hemoglobin A.

11. Answer: A. t(4;11)(q21;q23)

Translocation t(4;11)(q21;q23) is found in approximately 10% of acute lymphoblastic leukemia (ALL) in adult patients. Patients that demonstrate this chromosomal aberration have standard biological, immunophenotypic, and clinical characteristics. Translocation t(4;11) is a poor prognostic indicator. It shows violent behavior, hyperleukocytosis, organomegaly, and CNS involvement.

12. Answer: A. Megaloblastic anemia

Megaloblastic anemia is due to a deficiency in vitamin B12 or folate (coenzymes in DNA synthesis). This leads to delayed DNA replication. Patients usually present with anemia, and glossitis. Subacute combined degeneration occurs due to impaired myelination. Megaloblasts in bone marrow form macro-ovalocytes on peripheral blood. The giant metamyelocytes are found in bone marrow. White blood cells show hypersegmented neutrophils (>5 lobes) in peripheral blood.

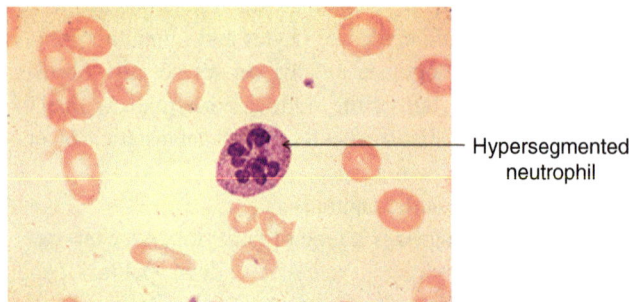

Hypersegmented neutrophil

13. Answer: D. Thrombotic thrombocytopenic purpura

Thrombotic thrombocytopenic purpura is commonly associated with a lack of metalloproteinase enzyme (ADAMTS13). This enzyme normally degrades von Willebrand factor (vWF). The multimeric form of vWF causes platelet aggregation. This usually leads to pentad of microangiopathic hemolytic anemia, thrombocytopenia, renal failure, fever, and neurologic deficits. It is commonly seen in adult females.

14. Answer: C. Multiple Myeloma

Multiple myeloma is a neoplastic proliferation that leads to clonal expansion of plasma cells. Characteristic presentation includes punched out bone lesions, hypercalcemia, myeloma kidney, marrow failure, frequent infection. Prognosis of multiple myeloma is poor and depends on the extent of disease.

15. Answer: E. Microangiopathic hemolytic anemia

Schistocytes (fragmented red blood cells) in peripheral blood cells smear is commonly found in microangiopathic hemolytic anemia (MAHA). Microangiopathic hemolytic anemia is a term used for nonimmune hemolytic anemia.

Schistocytes

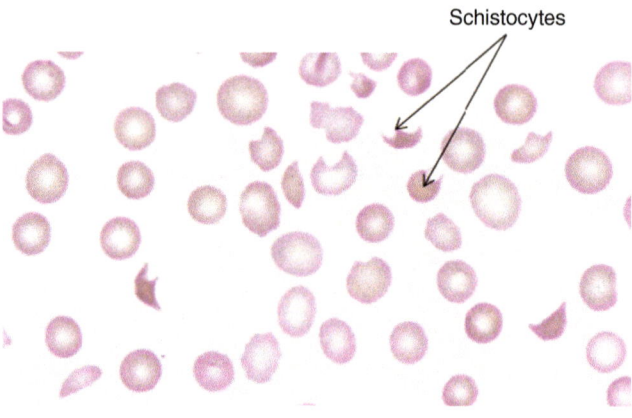

16. Answer: B. Iron

Pappenheimer bodies are dark blue granules found in red blood cells in sideroblastic anemia. The pappenheimer bodies are composed of iron. The red blood cells are usually hypochromic and show basophilic stippling that stains positive for iron.

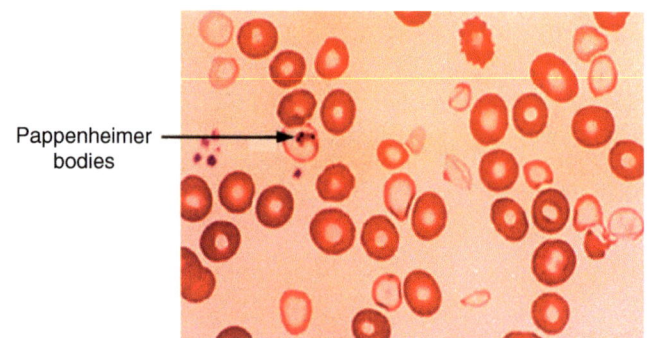

Pappenheimer bodies

17. Answer: A. Lead poisoning

Basophilic stippling is the presence of blue granules of different sizes found in the cytoplasm of the red blood cells. Basophilic stippling represent ribosomal precipitates. Common causes are lead poisoning, thalassemias, alcohol abuse, and heavy metal poisoning.

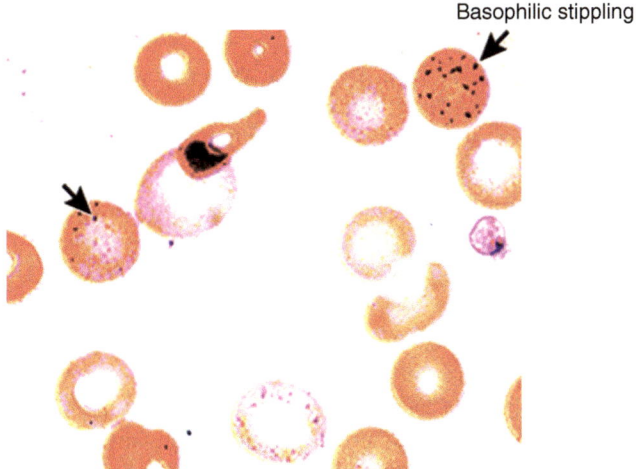

Basophilic stippling

18. Answer: A. G6PD deficiency

Bite cells are commonly found in G6PD deficiency. Intravascular hemolysis and splenic destruction occur following infection, or exposure to certain foods such as fava beans. Hemoglobin with an abnormal structure is removed by splenic macrophages causing bite cells.

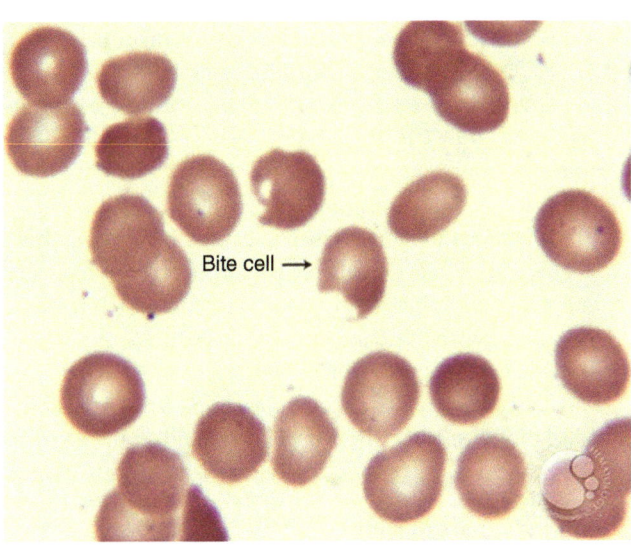

Bite cell →

19. Answer: B. Von Willebrand disease

A common inherited bleeding condition is Willebrand's disease (VWD). There are three types of VWD. Type 3 is due to absent or severely reduced vWF. There is a deficiency of vWF, which normally carries and stabilizes factor VIII. Patients present with mild mucosal skin bleeding. Patients usually have increased activated partial thromboplastin time (aPTT). Bleeding time is also increased.

20. Answer: D. Sickle cell anemia

In sickle cell disease, there is a single nucleotide change in codon causing valine to replace normal glu-

tamic acid at the sixth position of the Beta-globin chain. Peripheral blood smear shows multiple sickle cells. Howell–Jolly bodies and target cells may also be seen in peripheral blood smears. Common complications of sickle cell disease include infections, severe anemia, and vaso-occlusive phenomena.

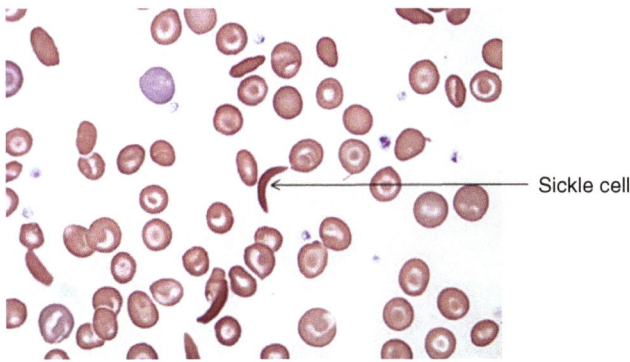

Sickle cell

21. Answer: A. Vitamin K

Prothrombin (factor II) and factors VII, IX, and X as well as proteins C and S are factors which require Gla for their function. Gla is an amino acid which gives the vitamin K-dependent proteins metal-binding properties. These proteins undergo a structural transformation with the addition of calcium ions which results in the exposure of a phospholipid binding site. As an enzyme cofactor, the requirement for vitamin K is unique to vitamin K-dependent gamma-glutamyl carboxylase and gamma-carboxyglutamic acid (Gla) biosynthesis. The vitamin K-dependent carboxylase is an integral membrane protein which requires carbon dioxide, molecular oxygen, and vitamin K of the hydroquinone to convert residues of glutamic acid (Glu) to Gla.

22. Answer: D. Von Willebrand factor activity is higher in newborns than adults

Newborns have higher vWF compared to adults. vWF is a glycoprotein present in endothelial cells, endothelial tissue and megakaryocytes. vWF binds exposed collagen and platelets at sites of injury.

23. Answer: D. Chronic lymphocytic leukemia

Chronic lymphocytic leukemia (CLL) is a neoplastic proliferation of lymphoid cells. It is more common in males, an average of presentation is 60 years. Patients may be asymptomatic. They may present with the symptoms of fatigue and weight loss. Physical examination shows lymphadenopathy and hepatosplenomegaly. CLL is associated with warm antibody autoimmune hemolytic anemia. Common complication is a bacterial infection due to hypogammaglobulinemia and neutropenia. Peripheral blood smears show increased number of normal appearing lymphocytes. Numerous smudge cells are present due to the fragility of the neoplastic cells. Bone marrow findings include numerous normal-appearing neoplastic lymphocytes. CLL rarely transforms into large cell lymphoma.

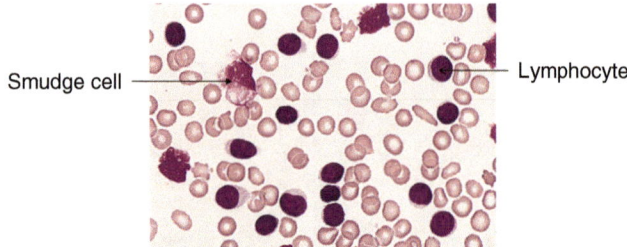

24. Answer: E. Emperipolesis

Emperipolesis is presence of one intact cell within another cell cytoplasm. The microscopic picture of question shows neutrophils in the cytoplasm of megakaryocytes. It may occur in reactive or myeloproliferative disorders (MPD) conditions, most commonly in polycythemia vera.

25. Answer: C. Platelet count

The platelet count is the most consistently abnormal laboratory test in Thrombotic thrombocytopenic purpura (TTP). Few experts use lactate dehydrogenase levels and creatinine levels to monitor a patient with TTP but the platelet count is the best indicator of response to therapy.

26. Answer: C. Factor X deficiency

Amyloidosis is associated with acquired factor Xa deficiency because of its heavy amyloid affinity. Patients usually present with easy bruisability. Laboratory findings show elevated PT and aPTT.

27. Answer: C. Hyperdiploidy

Hyperdiploidy carries a good prognosis for pre-B Childhood ALL. Other good indicators of B-ALL prognosis are t(12, 21), younger diagnostic age (1–9 years), female gender, and low white blood cells count (less than 50,000).

28. Answer: A. 20–24 °C

Platelets require careful handling while collection, preparation, and transfusion. The bags in which platelets are stored are made from gas-permeable plastic to allow sufficient oxygen to maintain aerobic respiration. Platelets should be stored at 20–24°C. Storage at low temperature leads to irreversible changes on the platelet membrane, resulting in phagocytosis. Higher temperature may lead to an increase in bacterial infections.

29. Answer: C. IgM

Waldenström macroglobulinemia (WM) is a neoplasm of plasmacytoid lymphocytes. It is monoclonal IgM gammopathy in the blood. Patients usually present with anemia, fever, night sweats, weight loss. Physical examination reveals enlarged lymph nodes and hepatosplenomegaly. Hyperviscosity syndrome may involve central nervous system causing blurring or loss of vision, headache, ataxia, dementia and stroke. Bone marrow biopsy must show more than 10% infiltration by small lymphocytes displaying differentiation of plasmacytoid cells or plasma cells.

30. Answer: D. Factor VII deficiency

Factor VII deficiency is an inherited autosomal recessive bleeding disorder. In Factor VII deficiency, prothrombin time is increased while aPTT remains normal. Patients present with bleeding episode after injury or surgery.

31. Answer: A. 35 days

The most common anticoagulant-preservative solution used for whole blood preservation in blood bank is CPDA-1 (citrate phosphate dextrose adenine). Other solutions are:

CPD (citrate phosphate dextrose)

CP2D (citrate phosphate dextrose dextrose)

ACD-A (citrate dextrose anticoagulant A)

CDPA-1 has a shelf life of 35 days while other products like CPD, CP2D, and ACD-A have a shelf life of 21 days.

32. Answer: A. Infectious mononucleosis

Infectious mononucleosis is caused by Epstein–Barr virus. The patient usually presents with fever, lymphadenopathy, and pharyngitis with symptoms of infectious mononucleosis. Monospot test is positive. Peripheral blood smear shows atypical lymphocytes. Atypical lymphocytes have abundant cytoplasm and irregular nuclei. Red blood cells usually surround and indent the atypical lymphocytes. Infectious mononucleosis is a self-limited condition.

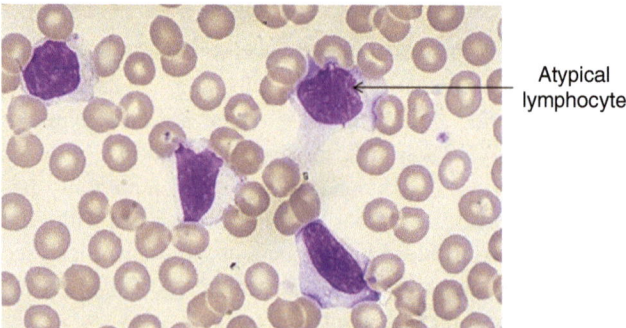

33. Answer: D. After splenectomy

Red cell inclusions (figure of eight) are called Cabot's rings. They are usually thread like red to violet rings and are remnants from the mitotic spindle. They are usually found in megaloblastic anemia and after splenectomy.

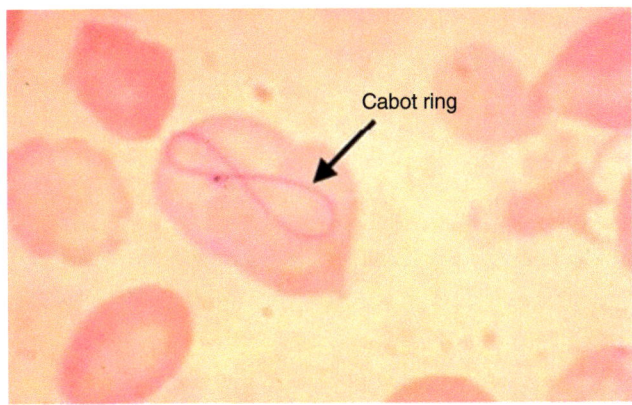

Cabot ring

34. Answer: C. Ankyrin

Hereditary spherocytosis (HS) is an autosomal dominant disease showing deficiency of spectrin, ankyrin leading to red blood cell fragility. It forces the red blood cells in a spherical shape. Spherical cells are less deformable, become trapped within the spleen and are then phagocytosed. Patients present with anemia, splenomegaly, and jaundice. Patients may develop cholelithiasis (bilirubin gallstones). Osmotic fragility test is positive (RBCs get lysis in hypotonic salt). Mean corpuscular hemoglobin concentration (MCHC) is increased. Peripheral blood smear shows spherocytes.

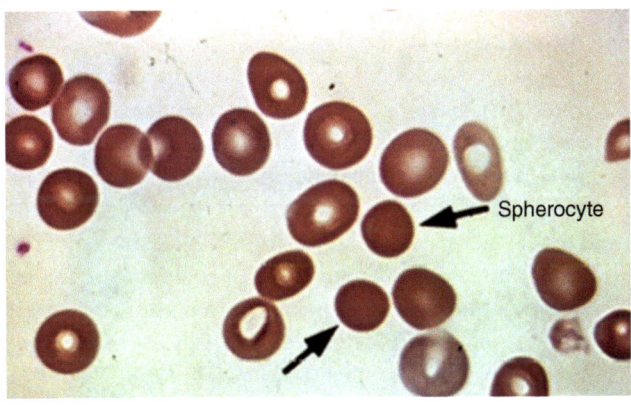

Spherocyte

35. Answer: B. Acute monocytic leukemia

Acute monocytic leukemia (AML-M5a) involves extramedullary sites, such as gums, skin, and central nervous system. Cells usually seen are malignant promonocytes, which are recognized by their delicately creased tissue-paper nuclei.

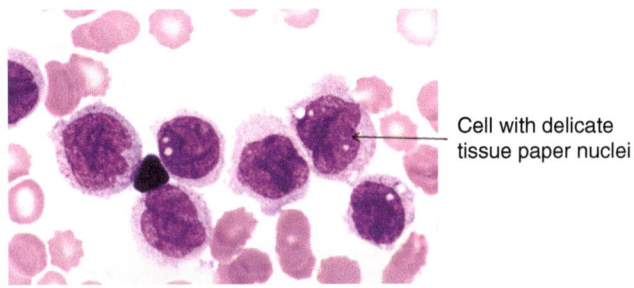

Cell with delicate tissue paper nuclei

36. Answer: D TdT positivity

Terminal deoxynucleotidyl transferase (TdT) is a nuclear enzyme that polymerizes triphosphate deoxynucleoside commonly found in immature pre-B, and pre-T lymphoid cells. TdT staining is positive in both B and T cell ALL (T-ALL), thus helping to distinguish ALL from mature lymphoid malignancies.

37. Answer: B. Brilliant cresyl blue

Reticulocytes are precursors to red blood cells, released from the bone marrow into the bloodstream and that contain remnants of ribonucleic acid (RNA) and ribosomes but no nucleus. A reticulocyte test is used to help evaluate conditions that affect red blood cells such as anemia or bone marrow disorders. It indicates the amount of red blood cell production taking place in the bone marrow. Supravital stain (methylene blue or brilliant cresyl blue is commonly used to stain reticulocytes, RNA appears as blue precipitating granules or filaments within the red cells.

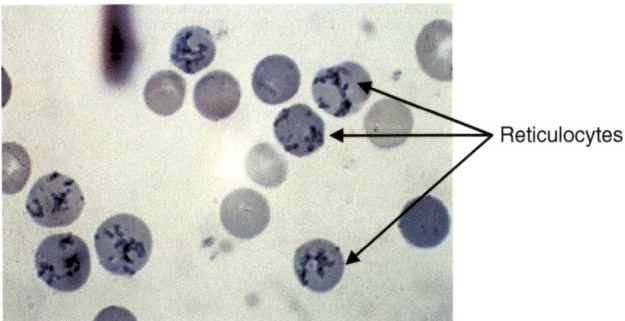

Reticulocytes

38. Answer: A. Decreased MCV, Increased RDW

Iron deficiency anemia is present with a decreased mean corpuscular volume (MCV) because the red blood cells are smaller. Anemia is considered microcytic when the MCV is less than 80 fL. Microcytosis is associated with decreased hemoglobin content within the RBC (mean corpuscular hemoglobin, MCH). This results in a microcytic and hypochromic appearance on the blood smear. RBCs are also variably sized, ranging from small to normal increasing red blood cell distribution width (RDW).

39. Answer: C. Fibrinogen Degradation Products (FDP)

Disseminated intravascular coagulation is the activation of the coagulation cascade, which leads to microthrombi and consumption of platelets and coagulation factors (II, V, VIII, and fibrinogen). DIC results from the release of tissue thromboplastin or activation of the intrinsic pathway. Common causes include obstetric complications (preeclampsia, retained fetus or abruptio placentae) gram-negative sepsis malignancy and acute promyelocytic leukemia). Period of prothrombin (PT), aPTT, prothrombin time and bleeding time is increased. Fibrinogen platelet counts are decreased. Fibrinogen degradation products are the most sensitive test for disseminated intravascular coagulation (DIC).

40. Answer: A. Acute lymphoblastic leukemia

Cytochemical studies help in differentiating types of leukemias. Lymphoblasts usually reveal PAS-positive granules. Myeloperoxidase cytochemical stain is used to differentiate myeloid leukemia from acute lymphoblastic leukemia.

41. Answer: C. Myeloperoxidase

Either the existence of Auer rods, cytochemical positivity for myeloperoxidase, or the presence of ample myeloid/monocytic markers detected by immunophenotyping indicate the leukemic cells of myeloid origin.

Myeloperoxidase (MPO) is found in myeloid and monocytic cell granules but is absent from lymphocytes. Therefore, it is an important marker for distinguishing myeloid from lymphoid blasts. Staining is used to differentiate acute myeloid leukemia (AML) and other myeloid leukemias from lymphoid disorders.

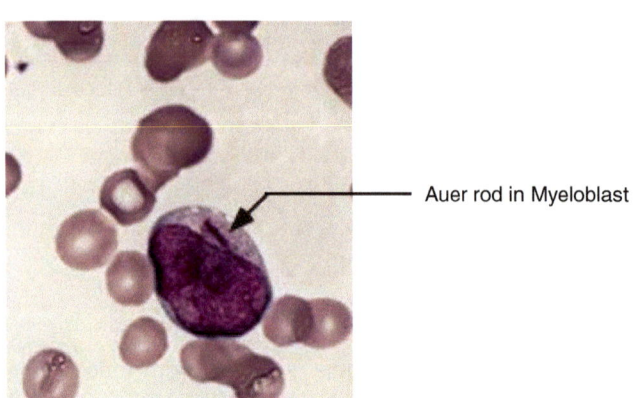

Auer rod in Myeloblast

42. Answer: D. Mixed phenotype acute leukemia

Mixed phenotype acute leukemia (MPAL) is a rare type of leukemia where more than one type of leukemia occurs at the same time. In MPAL, either both acute lymphoblastic leukemia (ALL) blasts (cancer cells) and acute myeloblastic leukemia (AML) blasts at the same time or leukemic blasts exhibit the features of both ALL and AML on the same cell. Symptoms of MPAL include anemia, fatigue, bleeding or bruising, recurrent infections, bone and joint pain, abdominal distress, weight loss, swollen lymph nodes, and trouble breathing.

43. Answer: D. Chronic myeloid leukemia

Chronic myeloid leukemia is characterized by a marked neutrophilic leukocytosis and basophilia in the peripheral blood. Patients usually present with fatigue, malaise, weight loss and tenderness over the lower sternum. Physical examination may show hepatosplenomegaly. Laboratory findings show mild anemia and thrombocytosis. Bone marrow is hypercellular with a marked granulocytic hyperplasia. Bone marrow contains numerous myelocytes, segmented neutrophils, and basophils. Abnormal tyrosine kinase is produced due to translocation between chromosomes 9 and 22. Philadelphia chromosome is characteristic of chronic myeloid leukemia. Chronic myeloid leukemia usually has BCR-ABL fusion gene.

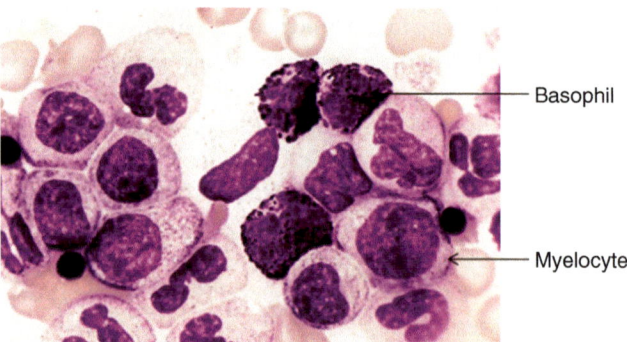

Basophil

Myelocyte

44. Answer: E. All of the above

Macrocytosis refers to a condition when the red blood cells (RBCs) are larger than the normal their size.

Common causes of macrocytosis include vitamin B-12 deficiency, folate deficiency, liver disease, alcoholism, hypothyroidism, medications that interfere with DNA synthesis, reticulocytosis, gastrointestinal diseases (celiac disease and Crohn's disease), and myelodysplastic syndrome. A patient is known to have macrocytosis when a mean corpuscular volume (MCV) of their red blood cells is greater than 100fl (femtolitre).

45. Answer: D. Monoclonal gammopathy of undetermined significance (MGUS)

Monoclonal gammopathy of undetermined significance (MGUS) is a clinically asymptomatic premalignant clonal plasma cell or lymphoplasmacytic proliferative disorder. It is defined by the presence of a serum monoclonal protein (M-protein) at a concentration <3 g/dL, a bone marrow with <10% monoclonal plasma cells, and absence of end-organ damage (lytic bone lesions, anemia, hypercalcemia, renal insufficiency, hyperviscosity) related to the proliferative process.

46. Answer: A. Hairy cell leukemia

Hairy cell leukemia is an uncommon leukemia distinguished by the presence of leukemic cells that have fine hair like cytoplasmic projection. It is rare B cell neoplasm that affects middle age males (M:F = 5:1). Hairy cells can be seen in the peripheral blood smear. Patients usually present with fever, bleeding, peripheral pancytopenia, and splenomegaly. Marked monocytopenia is characteristic. Hairy cells infiltrate the bone marrow and induce marrow fibrosis. Therefore, there is dry tap on bone marrow aspiration. Flow cytometry demonstrates B cell population that expresses CD25, CD103, and Annexin A1 and CD11c. Annexin A1 is the most specific marker. BRAFV600E is a characteristic mutation in hairy cell leukemia.

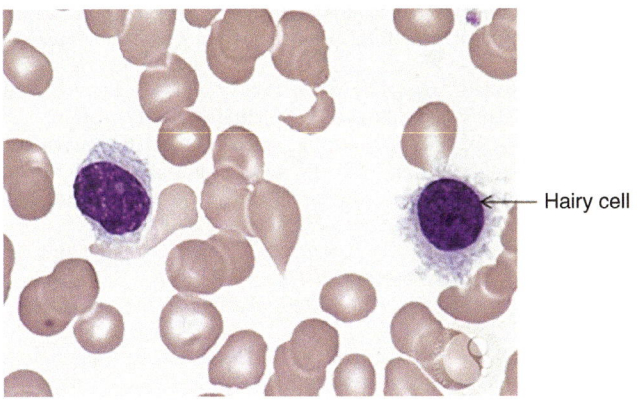

Hairy cell

47. Answer: A. Multiple myeloma

Multiple myeloma is the most common primary tumor arising in the bones of adults. Laboratory diagnosis shows M-spike: monoclonal immunoglobulin spike. The M-spike is broken down into heavy and light chains. Light chains are identical to Bence Jones proteins. Bence Jones proteins are found in the urine once tubular absorption capacity becomes saturated.

48. Answer: D. Chronic myelofibrosis

In chronic myelofibrosis, blood smear shows teardrop-shaped red cells and normoblast. JAK-2 mutations are commonly seen in chronic myelofibrosis. This

mutation is also seen in other chronic myeloproliferative disorders (polycythemia vera and essential thrombocythemia).

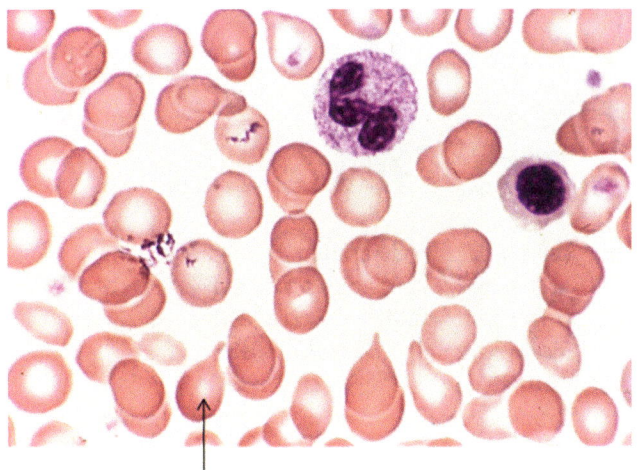

Teardrop-shaped red cell

49. Answer: E. Polycythemia vera

Polycythemia vera (PV) is neoplasm myeloid stem cells leading to excessive production of erythrocytes granulocytes, and megakaryocytes. There is increased red cell mass, increased hematocrit, and viscosity. Arterial oxygen saturation is more than 92%. There is decreased erythropoietin (EPO). Patients usually present with splenomegaly, thrombocytosis and leukocytosis, and pruritus. Other common clinical manifestations are plethora (redness) and cyanosis. Leukocyte alkaline phosphatase (LAP) score is increased in leukemoid reaction and polycythemia vera. Increased blood viscosity can cause deep vein thrombosis and infarcts. High cell turnover causes hyperuricemia resulting in gout. There is increased risk for acute leukemia.

50. Answer: A. Myelodysplastic syndrome

Myelodysplastic syndrome is a clonal disorder of the blood and marrow. It is more common in older adults. Patients presents with persistent cytopenias and dysplastic cells. Unexplained cytopenias (anemia, neutropenia, thrombocytopenia) or monocytosis and significant dysplasia in the cell lines (erythroid, myeloid, and megakaryocytes) should be further evaluated for Myelodysplastic syndrome. Common dysplastic changes found in MDS patients are Pelger-Huet cells and pawn ball megakaryocytes. MDS patients have an increased risk of developing acute leukemia.

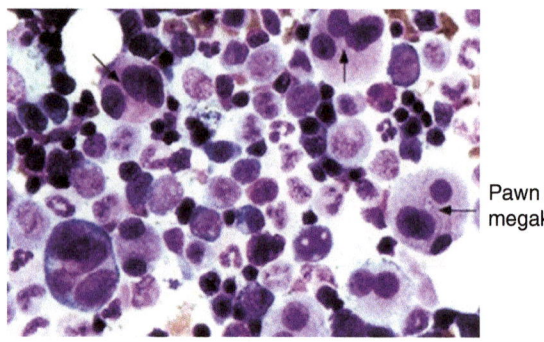

Pawn ball megakaryocyte

51. Answer: C. Elevated serum ferritin

Anemia of chronic disease (ACD) is suspected in a patient with a mild to moderate normocytic, normochromic hypoproliferative anemia with chronic infectious, inflammatory, or malignant condition. In anemia of chronic disease, there is elevated serum ferritin. Laboratory findings in anemia of chronic disease show low serum iron, normal to low serum transferrin (total iron binding capacity), elevated erythrocyte sedimentation rate and/or C-reactive protein.

52. Answer: A. Acute myeloblastic leukemia without maturation (AML-M1)

AML without maturation (AML-M1) accounts for 5–10% of AML. Acute myeloid leukemia without maturation (AML-M1) usually has a thin linear structure on the side of the nucleus. This linear structure is called Auer rod. Auer rods are large inclusion bodies and consist of fused lysosomes. AML without maturation (AML-M1) accounts for 5 to 10% of AML. AML-M1 is characterized by a high percentage of blasts.

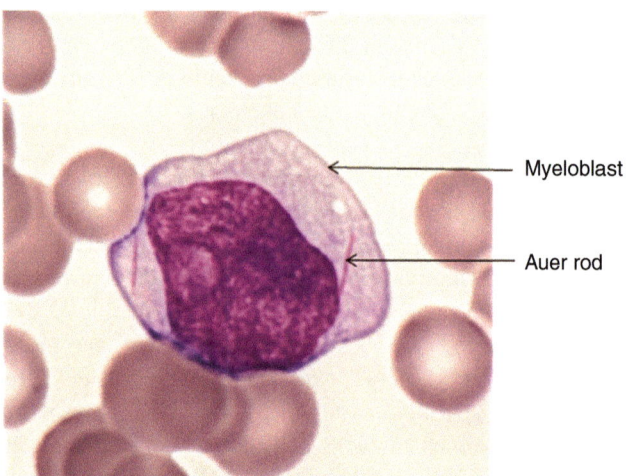

Myeloblast

Auer rod

53. Answer: C. Acute erythroid leukemia

Periodic-acid-Schiff (PAS) staining reactions are usually positive in acute erythroid leukemia (AEL). It may also show a diffuse cytoplasmic positivity in the erythroblasts. Erythroblasts comprise more than 80% in the pure erythroid leukemia. Erythroblasts are usually more than 50% in the erythroid/myeloid subtype. Erythroblasts in AEL are positive for CD71, CD36, hemoglobin A, MDR1, P-glycoprotein, and glycophorin A. Prognosis of acute erythroid leukemia is poor.

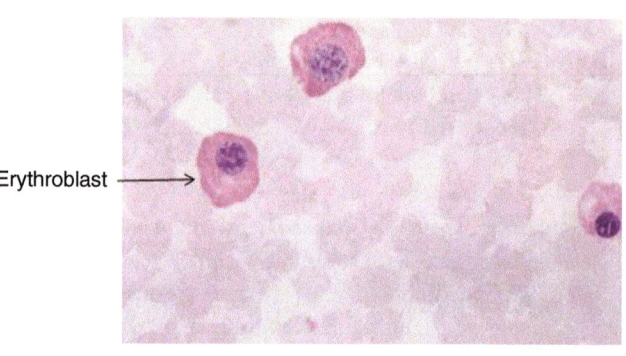

Erythroblast

Bibliography

1. Brodsky RA, Larson RA, Rosmarin AG. Clinical manifestations and diagnosis of paroxysmal nocturnal hemoglobinuria. 2019.
2. George JN, et al. Immune thrombocytopenia (ITP) in adults: clinical manifestations and diagnosis 2019.
3. Yates AM, et al. Prenatal screening and testing for hemoglobinopathy. 2019.
4. Tefferi A, et al. Approach to the patient with thrombocytosis. 2019
5. RBC Products: general transfusion indications. 2011.
6. Larson RA, et al. Clinical manifestations, pathologic features, and diagnosis of acute promyelocytic leukemia in adults. 2019.
7. Olson TS, Mentzer WC, Rosmarin AG. Aplastic anemia: pathogenesis, clinical manifestations, and diagnosis. 2019.
8. Benz EJ, Vichinsky EP, Tirnauer JS. Clinical manifestations and diagnosis of the thalassemias. 2019.
9. George JN, et al. Acquired TTP: Clinical manifestations and diagnosis. 2019.
10. Fairfield KM, Motil KJ, Tirnauer JS. Causes and pathophysiology of vitamin B12 and folate deficiencies. 2019.
11. George JN, et al. Approach to the patient with suspected TTP, HUS, or other thrombotic microangiopathy (TMA). 2019.
12. Rosenthal DS et al. Evaluation of the peripheral blood smear. 2019.
13. Glader B, Leung LLK, Tirnauer JS. Disorders of the hexose monophosphate shunt and glutathione metabolism other than glucose-6-phosphate dehydrogenase deficiency. 2019.
14. Rick ME, Leung LLK, Tirnauer JS. Clinical presentation and diagnosis of von Willebrand disease. 2019.
15. Vichinsky EP, DeBaun MR, Tirnauer JS. Overview of the clinical manifestations of sickle cell disease. 2019.
16. Furie B, et al. Vitamin K and the synthesis and function of gamma-carboxyglutamic acid. 2019.
17. Roth CG. Educational case: chronic lymphocytic leukemia. Acad Pathol. 2018;5:6011.
18. Cho MS, Sharma S. Transfusion-related acute lung injury (TRALI). 2019.
19. Cheung AT, et al. Cardiopulmonary bypass: management. 2019.
20. Leung LLK, et al. Clinical features, diagnosis, and treatment of disseminated intravascular coagulation in adults. 2019.
21. Thomas S. Platelets: handle with care. Transfus Med. 2016;26(5):330–8.
22. Rajkumar SV, et al. Epidemiology, pathogenesis, clinical manifestations, and diagnosis of Waldenström macroglobulinemia. 2019.

23. Mannucci PM, et al. Rare inherited coagulation disorders. 2019.

24. Teruya J, et al. Red blood cell transfusion in infants and children: selection of blood products. 2019.

25. Goldfinger D, et al. Granulocyte transfusions. 2019.

26. Rosenthal DS, Leung LLK, Tirnauer JS. Evaluation of the peripheral blood smear. 2019.

27. He B-J, Liao L, Deng Z-F, Tao Y-F, Xu Y-C, Lin F-Q. Molecular genetic mechanisms of hereditary spherocytosis: current perspectives. Acta Haematol. 2018;139:60–6.

28. Lawrence SM, Corriden R, Nizet V. The ontogeny of a neutrophil: mechanisms of granulopoiesis and homeostasis. Microbiol Mol Biol Rev. 2018;82(1):e00057.

29. Mare TA, et al. The diagnostic and prognostic significance of monitoring blood levels of immature neutrophils in patients with systemic inflammation. Crit Care. 2015;19(1):57.

30. Heath CW, Geneva A, Daland SB. Staining of reticulocytes by brilliant Cresyl blue influence of solutions of substances. Arch Intern Med. 1931;48(1):133–45.

31. He X, Zou R, Zhang B, You Y, Yang Y, Tian X. Whole Wiskott-Aldrich syndrome protein gene deletion identified by high throughput sequencing. Athens: Spandidos Publications; 1838.

32. Levi MM. Disseminated intravascular coagulation workup. 2018.

33. Braden CD, Besa EC. Which conditions are associated with eosinopenia? 2018.

34. Lippi G, Salvagno GL, Montagnana M, Lima-Oliveira G, Guidi GC, Favaloro EJ. Quality standards for sample collection in coagulation testing. Semin Thromb Hemost. 2012;38:565–75.

35. Giovanna Clavarino et al. Novel strategy for phenotypic characterization of human B lymphocytes from precursors to effector cells by flow cytometry. 2016.

36. Zhu F, et al. Screening for genes that regulate the differentiation of human megakaryocytic lineage cells. PNAS. 2018;115(40):9308–16.

37. Horton TM, et al. Overview of the clinical presentation and diagnosis of acute lymphoblastic leukemia/lymphoma in children. 2019.

38. Gurbuxani S, et al. Mixed phenotype acute leukemia. 2019.

39. Van Etten RA, Larson RA, Rosmarin AG. Clinical manifestations and diagnosis of chronic myeloid leukemia. 2019.

40. Tefferi A, Larson RA, Rosmarin AG. Clinical manifestations and diagnosis of primary myelofibrosis. 2019.

41. Leung LLK, Mentzer WC, Tirnauer JS. Macrocytosis/macrocytic anemia. 2019.

42. Schiffer CA, et al. Clinical manifestations, pathologic features, and diagnosis of acute myeloid leukemia. 2019.

43. Gundesen MT, et al. Plasma cell leukemia: definition, presentation, and treatment. Curr Oncol Rep. 2019;21(1):8.

44. Van Etten RA, Larson RA, Rosmarin AG. Molecular genetics of chronic myeloid leukemia. 2019.

45. Maitre E, et al. Hairy cell leukemia. Presse Med. 2019;48(1):842–9.

46. Ramakrishnan N, Jialal I. Bence-Jones protein. StatPearls. Treasure Island: StatPearls Publishing; 2019.

47. Chuzi S, Stein BL. Essential thrombocythemia: a review of the clinical features, diagnostic challenges, and treatment modalities in the era of molecular discovery. Leuk Lymphoma. 2017;58(12):2786–98.

48. Crispino SM, JD and Stein B. Myelofibrosis in 2019: moving beyond JAK2 inhibition. Blood. Cancer J. 2019;9(9):74.

49. Tefferi A, Larson RA, Rosmarin AG. Clinical manifestations and diagnosis of polycythemia vera. 2019.

50. Aster JC, et al. Clinical manifestations and diagnosis of the myelodysplastic syndromes. 2019.

51. Klepin HD. Myelodysplastic syndromes and acute myeloid leukemia in the elderly. Clin Geriatr Med. 2016;32(1):155–73.

52. Advani AS, et al. Clinical manifestations, pathologic features, and diagnosis of B cell acute lymphoblastic leukemia/lymphoma. 2019.

Lungs

9

Multiple Choice Questions

1. Superior vena cava (SVC) syndrome is a collection of clinical signs and symptoms resulting from either partial or complete obstruction of blood flow through the SVC. What is the commonest cause of superior vena cava (SVC) obstruction?
   A. Fibrosis of superior vena cava
   B. Bronchogenic carcinoma
   C. Pericardial fibrosis
   D. Hepatocellular carcinoma
   E. Bronchiectasis

2. Which of the following is the underlying lesion of the acute respiratory distress syndrome?
   A. Organizing pneumonia
   B. Bronchiolitis
   C. Diffuse alveolar damage
   D. Usual interstitial pneumonitis
   E. Bronchopneumonia

3. A 2-year-old male child is brought to the pediatrician office by his mother with symptoms of fever, shortness of breath, and rapid breathing. X-ray of the chest is done which shows patchy appearance with peribronchial thickening and poorly defined air space opacities. What is the diagnosis?
   A. Atypical pneumonia
   B. Tuberculosis
   C. Bronchopneumonia
   D. Atelectasis
   E. Lobar pneumonia

4. A 40-year-old male patient has clinical presentation fevers, night sweats, weight loss, cough, and hemoptysis for the last 4 weeks. Physical examination shows lymphadenopathy. Another family member of the patient is taking medications for similar symptoms. What is the diagnosis?

   A. Sarcoidosis
   B. Tuberculosis
   C. Bronchopneumonia
   D. Atypical pneumonia
   E. Bronchiectasis

5. A 35-year-old female come to the office with symptoms of fatigue, malaise, shortness of breath, skin lesions, eye irritation, fever, and night sweats. Lung biopsy shows noncaseating granulomas. What is the diagnosis?
   A. Tuberculosis
   B. Bronchopneumonia
   C. Sarcoidosis
   D. Lobar pneumonia
   E. Bronchogenic carcinoma

6. Microscopic pictures of the lung of a patient with a history of smoking for the last 25 years is shown below. What is the diagnosis?

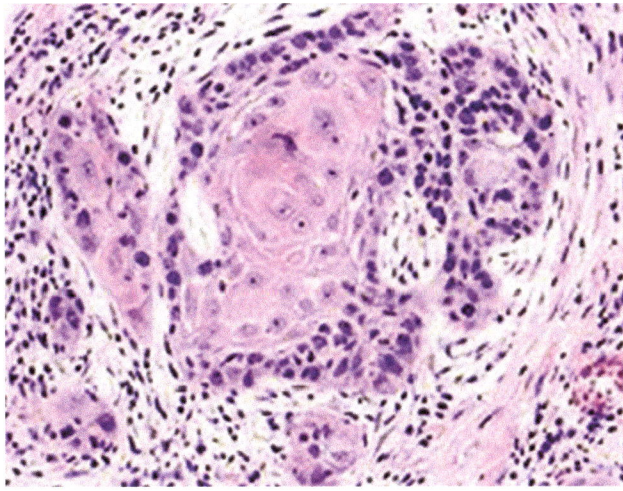

   A. Large cell carcinoma
   B. Squamous cell carcinoma

V. K. Kohli et al., *Comprehensive Multiple-Choice Questions in Pathology*, https://doi.org/10.1007/978-3-031-08767-7_9

C. Large cell anaplastic carcinoma

D. Malignant mesothelioma

E. Adenocarcinoma

7. A 50-year-old woman with α1-antitrypsin deficiency and no history of smoking requires a double lung transplant for severe emphysema. Which type of emphysema would most likely predominate in this patient's lung?

A. Paraseptal emphysema

B. Panacinar emphysema

C. Interstitial emphysema

D. Centriacinar emphysema

E. Proximal acinar emphysema

8. A 51-year-old male patient presents with shortness of breath, fever, and weight loss. He is a nonsmoker. He worked in restoring building for most of his life. Imaging studies show bilateral pleural effusions. Pleural biopsy is performed and shows discohesive aggregates of round tumor cells with abundant cytoplasm in a fuzzy cell borders. What is the diagnosis?

A. Small cell lung cancer

B. Malignant mesothelioma

C. Squamous cell carcinoma of the lung

D. Nonsmall cell lung cancer (NSCLC)

E. Adenocarcinoma of the lung

9. A 39-year-old man presents with symptoms of chest pain, wheezing, shortness of breath, diarrhea. He also complains of redness/feeling of warmth in the face and the neck. Imaging studies show an area of consolidation in the right upper lobe. What is the appropriate diagnosis?

A. Adenocarcinoma

B. Carcinoid tumor

C. Squamous cell carcinoma

D. Malignant mesothelioma

E. Hamartoma

10. Consolidation of the lung is a common pathological reaction pattern to broad category of etiologic agents and pulmonary disease. Which of the following etiologic agents is commonly responsible for alveolar exudative solidification?

A. Viral pneumonia

B. Bacterial pneumonia

C. Chlamydial pneumonia

D. Mycoplasma pneumonia

E. Mycobacterium tuberculosis

11. Which oncogene is found in the small cell lung carcinoma?

A. Ki-ras

B. L-myc

C. c-myc

D. n-myc

E. Cyclin D

12. Although most cases of lung cancer are due to tobacco smoking, lung cancer among never smokers is an important problem. Which of the following fusion oncogene is seen in nonsmall cell lung cancer?

A. Anaplastic lymphoma kinase (ALK) fusion oncogene

B. BCAM-AKT2

C. BCR-ABL

D. EWSR1-CREB1 and EWSR1-ATF1

E. ETV6-NTRK3

13. Exposure to which of the following substances causes calcification of the rim of hilar nodes (eggshell calcification)?

A. Beryllium

B. Silica

C. Coal dust

D. Organic dust

E. Nylon flock exposure

14. A 19-year-old patient comes to the physician office with symptoms of fever, sore throat, and hoarseness and shortness of breath. Chest imaging shows reticulonodular opacities. Laboratory investigation shows elevated cold agglutinin titer. Which of the following organisms is responsible for this patient's condition?

A. Mycoplasma pneumoniae

B. Pseudomonas aeruginosa

C. Staphylococcus aureus

D. Streptococcus pneumoniae

E. Streptococcus pyogenes

15. Pulmonary nodules may be detected on cross sectional imaging studies performed for an unrelated reason. Which of the following is the benign tumor of the lung?

A. Hamartoma

B. Adenocarcinoma

C. Squamous cell carcinoma

D. Large cell carcinoma

E. Small cell carcinoma

16. Gross appearance of the affected lung is shown in the figure below. Which of the following pathogen is a cause of this appearance of lung?

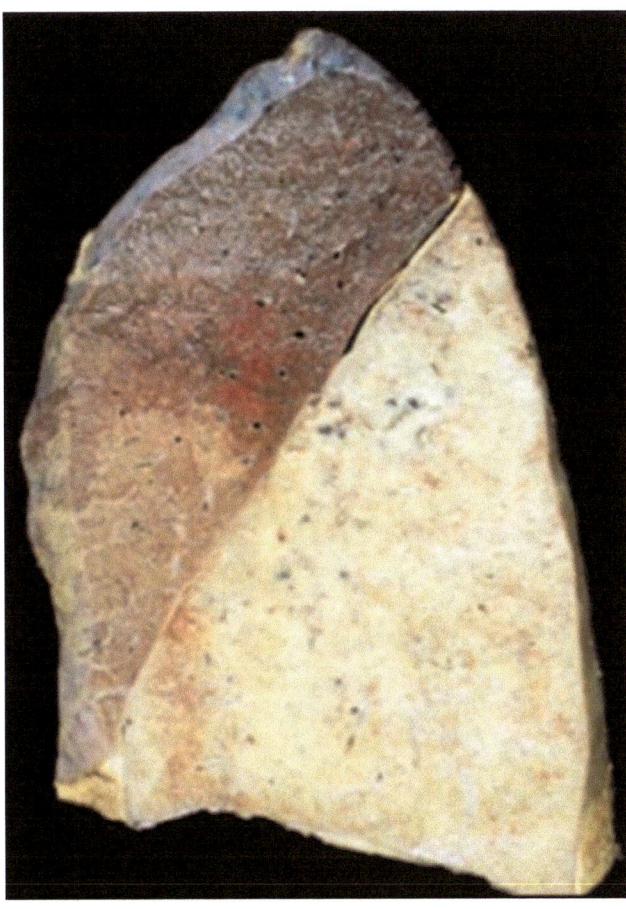

A. Streptococcus pneumoniae
B. Mycoplasma pneumoniae
C. Pneumocystis jiroveci
D. Streptococcus aureus
E. Pseudomonas aeruginosa

17. A 35-year-old man presents with symptoms of chronic obstructive pulmonary disease. X-ray shows vague reticulonodular pattern. Bronchoscopy is done and a methenamine silver stain highlights the cysts. Which additional testing should be performed?
    A. Blood culture
    B. Sputum gram stain and culture
    C. HIV antibody testing
    D. Mycobacterial culture
    E. Pulmonary function testing

18. All of the following paraneoplstic syndromes are seen in carcinoma lung except:
    A. Hypertrophic osteoarthropathy
    B. Myasthenia gravis
    C. Cushing's syndrome
    D. Hypoglycemia
    E. Hypercalcemia

19. Which of the following organisms is most likely responsible for lung abscess?
    A. Pseudomonas aeruginosa
    B. Peptostreptococcus
    C. Escherichia coli
    D. Streptococcus pneumoniae
    E. Streptococcus pyogenes

20. Shoulder and arm pain, atrophy of muscles of the hand and Horner syndrome are because of which of the following condition?
    A. Multiple myeloma
    B. Adenoid cystic carcinoma
    C. Pancoast tumor
    D. Mesothelioma
    E. Lymphoma

21. Which of the following pulmonary infections does not result in granuloma formation?
    A. Mycobacterium tuberculae
    B. Histoplasma capsulatum
    C. Blastomyces dermatitidis
    D. Coccidioides immitis
    E. Legionella pneumophila

Answers and Explanations

1. Answer: B. Bronchogenic carcinoma
   Bronchogenic carcinoma occurs most commonly between 50 and 80 years of age. Risk factors include cigarette smoking, air pollution, and occupational exposure (asbestosis, radiation, etc.). Small cell lung cancer causes more commonly superior vena cava syndrome. Patients of superior vena cava syndrome present with cough, pain, and dyspnea. There may be dysphagia and the sensation of fullness in the head. Physical examination usually shows a prominent venous pattern on the chest, facial edema and plethoric appearance. Imaging studies usually show widening of the mediastinum.

2. Answer: C. Diffuse alveolar damage
   In Acute respiratory distress syndrome (ARDS) there is diffuse damage of alveolar epithelium and capillaries. Histologically, there is interstitial and intra-alveolar edema, loss of type 1 pneumocytes, and hyaline membrane formation. Common causes of diffuse alveolar damage are usually shock, sepsis, trauma, oxygen toxicity, and pulmonary infections. Patients usually present with dyspnea, tachypnea, hypoxemia. There may be cyanosis and use of accessory respiratory muscles. X-ray shows bilateral diffuse opacities.

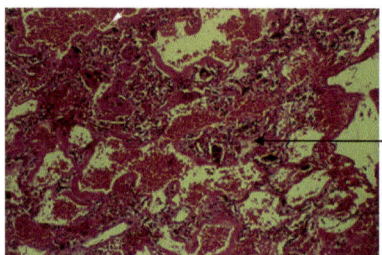
Diffuse alveolar damage with alveolar hemorrhage

3. Answer: C. Bronchopneumonia

Bronchopneumonia is patchy consolidation distributed around bronchioles and adjacent alveoli. It tends to be multilobar, basilar, and bilateral. Most common organisms causing bronchopneumonia are *Streptococcus pyogenes*, *Staphylococcus aureus*, and *Haemophilus influenzae*. Histologically, there is acute inflammation of bronchioles and surrounding alveoli. Diagnosis is usually made by blood cultures, sputum gram stain, and culture. It usually affects young, old, and terminally ill patients.

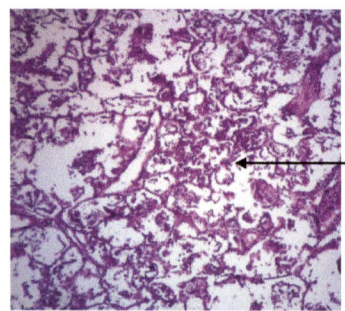
Acute inflammation of bronchioles and surrounding alveoli in Bronchopneumonia

4. Answer: B. Tuberculosis

Tuberculosis is primarily caused by *Mycobacterium tuberculosis* and lung is the most common site of primary infection. Patients usually present with fever, night sweats, weight loss, cough, and hemoptysis. There are three forms of tuberculosis: primary, secondary, and miliary. Primary tuberculosis consists of a peripheral parenchymal lesion called a Ghon focus and granulomas in involved hilar lymph nodes. Secondary (reactivation) tuberculosis results from the reactivation of a prior site of infection. Miliary tuberculosis is disseminated disease caused by hematogenous spread of bacteria. Tuberculosis is transmitted by airborne droplets from infected patients. Imaging studies help in the diagnosis of tuberculosis. In secondary tuberculosis lesions are located in the apices or superior segment of lower lobe. Culture of the organism from sputum is needed for a definitive diagnosis. Acid-fast staining is useful for identifying the bacteria. Light microscopy shows caseating granulomas with acid-fast bacilli.

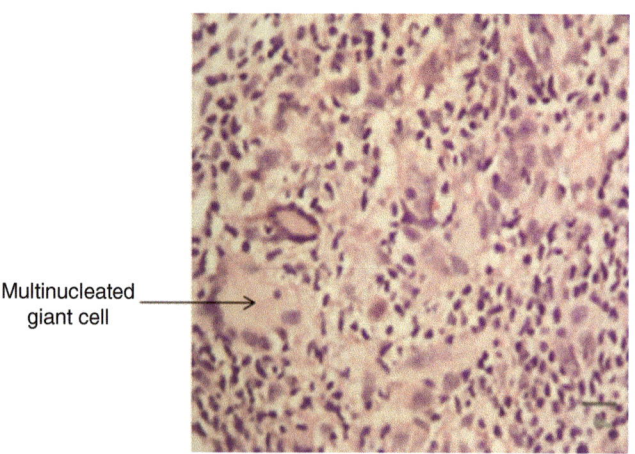
Multinucleated giant cell

5. Answer: C. Sarcoidosis

Sarcoidosis is more common in females between the second and sixth decades of life. It is a chronic disorder of waxing and waning course. Patients usually present with cough, shortness of breath, fatigue, malaise, skin lesions. There may be eye irritation or pain, fever/night sweats. It is characterized by immune-mediated noncaseating granulomas and elevated serum angiotensin-converting enzymes. X-ray shows bilateral hilar lymphadenopathy. Light microscopy shows noncaseating granulomas, Schaumann bodies (laminated calcifications), asteroid bodies (stellate giant cell cytoplasmic inclusions).

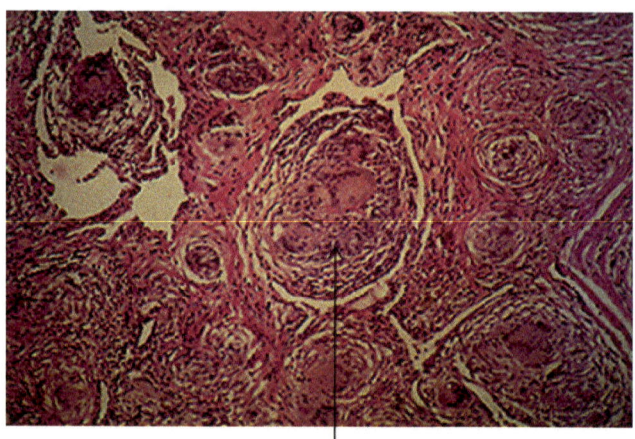
Noncaseating granuloma with multinucleated giant cell

6. Answer: B. Squamous cell carcinoma

Squamous cell carcinoma is more common in males and strongly related to smoking. Grossly, the tumors are centrally located, gray-white bronchial mass. Light microscopy shows invasive nests of squamous cells, intercellular desmosomes (intercellular bridges), and keratin production (squamous pearls). Common immunohistochemistry stains which help in the diagnosis of squamous cell carcinoma are p40, p63, CK5, or CK5/6.

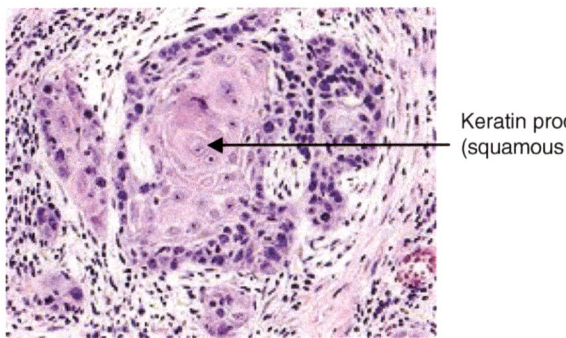

Keratin production (squamous pearls)

7. Answer: B. Panacinar emphysema

Emphysema is abnormal and permanent airway enlargement distal to the terminal bronchiole. This leads to progressive destruction of alveolar walls and surrounding interstitium leading to loss of elastic recoil. Major causes of emphysema are smoking and hereditary α1-antitrypsin deficiency. It is an autosomal dominant and accounts for 1% of emphysema cases. Patients with α1-antitrypsin deficiency often develop emphysema at a much younger age than smokers. In α1-antitrypsin deficiency, the entire acinus is involved leading to Panacinar (Panlobular) emphysema.

8. Answer: B. Malignant mesothelioma

Mesothelioma is a neoplasm of serosal surfaces that has been associated with exposure to asbestos. Patients present with pleural thickening and recurrent pleural effusions (often hemorrhagic) on imaging. There are three variants: epithelial, diffuse fibrous, and mixed. Immunohistochemistry (IHC) profile for malignant mesothelioma is positive for WT-1 and calretinin. Histologically tumor is composed of cell clusters, cytoplasmic vacuolization, and presence of abundant microvilli. These vacuoles contain crystallized hyaluronic acid when seen by electron microscopy.

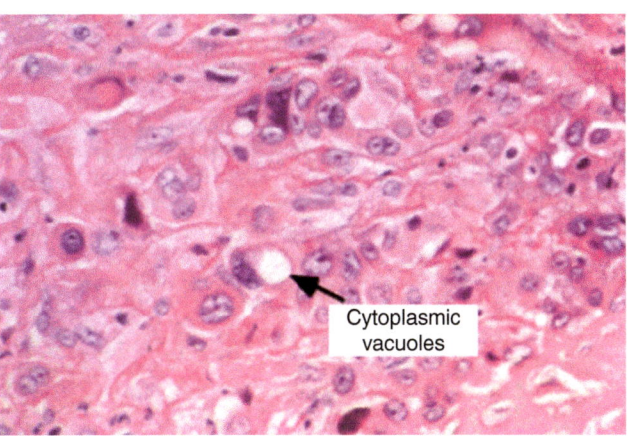

Cytoplasmic vacuoles

9. Answer: B. Carcinoid tumor

Bronchial carcinoids (lung neuroendocrine tumors) are common in a younger age group, usually below the age of 40 years. Patients present with wheezing, shortness of breath, chest pain, and diarrhea. There may be redness or a feeling of warmth in the face and neck. Grossly, bronchial carcinoids show polypoid intrabronchial mass. Light microscopy shows small round, uniform cells which are arranged in nests. CT/MRI can be used to locate the carcinoid tumor. Laboratory diagnosis shows elevated levels of 5-hydroxyindoleacetic acid (5-HIAA) in the urine.

10. Answer: B. Bacterial pneumonia

Bacterial infection causes an acute inflammatory response. They attract neutrophils which release bactericidal granules through opsonization, protease destruction. Macrophages eventually cause the phagocytosis of bacteria. The accumulation of bacterial debris, macrophages, and granulocytes creates a thick exudate. Thick exudate fills up the alveolar space and causes consolidation.

11. Answer: B. L-Myc

MYC family members are usually amplified in small cell lung carcinoma (SCLC). Amplifications and elevated expression of the L-myc gene is seen in small cell lung carcinoma. It is commonly seen in the central airways of smokers. Along with L-myc, SCLCs are also positive for keratin and TTF-1.

12. Answer: A. Anaplastic lymphoma kinase (ALK) fusion oncogene

Anaplastic lymphoma kinase (ALK) fusion oncogene is commonly seen in nonsmall cell lung cancer. It is commonly seen in nonsmokers. Patients are relatively young and type of lung carcinoma is usually adenocarcinoma.

13. Answer: B. Silica

Hilar and mediastinal lymph node enlargement due to reactive lymph node hyperplasia is relatively common in patients with silicosis. Punctate calcification in the lymph nodes is common. Also, calcium salt deposits in the sinus of the marginal lymph node result in the characteristic eggshell calcification of lymph nodes. This development can be seen in up to 5% of workers with silicosis. Eggshell calcifications can also be found in coal worker's pneumoconiosis, long standing sarcoidosis or treated lymphoma.

14. Answer: A. *Mycoplasma pneumoniae*

Pneumonia is caused by Mycoplasma pneumonia is community acquired. Patients usually present with fever, sore throat, hoarseness, and pharyngitis. X-ray chest usually shows reticulonodular opacities. Mycoplasma leads to the development of IgM autoantibody. This autoantibody causes immune mediated hemolysis (cold agglutinin disease).

15. Answer: A. Hamartoma

Pulmonary hamartoma is a common benign tumor of the lung. It is a mass of disorganized tissue elements composed of cartilage, connective tissue, muscle, and fat. It accounts for about 8% of lung neoplasms.

16. Answer: A. *Streptococcus pneumoniae*

Bacterial pneumonia is commonly caused by *Streptococcus pneumoniae*. The patient usually presents with fever, cough, pleuritic chest pain, dyspnea, and sputum production. Chest radiograph is the gold standard test for diagnosing pneumonia.

17. Answer: C. HIV antibody testing

Pneumocystis jirovecii pneumonia (PCP) is common in HIV positive patients. It is a fungal infection (formerly classified as a protozoan) seen usually immunocompromised patients. Imaging studies show diffuse infiltrates. Histologically shows alveolar spaces filled with pink, foamy amorphous material. There may be cell debris, mild inflammatory reaction with fibrin exudate. Methenamine silver stains highlight the cysts of PCP.

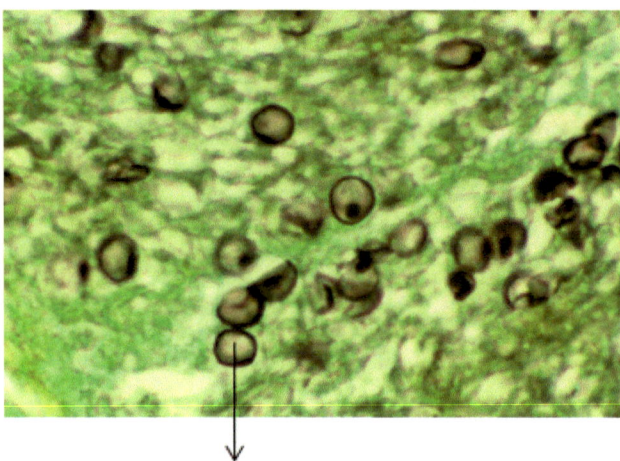

Cyst of Pneumocystis jirovecii pneumonia (PCP)

18. Answer: D. Hypoglycemia

Common paraneoplastic syndromes of carcinoma of the lung include hypercalcemia and syndrome of inappropriate antidiuretic hormone (SIADH) secretion. Other important paraneoplastic syndrome includes disseminated intravascular coagulopathy, myasthenia gravis, Cushing's syndrome, hypertrophic osteoarthropathy, and dermatomyositis.

19. Answer: B. Peptostreptococcus

Localized pus collection within the lung parenchyma is called lung abscess. It is common complication of aspiration pneumonia or bronchial obstruction (e.g. tumor). It tends to involve right lower lobe. Common organisms which cause lung abscess include anaerobic

oral flora. These organisms include bacteroides, fusobacterium, and peptostreptococcus. Patients are usually unresponsive to antibiotics. Imaging studies shows cavitation with air fluid levels.

20. Answer: C. Pancoast tumor

Pancoast tumor is also called superior sulcus tumor. It is a carcinoma that arises in apex of the lung. This tumor can involve surrounding structures causing a variety of syndromes. These syndromes can coexist in a variety of combinations, collectively referred to as pancoast syndrome. Pancoast tumor causes Horner's syndrome. Common findings in Horner's syndrome are ptosis, miosis, anhidrosis, and enophthalmos.

21. Answer: E. *Legionella pneumophila*

Several pulmonary infectious agents can cause granuloma formation. Common infectious agents include *Blastomyces dermatitidis*, Mycobacterium tuberculae, *Coccidioides immitis*, and *Histoplasma capsulatum*. Legionella pneumonia does not cause granuloma formation. Usually, it consists of neutrophils and macrophages.

Bibliography

1. Midthun DE, Lilenbaum RC, Vora SR. Overview of the risk factors, pathology, and clinical manifestations of lung cancer. Baltimore: Wolters Kluwer; 2019.
2. Tazelaar HD, et al. Pathology of lung malignancies. Waltham: UpToDate; 2019.
3. Schwarz MI, King TE, Hollingsworth H Jr. The diffuse alveolar hemorrhage syndromes. Waltham: UpToDate; 2019.
4. Barson WJ, Kaplan S, Torchia M. Pneumonia in children: epidemiology, pathogenesis, and etiology. Waltham: UpToDate; 2019.
5. Bernardo J, von Reyn CF, Baron EL. Diagnosis of pulmonary tuberculosis in adults. Waltham: UpToDate; 2019.
6. King TE, Flaherty KR, Hollingsworth H. Clinical manifestations and diagnosis of pulmonary sarcoidosis. Waltham: UpToDate; 2019.
7. Bernardo J, von Reyn CF, Baron EL. Clinical manifestations, diagnosis, and treatment of miliary tuberculosis. Waltham: UpToDate; 2019.
8. Pahal P, Avula A, Sharma S. Emphysema. Treasure Island: StatPearls; 2019.
9. Litzky LA, et al. Pathology of malignant pleural mesothelioma. Waltham: UpToDate; 2019.
10. Thomas CF, et al. Lung neuroendocrine (carcinoid) tumors: epidemiology, risk factors, classification, histology, diagnosis, and staging. Waltham: UpToDate; 2019.
11. Sax PE, Bartlett JG, Sullivan M. Clinical presentation and diagnosis of pneumocystis pulmonary infection in HIV-infected patients. Waltham: UpToDate; 2019.
12. Glisson BS, et al. Pathobiology and staging of small cell carcinoma of the lung. Waltham: UpToDate; 2019.
13. Wakelee H, Lilenbaum RC, Vora SR. Lung cancer in never smokers. Waltham: UpToDate; 2019.
14. Stark P, et al. Imaging of occupational lung diseases. Waltham: UpToDate; 2019.
15. Horwitz MJ, Rosen CJ, Mulder JE. Hypercalcemia of malignancy: mechanisms. Waltham: UpToDate; 2019.

16. Baum SG, File TM Jr, Bond S. *Mycoplasma pneumoniae* infection in adults. Waltham: UpToDate; 2019.

17. Weinberger SE, et al. Diagnostic evaluation of the incidental pulmonary nodule. Waltham: UpToDate; 2019.

18. Martin R, et al. Pathophysiology, clinical manifestations, and diagnosis of respiratory distress syndrome in the newborn. Waltham: UpToDate; 2019.

19. Bartlett JG, et al. Diagnostic approach to community-acquired pneumonia in adults. Waltham: UpToDate; 2019.

20. Liou DZ, Berry MF. Diagnosis and management of mesothelioma. AME Med J. 2018;3(99):10–21037.

21. Barber CM, Fishwick D. Idiopathic pulmonary fibrosis and asbestos use. BMJ. 2019;364:l1041.

22. Midthun DE, et al. Overview of the risk factors, pathology, and clinical manifestations of lung cancer. Waltham: UpToDate; 2019.

23. Takayoshi S, Yoko S, Naomi H, Kiyoshi S, Il-Je Y, Hyun-Sul L, Hiroshige M, Hiroshi S, Fumio K, Eiji S. The association among ferruginous body, uncoated fibers, asbestos and non-asbestos fibers in lung tissue in terms of length. Ind Health. 2016;54(4):370–6.

24. Fakhoury K, et al. Causes of bronchiectasis in children. Waltham: UpToDate; 2019.

25. Bartlett JG, Calderwood SB, Bond S. Lung abscess. Waltham: UpToDate; 2019.

26. Pusey CD, et al. Pathogenesis and diagnosis of anti-GBM antibody (Goodpasture's) disease. Waltham: UpToDate; 2019.

27. Han MK, et al. Chronic obstructive pulmonary disease: definition, clinical manifestations, diagnosis, and staging. Waltham: UpToDate; 2019.

28. Arcasoy SM, et al. Superior pulmonary sulcus (Pancoast) tumors. Waltham: UpToDate; 2019.

Multiple Choice Questions

1. A middle-aged man comes to the physician office with a lump on the left side of face for the last 8 months. Physical examination shows a painless mass in the region of the left parotid gland. The mass is completely excised. Microscopically, there are spaces lined by a double layer of epithelial cells with a dense lymphoid stroma. What is the diagnosis?
   A. Warthin tumor
   B. Acinic cell carcinoma
   C. Squamous cell carcinoma
   D. Pleomorphic adenoma
   E. Mucoepidermoid carcinoma

2. Which salivary gland is the most frequent site of tumor involvement?
   A. Parotid gland
   B. Submaxillary gland
   C. Sublingual gland
   D. Minor salivary glands
   E. Submandibular gland

3. A 59-year-old male presents with symptoms of chronic nasal congestion, ear fullness, tinnitus, headaches, and dizziness for the last 6 months. There is a long history of smoking. Imaging studies demonstrate a left-sided, homogenous mass in the region of Rosenmuller's fossa. Resection of the mass is done that is EBER positive. What is the diagnosis?
   A. Granular cell tumor
   B. Non-Hodgkin lymphoma
   C. Rhabdomyosarcoma
   D. Nasopharyngeal carcinoma
   E. Paraganglioma

4. Which of the following mutations are seen in medullary carcinoma of thyroid?
   A. RET
   B. PAX8/PPARγ
   C. RET/PTC
   D. RAS
   E. BRAF

5. Viral Parotitis is caused by which organism?
   A. Herpes simplex
   B. Parvovirus B19
   C. Adenovirus
   D. Paramyxovirus
   E. Papillomavirus

6. Which of the following is the most common salivary gland neoplasm?
   A. Pleomorphic adenoma
   B. Adenoid cystic carcinoma
   C. Warthin tumor
   D. Oncocytoma
   E. Basal cell adenoma

7. A 49-year-old man presents with a neck mass involving the right submandibular gland. Biopsy of the mass shows interlobular fibrosis, periductal fibrosis with lymphoplasmacytic proliferation. What is the diagnosis?
   A. Chronic sclerosing sialadenitis
   B. Pleomorphic adenoma
   C. Adenoid cystic carcinoma
   D. Mucoepidermoid carcinoma
   E. Nodular sclerosis Hodgkin lymphoma

8. A 42-years-old female presents with symptoms of hypothyroidism. Biopsy shows diffuse lymphoid infiltrate with germinal center formation. What is the diagnosis?
   A. Hashimoto's thyroiditis
   B. Graves' disease
   C. Subacute thyroiditis
   D. Papillary carcinoma of thyroid
   E. Follicular thyroid carcinoma

9. Diagram of a 35-year-old male patient with white lesions on the mucosa of the floor of the mouth is shown below. Patient smoked one pack of cigarettes per day for the last 15 years. What is the diagnosis?

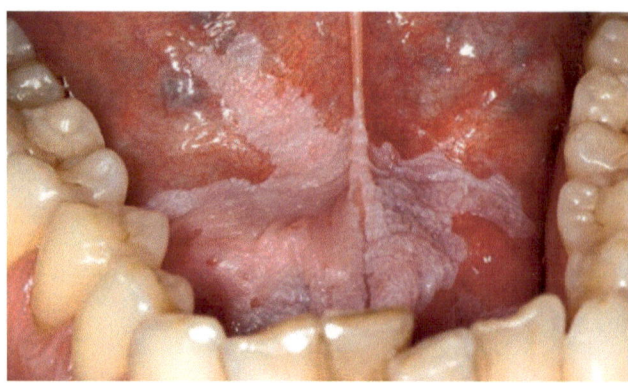

A. Frictional keratosis
B. Candidiasis
C. Leukoplakia
D. Lichen planus
E. White sponge nevus

10. A 21-year-old man presented with a 2 months history of swelling in his lower right back teeth region. On intra-oral examination, a solitary well-defined oval-shaped erythematous mass was noticed in the right retromolar area. Biopsy of the mass is done. H&E microscopic picture is shown below. What is the diagnosis?

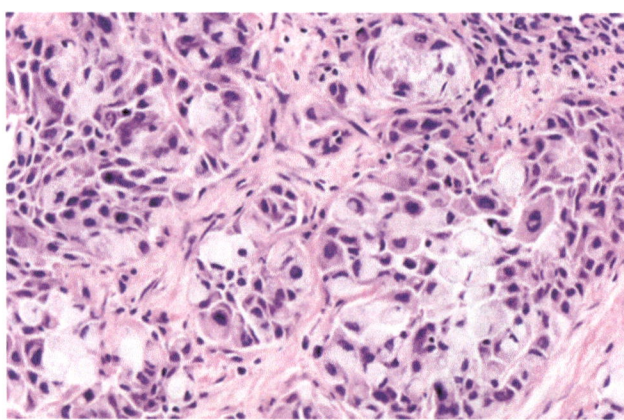

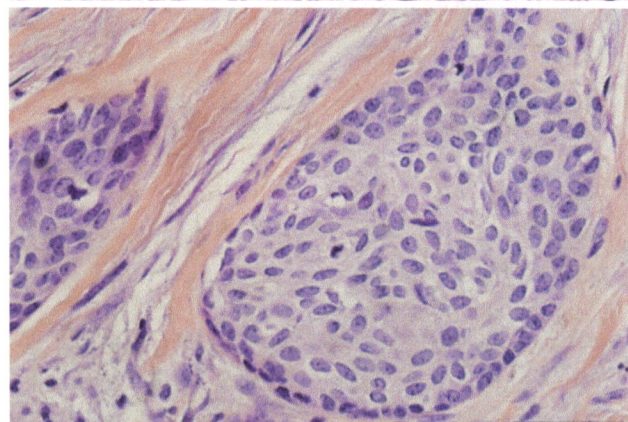

A. Mucoepidermoid carcinoma
B. Acinic cell carcinoma
C. Squamous cell carcinoma

D. Pleomorphic adenoma
E. Mucoepidermoid carcinoma

11. Fine needle aspiration of a painless cystic mass in the midline neck region shows degenerative debris. This debris is admixed with mature squamous epithelium, colloid cells, hemosiderin laden macrophages, and lymphocytes. What is the diagnosis?
A. Thyroglossal duct cyst
B. Epidermoid cyst
C. Branchial cyst
D. Squamous cell carcinoma
E. Metastatic thyroid carcinoma

12. A 12-year-old male boy is evaluated by an otolaryngologist for chronic nasal obstruction and purulent rhinorrhea for the last couple of months. Nasal endoscopy demonstrates a large multi-lobulated polyp herniating into the right vestibule. CT scan shows a large mass filling the right nasal cavity with post-obstructive pansinusitis and destructive invasion of bone by tumor cells. What is the diagnosis?
A. Rhabdomyosarcoma
B. Lymphoproliferative disorders
C. Nevoid basal cell carcinoma
D. Non-Hodgkin lymphoma
E. Olfactory neuroblastoma

13. A 13-year-old male presents with a 1.5 cm mass in the anterolateral neck. His mother states that she noticed the mass when the patient had a growth spurt. There is no change in the mass. Resection is done. Microscopic examination shows cells overly a stroma with a dense polymorphic lymphocytic infiltrate. What is the diagnosis?
A. Thyroglossal duct cyst
B. Hodgkin lymphoma
C. Marginal zone lymphoma
D. Mantle cell lymphoma
E. Branchial cleft cyst

14. A 62-year-old male, heavy smoker, presents with a large mass in the oral cavity. Physical examination shows large fungating mass in the oral cavity. Biopsies are taken and histology shows elongated fronds of surface growth with marked keratosis. Photograph of the oral cavity and microscopic picture are shown below. What is the diagnosis?

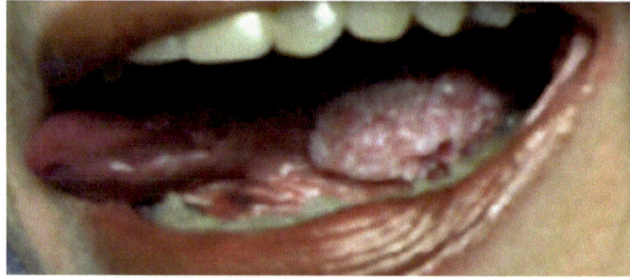

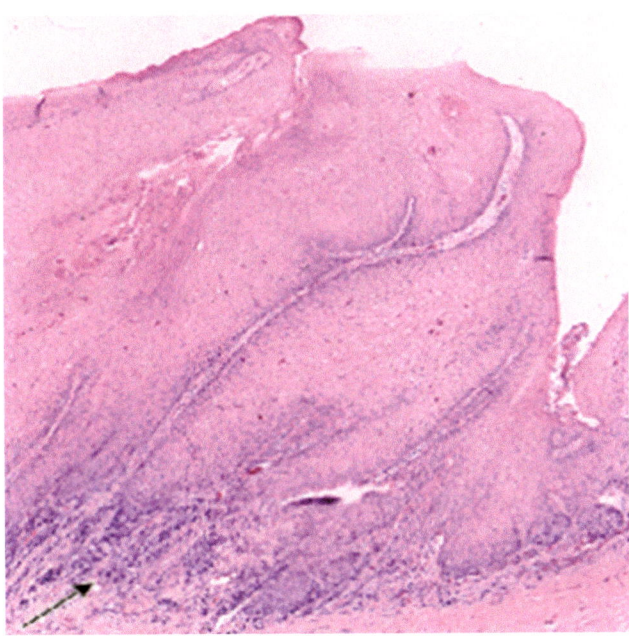

A. Squamous cell carcinoma
B. Verrucous carcinoma
C. Mucoepidermoid carcinoma
D. Low-grade adenocarcinoma
E. Adenoid cystic carcinoma

15. A 45-year-old male presents with small 4 cm right parotid mass. Histological features are composed of prominent layer of the basal cells arranged in a trabecular pattern. What is the diagnosis?
A. Warthin tumor
B. Mucoepidermoid carcinoma
C. Sebaceous hyperplasia
D. Adenoid cystic carcinoma
E. Basal cell adenoma

16. A 58-year-old female presents with a firm mass in the neck. Biopsies show massive fibrotic tissue with few entrapped thyroid follicles. What is the diagnosis?
A. Thyroid lymphoma
B. Papillary carcinoma of thyroid
C. Follicular carcinoma of thyroid
D. Fibrosing thyroiditis
E. Thyroid adenoma

17. There are different kinds of thyroid cancers. Which of the following thyroid cancer is characterized by Orphan Annie eye nuclei?
A. Papillary thyroid carcinoma
B. Follicular thyroid carcinoma
C. Hurthle cell carcinoma
D. Medullary thyroid carcinoma
E. Anaplastic thyroid carcinoma

18. A mass is removed from the middle ear of a 44-year-old man. What is the diagnosis?
A. Cholesteatoma
B. Squamous cell carcinoma
C. Adenoma of the middle ear
D. Cholesterol granuloma
E. Dermoid cyst

19. A 51-year-old man presents with facial palsy and a parotid mass undergoes a resection. Biopsy of the mass shows tumor cells in cribriform, tubular, and solid patterns. What is the diagnosis?
A. Acinic cell carcinoma
B. Warthin tumor
C. Adenoid cystic carcinoma
D. Salivary duct carcinoma
E. Mucoepidermoid carcinoma

20. Which of the following is the most common site of origin of minor salivary gland neoplasm?
A. Esophagus
B. Bronchi
C. Oral cavity including palate
D. Nasal cavity
E. Trachea

21. A 50-year-old woman presents with difficulty breathing. Physical examination shows nasal obstruction. A biopsy shows large vacuolated cells and plasma cells. PAS and Gram stain reveals Gram-negative coccobacilli. What is the diagnosis?
A. Wegner's granulomatosis
B. Tuberculosis
C. Myospherulosis
D. Rhinoscleroma
E. Rhinosporidiosis

22. A 27-year-old male with a history of Hodgkin lymphoma which is now in remission presents with lymphadenopathy in the neck. What is the diagnosis?
A. Reactive histiocytes
B. Recurrent/Persistent Hodgkin lymphoma
C. Anaplastic large cell lymphoma
D. Follicular lymphoma
E. Non-Hodgkin lymphoma

23. A 67-year-old man presents with pink-red lesion on the right side of the face. The lesion appears to be ulcerated and bleeding. Incisional biopsy is performed and shows nest of atypical squamous cells infiltrating the underlying dermis. What is the diagnosis?
A. Basal cell carcinoma
B. Adenoid cystic carcinoma
C. Non-Hodgkin lymphoma
D. Sebaceous carcinoma
E. Squamous cell carcinoma

Answers and Explanations

1. Answer: A. Warthin tumor

   Warthin tumor is a benign biphasic tumor of the parotid gland. It is also known as papillary cystadenoma lymphomatosum. Warthin tumors comprise 10% of parotid gland tumors. 5% of the tumor is bilateral. Patient presents with soft fluctuant parotid mass, often waxing and waning in size. Histologically, Warthin tumor is composed of a double layer of epithelial cells, with a dense lymphoid stroma. Cystic spaces are present with palisading oncocytic tumor cells. Oxyphilia is due to an abundance of mitochondria in epithelial cells. Squamous metaplasia may be present. Treatment is excision with facial nerve preservation.

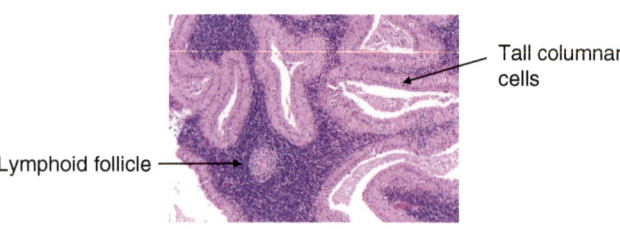

Tall columnar cells

Lymphoid follicle

2. Answer: A. Parotid gland

   Benign salivary gland tumors are common in parotid gland. Approximately 80% of all salivary gland neoplasms occur in parotid gland. Pleomorphic adenoma is the most common benign salivary gland tumor. Salivary gland tumors make up about 2–7% of the head and neck tumors.

3. Answer: D. Nasopharyngeal carcinoma

   Nasopharyngeal carcinoma is a squamous cell carcinoma of surface epithelial origin in the nasopharynx. WHO classifies as keratinizing (25%), nonkeratinizing (15%), and undifferentiated(60%). Nasopharyngeal carcinoma (NPC) arises near the eustachian tube in the region of Rosenmuller's fossa. All types have a male predilection. Elevated antibody titer of Epstein–Barr Virus is found in undifferentiated and nonkeratinizing types, but no clear causal relationship is established. They have been associated with HLA-A2 and HLA-BW46. Tumor cells are large cells with pale chromatin and prominent nucleoli. Background demonstrates lymphocytic infiltrate. Undifferentiated type has the best prognosis because it is most radiosensitive. Keratinizing type has the worst prognosis.

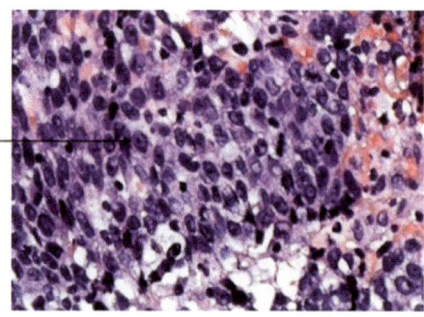

Large tumor cell with prominent nucleoli

4. Answer: A. RET

   Medullary carcinoma of thyroid (MTC) comprises 5–10% of all thyroid neoplasms. Two forms are seen, sporadic (nonfamilial) and familial (hereditary). 20% occur from germline mutations of the RET gene. Somatic mutations of the RET gene can be seen in 40–50% cases. 95% of MEN 2B cases are associated with a single amino acid substitution in the RET protein. MTC is seen in females between the fifth and sixth decades. Cervical nodal metastasis is common. Elevated basal serum calcitonin levels are present in patients with clinical evidence of disease. This is found in 80% of all medullary carcinomas. Histologically, polymorphism is the norm in MTC. Patterns include small cell neuroendocrine, plasmacytoid, spindle cell, insular trabecular, carcinoid-like, glandular, solid, oxyphilic, pigmented or melanotic.

5. Answer: D. Paramyxovirus

   Common viruses which cause viral parotitis are paramyxovirus (mumps), Epstein–Barr virus, coxsackie virus, and influenza A and parainfluenza viruses. Acute suppurative parotitis is usually caused by *Staphylococcus aureus*, streptococcus species.

6. Answer: A. Pleomorphic adenoma

   Pleomorphic adenoma (PA) is a benign tumor composed of mixed epithelial and myoepithelial elements. This tumor is the most common salivary gland tumor (40–70%). It is most common in every gland, including minor glands, except sublingual, where they are rare. It is common in females. Most common site is the tail of parotid. It usually does not involve facial nerve. Pain suggests malignancy. Grossly, the tumor is a firm, circumscribed, well-demarcated, relatively well-encapsulated, gray-white, myxoid, rubbery masses with solid cut surfaces. Microscopic pictures show the admixture of epithelial (sheets, tubules, acini) components with chondromyxoid or hyaline osseous matrix containing spindle myoepithelial cells. Treatment is complete resection with a rim of normal tissue. It may recur and malignant transformation is rare. Cytology is classic and shows large clumps of fibrillary eosinophilic material ("trol-hai") with background of epithelial and myoepithelial cells.

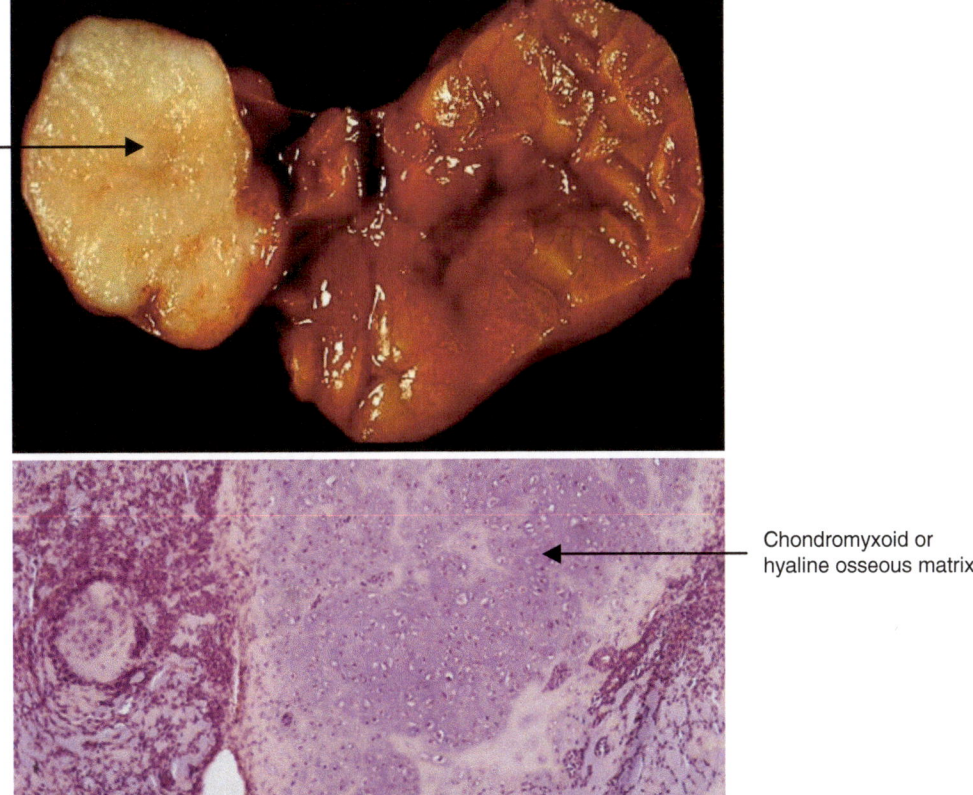

Well circumscribed mass of pleomorphic adenoma

Chondromyxoid or hyaline osseous matrix

7. Answer: A. Chronic sclerosing sialadenitis

Chronic sclerosing sialadenitis (CSS) is a tumor like inflammatory condition of the salivary glands. It commonly involves the submandibular gland either unilaterally or bilaterally. CSS usually occurs in middle-aged or older adults. It has a slight predominance in men. The basic lobular architecture of the gland is preserved. There is a substantial acinar atrophy. Extensive fibrosis is commonly seen in interlobular septae, periductal areas, and the central lobules. There is a dense lymphoplasmacytic infiltrate associated with reactive follicular hyperplasia. Histologically, there is interlobular fibrosis, periductal fibrosis, and lymphoplasmacytic proliferation. Many reactive appearing germinal centers are commonly seen with a loss of normal appearing salivary gland parenchyma.

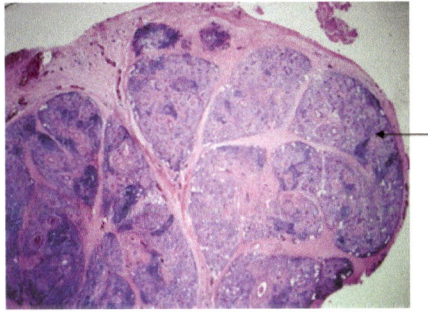

Lymphoplasmacytic proliferation

8. Answer: A. Hashimoto's thyroiditis

Hashimoto's thyroiditis is more common in women. Patients may present with an enlarged thyroid and features of hypothyroidism. Histologically, there is a diffuse lymphoid infiltrate usually with germinal center formation. Hurthle cell changes are present in follicular epithelium. Hurthle cells changes in epithelial cells include abundant eosinophilic granular cytoplasm. Squamous metaplasia is present in advanced cases. Hashimoto's thyroiditis is also known as chronic lymphocytic thyroiditis.

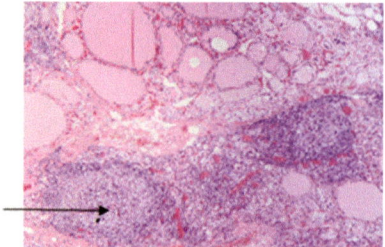

Diffuse lymphoid infiltrate with germinal center

9. Answer: C. Leukoplakia

Leukoplakia is a white lesion of the oral cavity. There is an increased risk of malignant transformation. Leukoplakia is common in smokers between the ages of 30–40 years. Microscopic findings include hyperkeratosis without epithelial dysplasia to various degrees of epithelial dysplasia. The lesions are described as white painless plaques that, unlike candida, cannot be scraped from the surface to which they adhere.

10. Answer: A. Mucoepidermoid carcinoma

Mucoepidermoid carcinoma is a malignant epithelial tumor with admixture of mucocytes, intermediate cells, and epidermoid cells. It is the most common malignant salivary gland tumor and occurs over a wide age range. It is common in females and patients present as painless mass, but some patients note tenderness, drainage, facial paralysis. Grossly, tumor may be circumscribed or infiltrative and cut surface often demonstrates small cysts. Microscopic examination shows mucus cells or cells without obvious mucin which are positive by mucin, such as mucicarmine. Mucus cells occur in small clusters or may be scattered singly among other cell types. Intermediate cells are usually predominant cell types. Low grade tumors metastasize to nodes in 2.5% while high grade tumor metastasis to nodes in about 55% of the cases.

11. Answer: A. Thyroglossal duct cyst

Thyroglossal duct cysts present as tender or nontender midline nodules. These cysts are present anywhere along the embryologic course of the thyroglossal duct from posterior tongue to below the cricoid cartilage. These cysts differ from branchial cleft cysts by their location. Branchial cysts never show thyroid tissue.

12. Answer: A. Rhabdomyosarcoma

Rhabdomyosarcoma (RMS) is the most common sarcoma of the head and neck. RMS the most common

malignancy to arise within the nasal cavity and paranasal sinuses in children. Males and females are equally affected and common in first and second decades. Most common sites are orbit, nasopharynx, ear, and sinonasal tract. Symptoms are site specific. The embryonal type is most common in the head and neck, but alveolar pattern may also be seen. Embryonal type shows variegated hypo and hypercellular areas. Cells are round to spindled, hyperchromatic, and may have brightly eosinophilic cytoplasm (rhabdomyoblasts). The background has a myxoid appearance. Alveolar type consists of non-cohesive round tumor cells that cling to a fibrovascular network giving an alveolar pattern. Common immunohistochemical stains which help in the diagnosis are desmin, myo D1, and myoglobin.

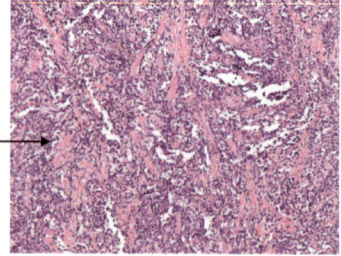

Round tumor cells in Alveolar Rhabdomyosarcoma

13. Answer: E. Branchial cleft cyst

Branchial cleft cyst is a congenital remnant of the first–fourth branch pouches. It presents as an anterolateral neck mass in children. It is not uncommon in adults. The epithelial cells that line the cyst cavity can be squamous, mucinous respiratory cells. These cells overly a stroma with a dense polymorphic lymphocytic infiltrate. This infiltrate contain reactive follicles containing tingle body macrophages. Metastatic squamous cell carcinoma should be excluded.

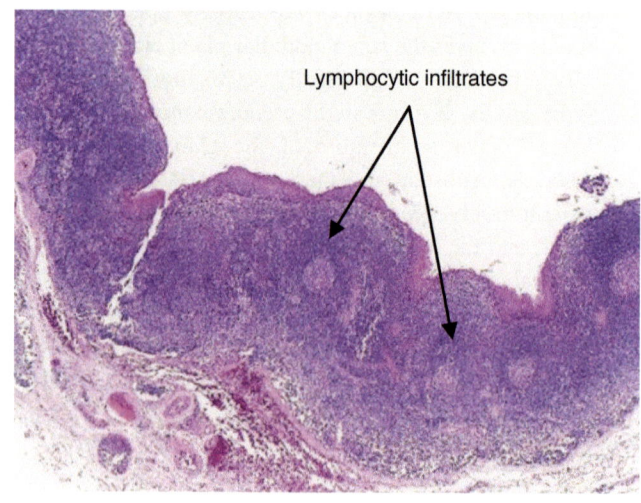

Lymphocytic infiltrates

14. Answer: B. Verrucous carcinoma

Verrucous carcinoma is a well-differentiated squamous cell carcinoma. It is a rare tumor, common in males between sixth and seventh decades of life. It may be related to smoking use. Most common sites are glottic larynx and buccal mucosa. Grossly, the tumor is warty appearing with lots of surface keratinization. Microscopic examination shows uniform cells without dysplasia or mitosis. There is also marked surface keratinization with broad or bulbous rete pegs with pushing border. Prognosis is excellent if completely excised.

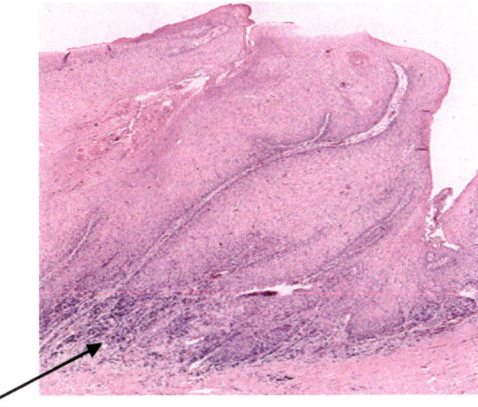

Broad Rete pegs in Verrucous carcinoma

15. Answer: E. Basal cell adenoma

Basal cell adenomas are well-circumscribed masses composed of a prominent layer of basal cells arranged in a trabecular pattern. Basal cell adenomas are benign tumors derived from either striated or intercalated ducts.

Patients present with a mass in the parotid gland. Warthin tumors are the second most common benign salivary gland neoplasm, and occur exclusively in the parotid gland. Warthin tumors can be bilateral.

16. Answer: D. Fibrosing thyroiditis

Fibrosing thyroiditis is sometimes called Riedel thyroiditis. It is most often seen in females. In this thyroiditis, fibroblasts proliferate and lay down collagen. Normal thyroid is replaced by dense fibrotic tissue. Thyroid biopsies show massive fibrotic tissue with few entrapped thyroid follicles. The thyroid becomes a rockhard, woody mass as the disease progresses. The hard woody mass may compress the trachea. Treatment is surgical removal.

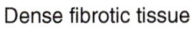

Dense fibrotic tissue

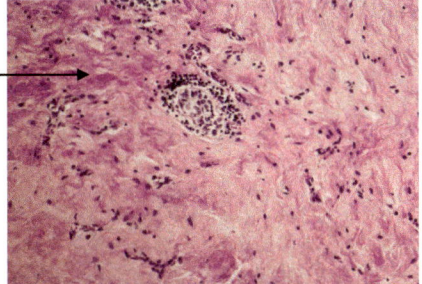

17. Answer: A. Papillary thyroid carcinoma

Papillary thyroid carcinoma is the most common malignant tumor of thyroid and accounts up to 80% of cancers of the thyroid. Papillary carcinoma presents usually as a solitary nodule. It is common in females and most common in the third to fifth decades of life. Histologically, there are several papillae lined by large tumor cells. The nuclei have clefts, grooves, nuclear pseudoinclusions, and with cleared out appearance. Such nuclei are called "Little Orphan Annie" nuclei. Nucleoli are prominent. Psammoma bodies are present in one-half of PTCs. Approximately half of the PTCs possess a BRAF V600E mutation. The mutation is associated with a more aggressive clinical course. RET gene has been identified in about 25% of PTCs. It carries a good prognosis.

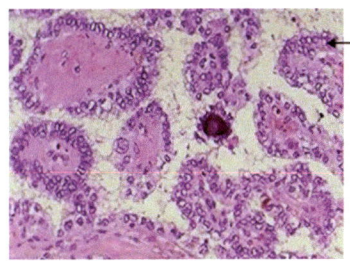

Cells with cleared-out nuclei (Orphan Annie eyes)

18. Answer: A. Cholesteatoma

Cholesteatomas are cysts containing keratin. They are common in men and are most common in the third or fourth decades of life. Middle ear is the usual site. Grossly, cholesteatoma resembles an epidermal cyst. Light microscopy shows keratinizing squamous epithelium, keratinous debris, fibrous connective tissue or granulation tissue. Cysts can be congenital or acquired. The congenital form is usually closed and arises from epidermoid cell rests. The most common acquired form is open and causes chronic otitis media and tympanic perforation.

Keratin layer

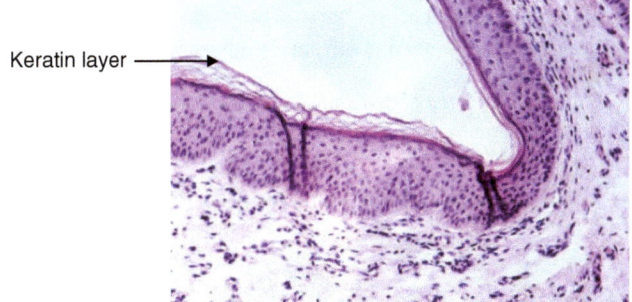

19. Answer: C. Adenoid cystic carcinoma

Adenoid cystic carcinoma (ACC) is a malignant epithelial tumor of the major and minor salivary glands. It is most common between the fourth and sixth decades of life. ACC is a slow growing mass. Tenderness, pain, nerve paralysis develops during the course of disease. Perineural invasion is almost always conspicuous.

Histologically, main patterns are cribriform, tubular, and solid. Cribriform is most common and solid is least common. Most tumors have a mixture of patterns. Cribriform pattern looks like Swiss cheese, with basophilic or hyalinized material in cyst-like spaces. Solid tumors have the worst prognosis. The p53 oncogene is a marker of recurrent tumors and late-stage disease.

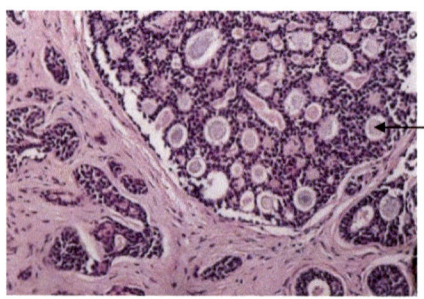

Basophilic or hyalinized material in cyst-like spaces

mous cell carcinoma shows nests of atypical squamous cells infiltrating the underlying dermis. There is an inflammatory background and characteristic keratin pearls.

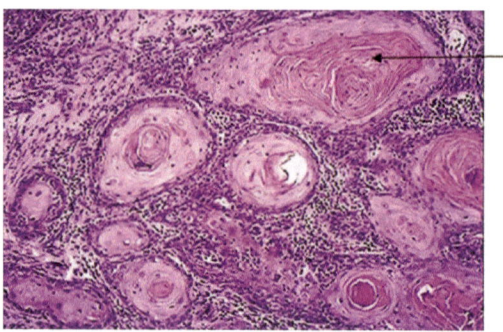

Keratin pearl

20. Answer: C. Oral cavity including palate

Parotid, submandibular, sublingual are the key salivary glands. Salivary gland tissue is also present in the nasal cavity, paranasal sinuses, nasopharynx, oral cavity, esophagus, trachea, and bronchi. Salivary gland neoplasms can occur in these minor sites. Oral cavity, especially the palate is the most common site for minor salivary gland neoplasms.

21. Answer: D. Rhinoscleroma

Rhinoscleroma is caused by *Klebsiella rhinoscleromatis*. This organism is a Gram-negative rod. Incidence of infection is increased in HIV positive individuals. Histologically, it shows granulomatous inflammation, pseudoepitheliomatous hyperplasia, Russell bodies, and Mikulicz cells. Mikulicz cells are composed of large macrophages with clear vacuolated cytoplasm.

22. Answer: B. Recurrent/persistent Hodgkin lymphoma

Cytology of recurrent/persistent Hodgkin lymphoma shows a background of lymphocytes, fat, RBCs, and binucleated Reed–Sternberg cells, with coarse, irregular, and marginated chromatin. There as other irregular Hodgkin cells seen, with large nuclei showing coarse chromatin.

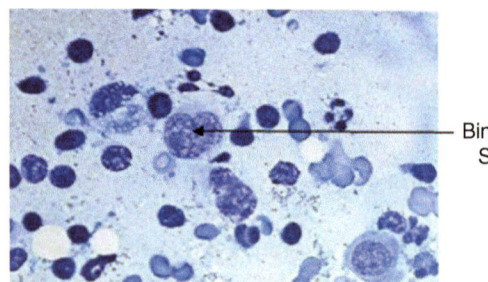

Binucleated Reed-Sternberg cells

23. Answer: E. Squamous cell carcinoma

Squamous cell carcinoma and basal cell carcinoma are common tumors of the face. Histologically, squa-

Bibliography

1. Yorita K, et al. Infarcted Warthin tumor with mucoepidermoid carcinoma-like metaplasia: a case report and review of the literature. J Med Case Reports. 2019;13:12.
2. Venkatesh S, Srinivas TN, Hariprasad S. Parotid gland tumors: 2-year prospective clinicopathological study. Ann Maxillofac Surg. 2019;9(1):103–9.
3. Charki S, et al. Experience of tracheo-esophageal fistula in neonates in a tertiary care center—case series. J Clin Neonatol. 2019;8(2):71–4.
4. Tuttle RM. Medullary thyroid cancer: clinical manifestations, diagnosis, and staging. Waltham: UptoDate; 2019.
5. https://www.cdc.gov/mumps/hcp.html. Accessed 15 Mar 2019.
6. Farhat F, Asnir RA, Yudhistira A, Daulay ER, Sagala IP. An uncommon occurrence of pleomorphic adenoma in the submandibular salivary gland: a case report. Open Access Maced J Med Sci. 2018;6(6):1101–3.
7. Peggy AW. Epidemiology, pathogenesis, and clinical features of basal cell carcinoma. Waltham: UptoDate; 2019.
8. Tan WW, Elston DM. Malignant melanoma. Waltham: UptoDate; 2019.
9. van der Waal I, Buduneli N. Oral leukoplakia: present views on diagnosis, management, communication with patients, and research. Curr Oral Health Rep. 2019;6(1):9–13.
10. Lin HH, Limesand KH, Anna DK. Current state of knowledge on salivary gland cancers. Crit Rev Oncog. 2018;23(3–4):139–51.
11. Zou H, Yang H, Zou Y, Lei L, Song L. Primary diffuse large B-cell lymphoma in the maxilla: a case report. Medicine (Baltimore). 2018;97(20):e10707.
12. Chen E, Ricciotti R, Oda D. Head and neck rhabdomyosarcoma: clinical and pathologic characterization of seven cases. Head Neck Pathol. 2017;11(3):321–6.
13. Graff-Radford NR, DeKosky ST, Wilterdink JL. Normal pressure hydrocephalus. Neurol Baltim. 2019;5:194–204.
14. Taxy JB, et al. Pathology of head and neck neoplasms. Waltham: UptoDate; 2019.
15. Sullivan JL, et al. Clinical manifestations and treatment of Epstein–Barr virus infection. Waltham: UptoDate; 2019.
16. Tuttle RM, et al. Papillary thyroid cancer. Treasure Island: StatPearls; 2019.
17. Young WF Jr, et al. Paragangliomas: epidemiology, clinical presentation, diagnosis, and histology. Waltham: UptoDate; 2019.
18. Tai P, et al. Sebaceous carcinoma. Waltham: UptoDate; 2019.

Gastrointestinal Tract

11

Multiple Choice Questions

1. The incidence and prevalence of regional enteritis are steadily increasing. Common site of regional enteritis is:
   A. Rectum
   B. Colon
   C. Caecum
   D. Distal ileum and colon
   E. Distal ileum

2. Which of the following diseases is associated with *Helicobacter pylori* infection?
   A. Esophagitis
   B. Diverticulitis
   C. Inflammatory bowel disease
   D. Duodenal peptic ulcer
   E. Celiac disease

3. Which of the following gastric neoplasm typically occurs at the junction of pyloric and corpus mucosa?
   A. Gastric adenoma
   B. Gastric xanthoma
   C. Gastric hyperplastic polyps
   D. Hamartomatous polyp
   E. Gastric carcinoid

4. A 48-year-old male with HIV presents with profuse, watery diarrhea of 7 days duration. What is the most likely cause of this patient's symptoms?
   A. Giardia
   B. Cryptosporidium
   C. Entamoeba histolytica
   D. Toxoplasma
   E. Histoplasma

5. A 25-year-old man presents to a rheumatologist with complaints of joint pain involving the large joints of the legs. On questioning, the patient indicates that exacerbations in the joint pain are frequently accompanied by diarrhea. Which of the following gastrointestinal disease is most likely to be implicated as the cause of the patient's joint problems?

   A. Amebic colitis
   B. Chronic appendicitis
   C. Diverticulosis
   D. Pseudomembranous colitis
   E. Ulcerative colitis

6. A 54-year-old man presents with abdominal pain, fever, and profuse diarrhea. There is a history of recent hospitalization where he was given clindamycin. What is the diagnosis?
   A. Ischemic colitis
   B. Diversion colitis
   C. Clostridium difficile colitis
   D. Irritable bowel syndrome
   E. Viral gastroenteritis

7. A biopsy of the GE junction is performed in a 60-year-old male. Biopsy shows Barrett's esophagus. The patient has an increased risk of which of the following disease?
   A. Adenocarcinoma
   B. Squamous cell carcinoma
   C. Leiomyoma
   D. Adenosquamous carcinoma
   E. Mucoepidermoid carcinoma

8. Which of the following disease is the most likely lifetime risk of colon cancer, if left untreated?
   A. Ulcerative colitis
   B. Familial juvenile polyposis
   C. Familial adenomatous polyposis
   D. Crohn disease
   E. Cowden disease

9. Gastrin-secreting tumors and elevated gastrin levels are characteristic findings of which of the following disease?
   A. Antral G cell hyperplasia
   B. Zollinger–Ellison syndrome
   C. Gastric antrum syndrome
   D. Retained antrum syndrome
   E. Menetrier disease

10. A 60-year-old woman presents to the emergency room with a 5 days of passing maroon, tarry stools. Endoscopy

© The Author(s), under exclusive license to Springer Nature Switzerland AG 2022
V. K. Kohli et al., *Comprehensive Multiple-Choice Questions in Pathology*, https://doi.org/10.1007/978-3-031-08767-7_11

is performed and shows thickening of the mucosal folds, irregular nodularity producing a cobblestone effect and ulceration. What is the diagnosis?

A. Extranodal lymphoma
B. MALToma
C. Diffuse large cell lymphoma
D. Gastric lymphoma
E. Non-Hodgkin lymphoma

11. A 65-year-old man complains of abdominal pain, thin caliber stools, and fatigue. His hematocrit is 32% and hemoglobin 9 g/dL. He underwent exploratory laparotomy and a 14 cm segment of his sigmoid colon is removed. What is the diagnosis?

A. Diverticulitis with perforation
B. Ulcerative colitis
C. Intussusception
D. Crohn's disease
E. Colorectal adenocarcinoma

12. A 3-year-old child is brought to the emergency room by her parents for 3 weeks of abdominal pain, vomiting, and weight loss. Pain is most severe after eating. On examination, the child appears well, until after she ingests some crackers. At this point, child cries inconsolably and grabs her abdomen. Esophageal pH monitoring reveals an abnormally high pH of gastric secretions. What is the diagnosis?

A. Inflammatory bowel disease
B. Malabsorption
C. Collagenous and lymphocytic colitis
D. Menetrier disease
E. Viral enteritis

13. A 52-year-old woman is undergoing endoscopy to evaluate persistent gastrointestinal reflux. In the stomach, there is a solitary, well-circumscribed fleshy mass covered with intact mucosa. Further studies show mutation in a gene that encodes tyrosine kinase c-KiT. What is the diagnosis?

A. Adenocarcinoma
B. Lymphoma
C. Epithelioid hemangioendothelioma
D. Gastrointestinal stromal tumor
E. Leiomyoma

14. A 2-week-old infant with Down syndrome presents with distended abdomen and history of no stools. Bowel sounds are absent. Abdominal X-rays shows megacolon. A sigmoid colon biopsy shows lack of mural ganglion cells. What is the most likely diagnosis?

A. Congenital pyloric stenosis
B. Chagas disease
C. Hirschsprung's disease
D. Cystic fibrosis
E. Rectal atresia

15. A 24-month-old girl presents with abdominal pain, diarrhea, vomiting, and weight loss. Duodenal biopsy reveals crypt hyperplasia, villous atrophy, and intraepithelial lymphocyte infiltration. What is the diagnosis?

A. Intussusception
B. Celiac disease
C. Hirschsprung's disease
D. Incarcerated hernia
E. Volvulus of bowel

16. A 40-year-old man comes to the physician office with severe upper abdominal pain. Upper gastrointestinal endoscopy reveals a small ulcer with a clean base in the duodenal bulb. Biopsy of which part of the stomach would demonstrate the infectious agent?

A. Gastric fundus
B. Gastric cardia
C. Pylorus
D. Gastric antrum
E. Body of the stomach

17. Which is a complication of long-standing GERD (gastroesophageal reflux disease) and is characterized by columnar metaplasia of the squamous epithelium that normally lines the esophagus?

A. Barrett esophagus
B. Leiomyoma
C. Squamous papilloma
D. Lipoma
E. Adenocarcinoma

18. A patient presents with diarrhea, cutaneous flushing, bronchospasm, and wheezing. Urine levels of 5-HIAA (5-hydroxyindoleacetic acid) is increased. What is the diagnosis?

A. Peutz–Jeghers syndrome
B. Turcot's syndrome
C. Carcinoid tumor
D. Gardner's syndrome
E. Familial adenomatous polyposis (FAP)

19. Which type of gastrointestinal disease is associated with pernicious anemia?

A. Acute hemorrhagic gastritis
B. Gastric cancer
C. Gastroesophageal reflux disease
D. Chronic atrophic gastritis
E. Chronic peptic ulcer

20. Left supraclavicular adenopathy and Krukenberg's tumor are usually found in which of the following disease?

A. Esophageal cancer
B. Gastric carcinoma
C. Malignant neoplasms of the small intestine
D. Non-Hodgkin lymphoma
E. Colonic adenocarcinoma

21. Four cardinal manifestations—arthralgias, diarrhea, abdominal pain, and weight loss are found in which of the following medical condition?
    A. Abdominal angina
    B. Celiac disease (Sprue)
    C. Malabsorption
    D. Whipple disease
    E. Tropical sprue

22. Failure of the lower esophageal sphincter to relax with swallowing is called as:
    A. Achalasia
    B. Gastroesophageal reflux disease
    C. Pseudoachalasia
    D. Esophageal spasm
    E. Jackhammer (nutcracker) esophagus

23. A 55-year-old male presented with a 6-month history of iron-deficiency anemia. Esophagogastroduodenoscopy (EGD) and colonoscopy were performed. Colonoscopy revealed a left sided polypoid colonic mass. Which of the following statements is most accurate regarding this kind of tumor?
    A. Associated with carcinoid tumors
    B. Most often presents in the left colon
    C. Most patients have favorable prognosis
    D. Associated with an overlying adenoma
    E. Most cases are positive for TTF-1

24. Which esophageal carcinoma presents mostly in the proximal-two third of the esophagus and frequently metastasizes to mediastinal lymph nodes?
    A. Adenocarcinoma
    B. Gastrointestinal stromal tumors
    C. Squamous cell carcinoma
    D. Leiomyosarcoma
    E. Barrett esophagus

25. Which is true for sessile serrated (SSA) polyp?
    A. Usually less than 1 mm in size
    B. More common in the left colon
    C. Always have cytological features of at least low-grade dysplasia
    D. Commonly have a high prevalence of KRAS mutations
    E. Associated with increased risk for colon cancer

26. Which of the following bacterial infections can histologically mimic ischemic colitis?
    A. Enteroadherent Escherichia coli
    B. Salmonella typhimurium
    C. Clostridium difficile
    D. Vibrio cholerae
    E. Yersinia pseudotuberculosis

27. Which of the following statements is most accurate regarding collagenous colitis?
    A. Often presents with bloody diarrhea
    B. Associated with autoimmune diseases

C. Neutrophils are prominent feature
D. Colonoscopic examination is often abnormal
E. Increased prevalence in men and smokers

Answers and Explanations

1. Answer: D. Distal ileum and colon
   Crohn's disease (CD) is an inflammatory bowel disease. It most commonly affects the terminal ileum but can occur throughout the entire gastrointestinal tract. Terminal ileum, ileocecal valve, and cecum are the most involved sites. Gross examination may show a cobblestone change of the mucosa.

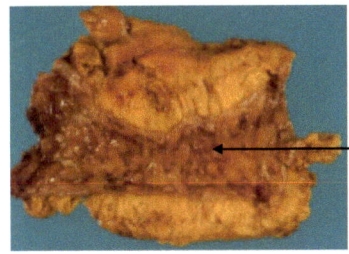

Cobblestone change of the mucosa of the terminal ileum

2. Answer: D. Duodenal peptic ulcer
   Duodenal peptic ulcers are etiologically related to *Helicobacter pylori* infection. Eradication of *H. pylori* infection increases the likelihood of healing and decreases infection. Peptic ulcers may also occur due to NSAID (nonsteroidal anti-inflammatory drug) use.

3. Answer: C. Gastric hyperplastic polyps
   Gastric hyperplastic polyps (HPP) typically occurs at the junction of pyloric and corpus mucosa. Hyperplastic polyps comprise about 70–90% of gastric polyps. 30% are multiple and are usually less than 2 cm. Histologically, these lesions contain branched gastric foveolae, with an edematous lamina propria, which is associated with a background of inflammation. The foveolar epithelium is often hypertrophic with prominent cystic changes. They are not usually associated with an increased risk of malignancy.

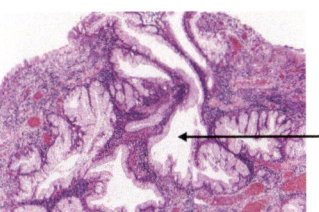

Branched gastric foveolae, with an edematous lamina propria

4. Answer: B. Cryptosporidium
   Cryptosporidium, a protozoan affects patients with AIDS and causes severe, chronic diarrhea. The organism

is highly infectious. Mode of spread is usually fecal-oral transmission. Diagnosis can be made by acid-fast examination of the stool which shows cryptosporidial oocysts as round, red-staining structures. Cryptosporidium are spherical and range from 4 to 6 mm. Treatment involves antiparasitic therapy and nutritional support.

5. Answer: E. Ulcerative colitis

    Ulcerative colitis is characterized by continuous and circumferential inflammation of the colon limited to mucosa and submucosa. It commonly involves the rectum. Polyps occurring in ulcerative colitis may be inflammatory polyps, adenomas, and dysplasia associated lesions/polyps. Non neoplastic pseudopolyps may be found which are areas of granulation tissue due to surrounding ulcerations. Endoscopy shows diffuse mucosal involvement with areas of granularity and friability. Light microscopy shows crypt abscesses, shortening, crypt atrophy, and inflammatory features of ulcerative colitis.

6. Answer: C. Clostridium difficile colitis

    Clostridium difficile colitis is reported most frequently with clindamycin, lincomycin, and ampicillin. Clostridium difficile produces enterotoxin (toxin A) that causes cell damage and inflammation, cytotoxin (toxin B) that causes cell death and a third toxin that stimulates colonic motor activity. This colitis presents as watery diarrhea, often associated with fever, colicky abdominal pain, and leukocytosis. Endoscopic appearance shows several 2–5 mm yellow raised plaques. Biopsy of the smaller plaque shows a small focus of superficial mucosal inflammation and necrosis from which the pseudomembranous inflammatory exudate mushroom out.

7. Answer: A. Adenocarcinoma

    Barrett esophagus is a pre-neoplastic clinic pathological condition. It is common in males. 6–12% of patients with GERD develop Barrett esophagus. Histological features show intestinal (goblet) metaplasia columnar mucosa. There is 30-fold increased risk of esophageal carcinoma. Common sites of the adenocarcinoma of the esophagus are the lower esophagus and gastroesophageal junction.

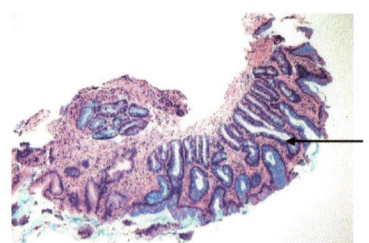
Intestinal (goblet) metaplasia

8. Answer: C. Familial adenomatous polyposis

    In familial adenomatous polyposis (FAP), there is an early onset of adenomatous polyps throughout the colon. In FAP, mutated gene is adenomatous polyposis coli (APC). All patients with FAP will develop colon cancer by the age of 35–40 years, if left untreated. FAP is inherited as an autosomal dominant.

9. Answer: B. Zollinger–Ellison syndrome

    Zollinger–Ellison syndrome is a clinical syndrome characterized by massive acid secretion and severe peptic ulcer disease, due to hypergastrinemia secondary to gastrinoma. Patients present with distal duodenal ulcers, heartburn, and diarrhea. Elevated gastrin levels are found in the patients. Gross examination shows massive hypertrophy of gastric rugal folds in the gastric body and fundus. Light microscopy shows parietal cell hypertrophy and hyperplasia with atrophy of overlying foveolar epithelium.

10. Answer: B. MALToma

    In the stomach, the development of MALT (mucosa-associated lymphoid tissue) lymphoma or MALToma is usually associated with *H. pylori* infection. Nearly 90% of gastric MALT lymphomas have evidence of *H. pylori* infection. A significant proportion of gastric MALT-lymphomas regress following the eradication of *H. pylori* by antibiotics. Low-grade MALT-lymphomas tend to occur in patients over 50 years old. Histology shows dense lymphocytic infiltrate in the mucosa that involves the submucosa. Monocytoid or centrocyte-like cells are also present. Lymphoepithelial lesions may be found. These tumors express both CD19 and CD 20.

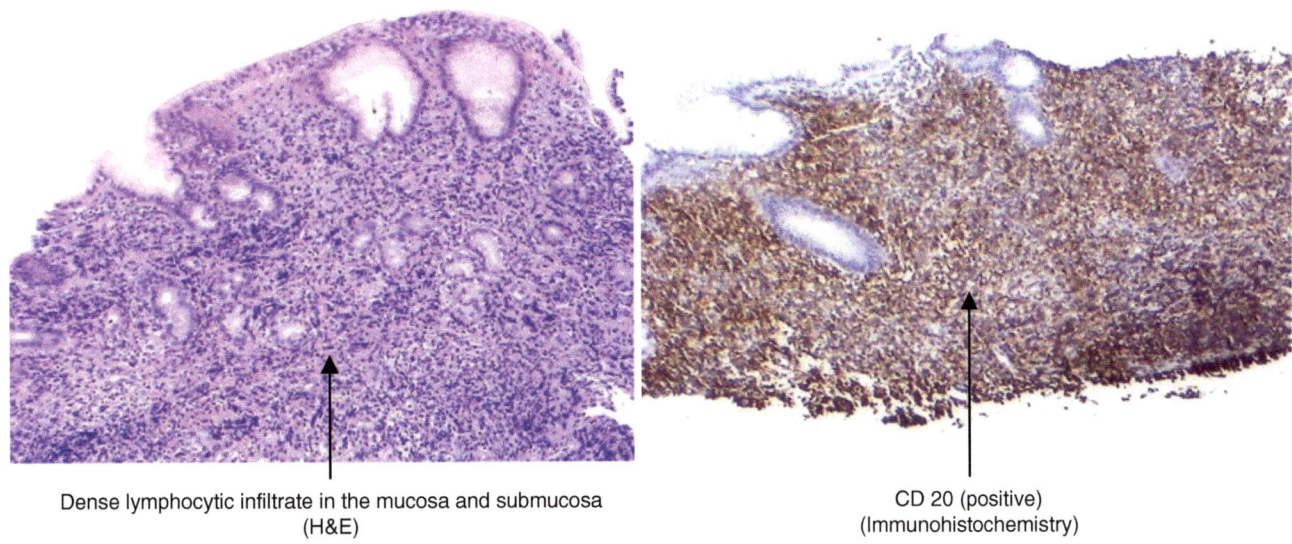

Dense lymphocytic infiltrate in the mucosa and submucosa
(H&E)

CD 20 (positive)
(Immunohistochemistry)

11. Answer: E. Colorectal adenocarcinoma

The vast majority of colorectal carcinoma passes through an adenoma phase and progress by enlargement and increasing dysplasia to carcinoma. In colorectal carcinoma, there is activation of proto-oncogene (KRAS) and inactivation of APC, p53, and loss of heterozygosity (LOH). Early features are alterations in bowel habits and anemia. Late features include overt rectal bleeding, weight loss, colonic obstruction, and the presence of a mass. Regular screening colonoscopy results in a reduction in the incidence of the disease. Genetic testing is recommended only for kindred of familial polyposis syndrome and HNPCC to see whether they have the inherited genetic defect. Diagnosis of colorectal carcinoma is established by biopsy. Histopathologically, the majority of cancers arising in the colon are adenocarcinomas. Prognosis depends on pathologic stage, histologic grade. A preoperative serum CEA value of more than 5 ng/mL is an adverse factor. Surgery is the primary treatment for colorectal carcinoma.

12. Answer: D. Menetrier disease

The patient presents with characteristic signs, symptoms and findings of Menetrier disease. Menetrier disease is a rare disease, characterized by hypertrophic gastropathy with hypoproteinemia and hypochlorhydria. Grossly, it shows giant polypoid mucosal folds/rugae. Histology, full thickness biopsy is required and shows marked foveolar hyperplasia with atrophy of oxyntic cells. In children, it is associated with CMV infection and is usually self-limited. Menetrier disease is associated with increased risk of gastric cancer. Immunohistochemistry is done by TGF-alpha.

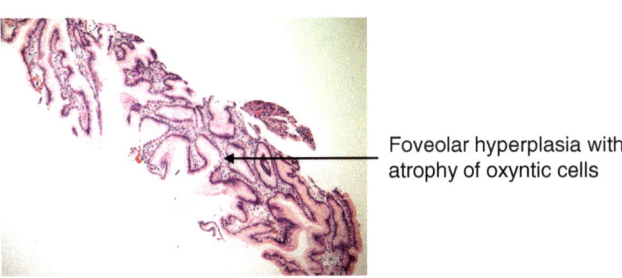

Foveolar hyperplasia with atrophy of oxyntic cells

13. Answer: D. Gastrointestinal stromal tumor

Gastrointestinal stromal tumors (GISTs) are usually submucosal spindle cells tumors. GISTs affect men and women roughly equally and about 75% of the cases occur in adults aged over 50. GISTs generally arise as solitary tumors of stomach, small intestine, large intestine or esophagus. Benign tumors are usually less than 5 cm and less than 5 mitotic counts/50 HPF. GISTs of size more than 5 cm and more than 5 mitotic counts/50 HPF favor malignancy. About 75–80% have a gain of function mutations in a gene that encodes tyrosine kinase c-KIT. GISTs are CD 117 and often CD 34 positive. There is an association with NF1 and GIST.

	Size (cm)	Mitotic counts/50 HPF
Low risk	2-5	<5
High risk	>5	>5

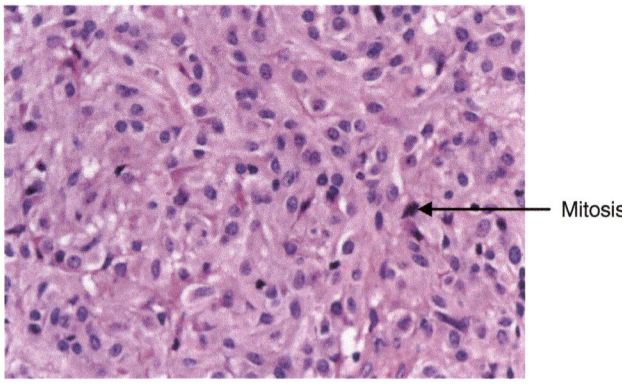

Mitosis

14. Answer: C. Hirschsprung's disease

Hirschsprung's disease is a common congenital disorder due to the absence of ganglion cells in the distal rectum. It is characterized by a lack of propulsive peristalsis in the distal colon resulting from aganglionosis. Hirschsprung's disease is most commonly diagnosed during infancy, after failure to pass meconium. The aganglionic segment begins in the distal rectumand extend proximally. Majority of cases have a short less than 40 cm aganglionic segment. The most serious complication is Hirschsprung associated enterocolitis (HAEC). Preoperative diagnosis is established by aganglionosis in the biopsy of the rectum taken at 2 cm or above the pectinate line. Children with trisomy 21 (Down syndrome) are at increased risk of Hirschsprung's disease.

15. Answer: B. Celiac disease

Celiac disease is the most common cause of malabsorption syndrome. It is also known as gluten-sensitive enteropathy. It is a systemic autoimmune disorder induced by exposure to gliadin or prolamin fraction of gluten proteins found in wheat, barley, and rye. Females affected are commonly twice as males. HLA-DQ2 or HLA-DQ8 is present in the vast majority of patients with celiac disease. Histology shows villous atrophy, crypt hyperplasia, an increased chronic infiltrate in the lamina propria, and increased intraepithelial lymphocytes.

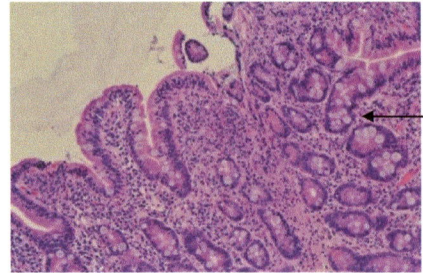

Mucosa is flat with complete loss of the normal villous architecture

16. Answer: D. Gastric antrum

Peptic ulcers are commonly caused by Helicobacter pylori. Heavy colonization in the gastric antrum occurs in duodenal ulcers.

17. Answer: A. Barrett esophagus

Barrett esophagus is common in adult to elderly male population and develops in the setting of GERD. Esophageal squamous metaplasia is replaced by glandular mucosa following erosion. There is excess risk of esophageal adenocarcinoma. Long segment has greater risk than short segment.

18. Answer: C. Carcinoid tumor

Carcinoid tumors are well-differentiated neuroendocrine tumors. They commonly originate in the digestive tract, lungs. Within the GI tract, jejunum, ileum, rectum, appendix are the most common locations. Urinary excretion of 5-HIAA in 24 h is the most important diagnostic test. There are increased levels of 5-hydroxyindoleacetic acid (5-HIAA) excretion in urine.

19. Answer: D. Chronic atrophic gastritis

Metaplastic (chronic) atrophic gastritis is also called gastric atrophy. There is mucosal thinning, loss of specialized cells along with metaplasia of epithelial cells. Chronic atrophic gastritis includes autoimmune and environmental subtypes. Chronic atrophic gastritis causes the replacement of normal oxyntic mucosa in gastric polyps by atrophic and metaplastic mucosa. This results in loss of intrinsic factor progressing to pernicious anemia (vitamin B12 deficiency).

20. Answer: B. Gastric carcinoma

Gastric carcinomas are most commonly located in the pyloric antrum and the incisura angularis. Gross appearance of advanced gastric carcinomas show polypoid lesions, malignant ulcers or fungating tumors with ulceration at the dome. There is a diffuse thickening of the gastric wall, the classic linitis plastic type. Approximately 70% of gastric carcinomas are intestinal and other 30% are diffuse, often with signet ring cells. Signet ring carcinoma occurs when there is abundant intracellular mucin which pushes aside the nucleus of the individual cells. The former have a better prognosis than the later. Lymphatics spread may reveal a left supraclavicular adenopathy. There may be enlarged ovary (Krukenberg's tumor) by peritoneal spread.

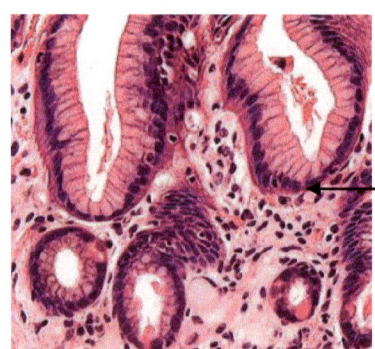

Signet ring cell carcinoma

21. Answer: D. Whipple disease

Whipple disease is a chronic multisystem disease resulting from infection with *Tropheryma whipplei*, a gram-positive rod shaped bacterium. The diagnosis is established by detecting the presence of *Tropheryma whipplei* DNA in affected tissues by polymerase chain reaction. Whipple disease manifests primarily in the intestine and mesenteric lymph nodes, but can involve central nervous system, eye, heart, skin, and bone. Small bowel biopsy shows thickened villi distended with PAS-positive foamy macrophages.

22. Answer: A. Achalasia

Achalasia is an esophageal motility disorder due to the degeneration of ganglion cells in the myenteric plexus. Achalasia causes a failure of relaxation of the lower esophageal sphincter and loss of peristalsis in the distal esophagus. The etiology of primary achalasia is unknown. The presentation of primary and secondary achalasia is identical and frequent symptoms are dysphagia for solids and liquids and regurgitation of bland undigested food or saliva. Patients may also present with chest pain, heartburn, and difficulty belching. Achalasia carries an increased risk of squamous carcinoma.

23. Answer: D. Associated with an overlying adenoma

Small cell carcinoma of the colon is frequently associated with an overlying adenoma, often villous/tubulo-villous (30–40% of cases). They are most often present in the right colon. Patients usually present with iron deficiency anemia due to occult blood loss. Right sided colon cancers grow as exophytic masses. The prognosis is poor due to early metastasis to lymph nodes and liver. Positive stains include neuron-specific enolase (84%), Synaptophysin (50%), chromogranin (37%), and CD56 (86%).

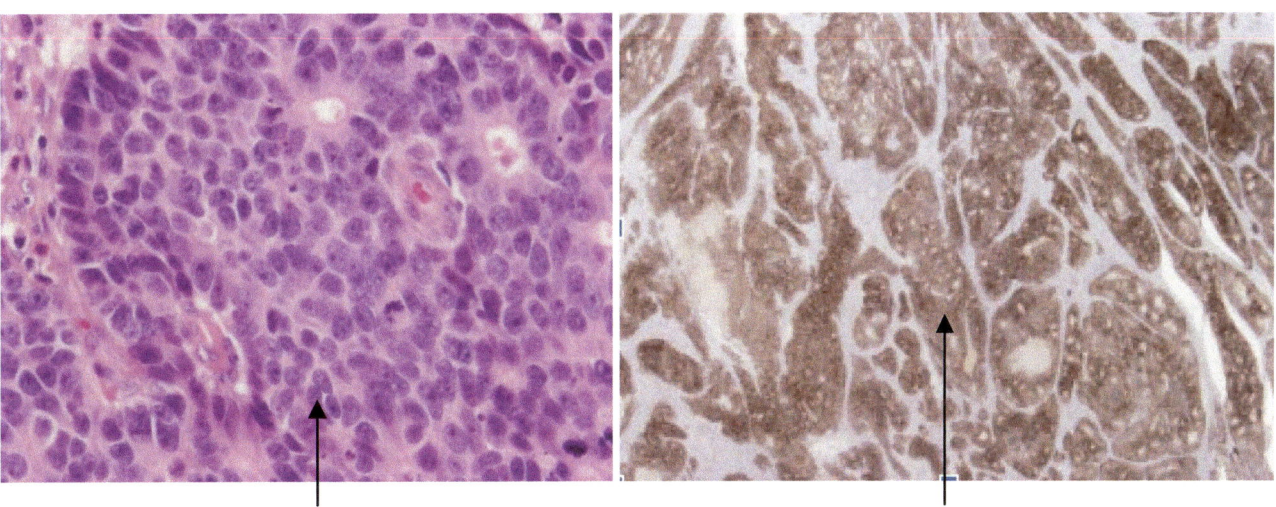

Small cell carcinoma of the colon (H&E)

Tumor cells positive for Synaptophysin (Immunohistochemistry)

24. Answer: C. Squamous cell carcinoma

Squamous cell carcinoma, accounts for the majority of cases of esophageal carcinoma. Approximately half of the esophageal squamous carcinomas occurs in the middle third; one-third on the lower esophagus; rest in the upper third. The major risk factors are cigarette smoking and alcohol use. Achalasia of the cardia is associated with a greater than 30-fold increase over the general population. Other risk factors are consumption of food rich in nitrates and nitrosamines. Plummer–Vinson syndrome, p53 point mutations may be present in over half of esophageal cancers. Other mutations such as mutation in p16, k-ras, and APC mutations may be found in these cancers. Patients present late with dysplasia. Grossly, there may be fungating masses, malignant ulcers or diffusely infiltrative lesions that are obvious at endoscopy. Diagnosis is done by biopsy.

25. Answer: E. Associated with increased risk for colon cancer

Sessile serrated adenoma (SSA) polyps can be found in any region of the colon and rectum but are more frequently found in the right colon. Most of the polyps are larger than 5 mm. Specific morphological features in sessile serrated polyps include expanded crypt proliferation zones, crypt basilar dilation, and decreased or absent cell maturation along the length of the crypt. 80% may demonstrate BRAF mutations.

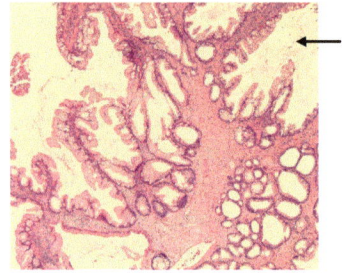

← Expanded crypt proliferation zones with crypt basilar dilation

26. Answer: C. *Clostridium difficile*

Bacterial infections of the gastrointestinal tract may histologically mimic inflammatory bowel diseases and ischemic colitis. Enterohemorrhagic *E. coli*, *Clostridium difficile*, and *Clostridium perfringens* are most commonly associated with an ischemic pattern of injury.

27. Answer: B. Associated with autoimmune diseases

Collagenous colitis is characterized by patch thickening of the subepithelial basement membrane. This condition is associated with some autoimmune diseases such as celiac sprue and autoimmune gastritis. It has increased prevalence in women and smokers, and often presents with watery diarrhea.

Bibliography

1. Rendi M, Younes M. Crohn disease pathology. Waltham: UptoDate; 2017.
2. Nakayama M, Oshima M. Mutant p53 in colon cancer. J Mol Cell Biol. 2019;11(4):267–76.
3. Waters AM, Der CJ. KRAS: the critical driver and therapeutic target for pancreatic cancer. Cold Spring Harb Perspect Med. 2018;8(9):a031435.
4. Ashley SW, et al. Postgastrectomy complications. New York: Springer; 2019.
5. Peppercorn MA, et al. Clinical manifestations, diagnosis, and prognosis of ulcerative colitis in adults. Baltimore: Wolters Kluwer; 2019.
6. Azer SA, Sun Y. Colitis. New York: Springer; 2019.
7. Anti-Saccharomyces cerevisiae Antibodies (ASCA). 2019.
8. Wehbi M, Anand BS. Familial adenomatous polyposis. Treasure Island: StatPearls; 2019.
9. Whiteman H, Collier J. Colorectal cancer: increasing fiber intake may lower death risk. New York: Springer; 2017.
10. Parzanese I, Qehajaj D, et al. Celiac disease: from pathophysiology to treatment. World J Gastrointest Pathophysiol. 2017;8(2):27–38.
11. Macrae FA, Bendell J, et al. Clinical presentation, diagnosis, and staging of colorectal cancer. Baltimore: Wolters Kluwer; 2019.
12. Kowdley KV. Primary sclerosing cholangitis in adults: clinical manifestations and diagnosis. Baltimore: Wolters Kluwer; 2019.
13. Perri G-A. Complications of end-stage liver disease. Can Fam Physician. 2016;62(1):44–50.
14. Ostermaier KK, et al. Down syndrome: clinical features and diagnosis. Baltimore: Wolters Kluwer; 2019.
15. Peppercorn MA, et al. Clinical manifestations, diagnosis and prognosis of Crohn disease in adults. Baltimore: Wolters Kluwer; 2019.
16. Tye-Din JA, Galipeau HJ, Agardh D. Celiac disease: a review of current concepts in pathogenesis, prevention, and novel therapies. Front Pediatr. 2018;6:350.
17. Narayanan M, Reddy KM, Marsicano E. Peptic ulcer disease and *Helicobacter pylori* infection. Mo Med. 2018;115(3):219–24.
18. Macrae FA, Goldberg RM, Seres D, Savarese DMF. Colorectal cancer: epidemiology, risk factors, and protective factors. Waltham: UptoDate; 2019.
19. Tebbi CK, Coppes MJ. Carcinoid tumor. New York: Springer; 2019.
20. Fletcher J, Sethi S. What to know about atrophic gastritis. Waltham: UptoDate; 2018.
21. Mansfield PF, et al. Clinical features, diagnosis, and staging of gastric cancer. Waltham: UptoDate; 2019.
22. Apstein MD, et al. Whipple's disease. Treasure Island: StatPearls Publishing; 2019.
23. Spechler SJ, et al. Achalasia: pathogenesis, clinical manifestations, and diagnosis. Baltimore: Wolters Kluwer; 2019.
24. Wesson DE, Lopez ME, et al. Congenital aganglionic megacolon (Hirschsprung disease). Baltimore: Wolters Kluwer; 2019.

Liver and Biliary Tract

12

Multiple Choice Questions

1. A middle-aged alcoholic man presents in the emergency department with nose bleed. Examination shows distended paraumbilical veins, ascites, and a flapping hand tremor on wrist extension. Which laboratory finding is the best indicator of poor prognosis in this alcoholic patient?
   A. Elevated level of serum glutamic oxaloacetic transaminase (SGOT)
   B. Elevated level of serum glutamic pyruvic transaminase (SGPT)
   C. Prolonged prothrombin time
   D. Elevated level of gamma-glutamyl transferase (GGT)
   E. Elevated level of alkaline phosphatase

2. Which of the following drug causes hepatocellular necrosis with inflammation?
   A. Acetaminophen
   B. Diclofenac sodium
   C. Ibuprofen
   D. Acetylsalicylic acid
   E. Sucralfate

3. A 10-year-old male child comes to the pediatrician office with symptoms of yellow appearance of the skin and sclera, foul-smelling, pale stools, poor weight gain, enlarged abdomen, loss of appetite. His father died of liver cirrhosis. Physical examination shows hepatomegaly. What is the diagnosis?
   A. Chronic viral hepatitis
   B. Alpha-1 antitrypsin deficiency
   C. Gilbert's syndrome
   D. Crigler–Najjar syndrome
   E. Dubin–Johnson syndrome

4. LDH 5 is found in which of the following organ?
   A. Kidney
   B. Heart
   C. Liver
   D. Prostate
   E. Brain

5. A 45-year-old woman presents with symptoms of pruritus, fatigue, right upper quadrant pain, recurrent cholangitis, and symptoms of portal hypertension. Laboratory findings show elevated alkaline phosphatase. Cholangiogram shows evidence of characteristic bile duct changes (multifocal strictures, segmental dilations). What is the diagnosis?
   A. Primary sclerosing cholangitis (PSC)
   B. Abdominal vascular Injuries
   C. Acalculous cholecystitis
   D. Autoimmune hepatitis
   E. Cholangiocarcinoma

6. Gross picture of a specimen is shown below. What is the diagnosis?

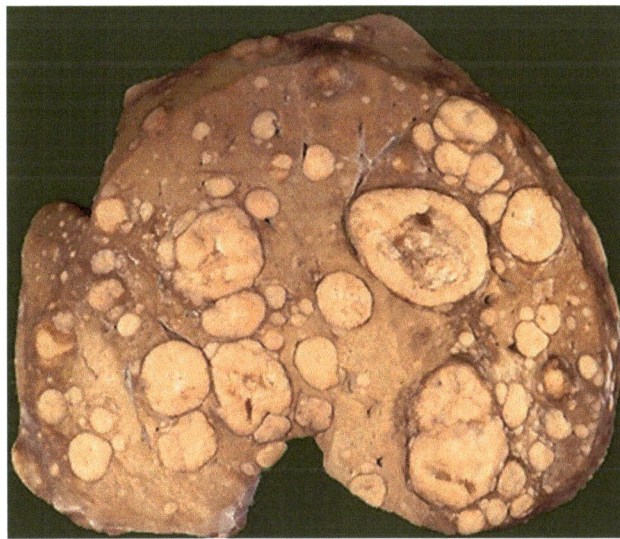

   A. Hemochromatosis
   B. Metastatic liver disease
   C. Fatty metamorphosis
   D. Micronodular cirrhosis
   E. Metabolic liver disease

V. K. Kohli et al., *Comprehensive Multiple-Choice Questions in Pathology*, https://doi.org/10.1007/978-3-031-08767-7_12

7. A 50-year-old woman presents with increasing abdominal girth and enlarging liver. Laboratory findings show elevated Alpha-fetoprotein in the serum. What is the diagnosis?
   A. Serous papillary cystadenocarcinoma
   B. Metastatic gastric adenocarcinoma
   C. Hepatocellular carcinoma
   D. Pancreatic carcinoma
   E. Endometrial carcinoma

8. What would be expected to be seen microscopically in a liver biopsy from a patient with typical acute hepatitis, if the biopsy was taken during the icteric phase?
   A. No pathologic changes
   B. Mononuclear inflammatory cells, ground glass hepatocytes and bridging necrosis
   C. Mononuclear inflammatory cells, swollen hepatocytes, and bile plugs in canaliculi
   D. Mononuclear inflammatory cells, especially a prominent Kupffer cell reaction
   E. Mononuclear inflammatory cells and piecemeal necrosis

9. A 52-year-old woman with a history of autoimmune thyroid disease (Hashimoto's thyroiditis) presents with severe pruritus, especially at night. Laboratory investigations show elevated alkaline phosphatase. What is the diagnosis?
   A. Alcoholic hepatitis
   B. Hemochromatosis
   C. Primary biliary cholangitis
   D. Hepatitis C
   E. Hepatitis A

10. Distant organ metastases in esophageal cancer is common in which of the following organ?
    A. Liver
    B. Lung
    C. Bone
    D. Brain
    E. Breast

11. A middle aged man with a history of abdominal swelling and pain, swelling in the legs and ankles, chronic fatigue, nausea, and vomiting. Histological picture is shown below. What is the diagnosis?

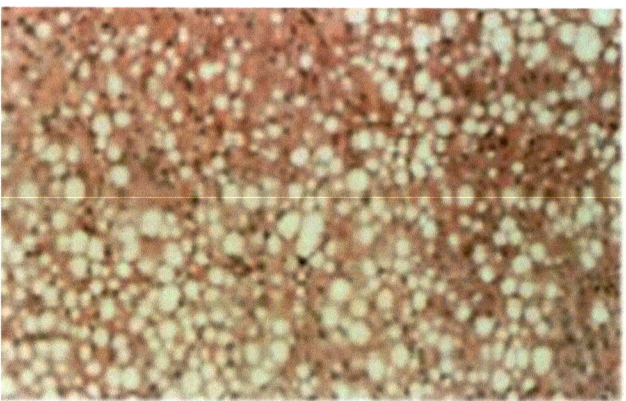

    A. Chronic viral hepatitis
    B. Metabolic liver disease
    C. Alcoholic fatty liver
    D. Hemochromatosis
    E. Hepatocellular carcinoma

12. Gross pictures of liver of middle aged male are shown below. What is the diagnosis?

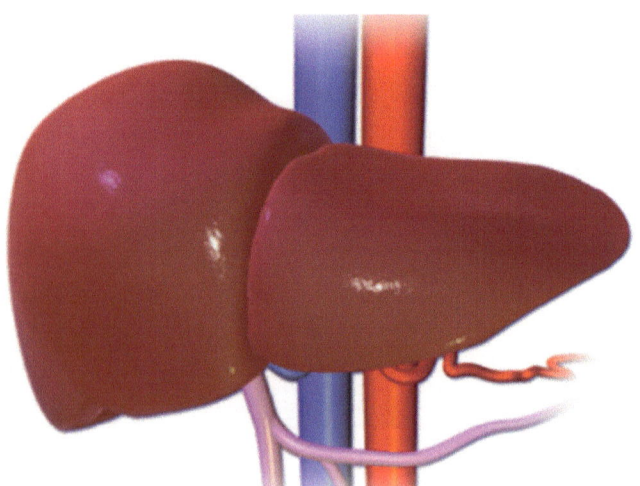

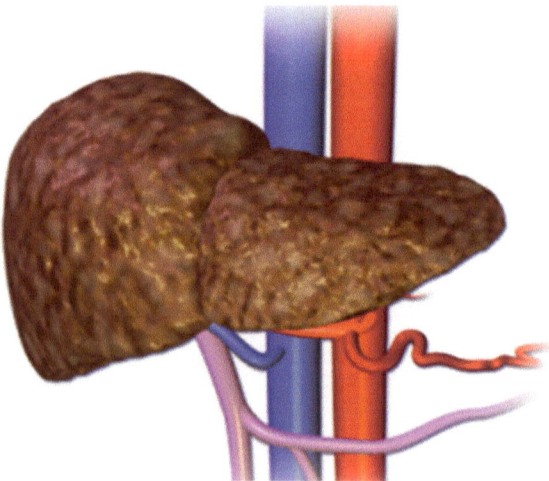

A. Cirrhosis of liver
B. Hemangioma of liver
C. Cholangiocarcinoma of liver
D. Angiosarcoma of liver
E. Metastatic tumors to the liver

13. Which of the following hepatitis viruses are responsible for hepatocellular carcinoma?
    A. Hepatitis A (HAV)
    B. Hepatitis B (HBV)
    C. Hepatitis C (HCV)
    D. Hepatitis D (HDV)
    E. Hepatitis B (HBV) and Hepatitis C (HCV)

14. Which of the following virus that replicates only in HBV-infected cells?
    A. Hepatitis A
    B. Hepatitis C
    C. Hepatitis D (Delta agent)
    D. Hepatitis E
    E. Epstein-Barr

15. A 40-year-old female patient comes to the physician office with symptoms of fever, nausea, vomiting, pain in the upper right side of the abdomen. Physical examination shows right upper quadrant tenderness on palpation. Laboratory investigations showed leukocytosis. What is the diagnosis?
    A. Acute cholecystitis
    B. Chronic cholecystitis
    C. Ascending cholangitis
    D. Acute pancreatitis
    E. Chronic pancreatitis

16. Microscopic findings of chronic inflammation and Rokitansky–Aschoff sinuses are found in which of the following medical conditions?
    A. Acute cholecystitis
    B. Chronic cholecystitis
    C. Ascending cholangitis
    D. Acute pancreatitis
    E. Chronic pancreatitis

17. A 30-year-old woman presents with sudden onset of severe abdominal pain. She is using oral contraceptives regularly. Ultrasound of abdomen shows a small hepatic mass. What is the diagnosis?
    A. Focal nodular hyperplasia
    B. Hepatic adenoma
    C. Nodular regenerative hyperplasia
    D. Adenomatous hyperplasia
    E. Cavernous hemangioma

18. Strawberry gallbladder is found in which of the following medical conditions?
    A. Cholesterolosis
    B. Hydrops of the gallbladder mucocele
    C. Ascending cholangitis
    D. Gallbladder cancer
    E. Bile duct cancer

19. Carcinoma of the intrahepatic bile ducts is found in which of the following medical conditions?
    A. Bile duct carcinoma
    B. Cholangiocarcinoma
    C. Klatskin's tumor
    D. Gallbladder cancer
    E. Hepatocellular carcinoma

20. Which parasite causes amoebic liver abscess?
    A. Entamoeba histolytica
    B. Hookworm (Necator americanus)
    C. Roundworm (Ascaris lumbricoides)
    D. Schistosoma mansoni
    E. Taenia solium

21. Which of the following is the most common benign liver tumor?
    A. Cavernous hemangioma
    B. Hepatoblastoma
    C. Choledochal cyst
    D. Hepatic adenomas
    E. Focal nodular hyperplasia

22. Which is the commonest type of gallbladder cancer?
    A. Squamous cell carcinoma of gallbladder
    B. Adenosquamous carcinoma of gallbladder
    C. Adenocarcinoma of gallbladder
    D. Small cell carcinoma of gallbladder
    E. Lymphoma

23. Industrial exposure to polyvinyl chloride is associated with which kind of liver cancer?
    A. Hepatocellular carcinoma
    B. Angiosarcoma of the liver
    C. Hepatic metastases
    D. Hepatoblastoma
    E. Cholangiocarcinoma

24. Transient unconjugated hyperbilirubinemia due to the immaturity of the liver is defined as which of the following medical conditions?
    A. Hereditary hyperbilirubinemias
    B. Biliary tract obstruction
    C. Choledochal cyst
    D. Physiologic jaundice of the newborn
    E. Nonimmune hemolytic anemia

25. A middle-aged man presents to the emergency department after an episode of vomiting of large volume of blood. There is also history of spiking fevers, chills, bloody, and tarry stools. Physical examination shows tender liver. Endoscopy shows bleeding esophageal varices. What is the diagnosis?
    A. Portal vein thrombosis
    B. Granulomatous hepatitis
    C. Hepatoportal sclerosis

D. Primary biliary cirrhosis

E. Budd–Chiari syndrome

26. A 22-year-old male comes to the physician office with symptoms of mild jaundice after fasting for 3 days. He has similar episodes in the past. Laboratory findings show total bilirubin 2.7 mg/dL, while liver enzymes (SGOT, SGPT) are within normal limits. What is the diagnosis?

A. Gilbert syndrome

B. Crigler–Najjar syndrome

C. Dubin–Johnson syndrome

D. Acetaminophen ingestion

E. Acute alcoholic hepatitis

27. Which is a common complication of chronic cholecystitis with porcelain gallbladder?

A. Squamous cell carcinoma

B. Adenosquamous carcinoma

C. Cholangiocarcinoma

D. Gallbladder adenocarcinoma

E. Lymphoma of gallbladder

28. SGOT (AST) SGPT (ALT) ratio greater than 1.5 is found in which of the following medical conditions?

A. Chronic pancreatitis

B. Alcoholic hepatitis

C. Hepatitis B

D. Hepatitis C

E. Hepatitis A virus infection

29. A 36-year-old male patient comes to the physician office with symptoms of abdominal pain, ascites, and liver enlargement. What is the diagnosis?

A. Alpha1-antitrypsin deficiency

B. Granulomatous liver disease

C. Cirrhosis

D. Budd–Chiari syndrome

E. Infectious hepatitis

30. A 35-year-old female presents with abdominal pain and weight loss over the last 6 months. On physical examination, the patient has scleral icterus, hepatomegaly, and a palpable hepatic mass. Imaging studies show a central scar in the left lobe with calcifications. Biopsy is done and shows large polygonal cells with abundant granular, eosinophilic cytoplasm separated into nests by hyalinized bands of acellular collagen. What is the diagnosis?

A. Angiosarcoma of liver

B. Neuroendocrine hepatic neoplasm

C. Metastatic carcinoma of liver

D. Fibrolamellar hepatocellular carcinoma

E. Classic hepatocellular carcinoma

31. A 29-year-old man has used illicit intravenous drugs in the past. He comes to the clinic with complaints of fatigue and weight loss. He drinks regularly. A liver biopsy is obtained, and light microscopy shows ground glass hepatocytes. Which of the following is the most likely diagnosis in this patient?

A. Hepatitis A infection

B. Cirrhosis of liver

C. Chronic hepatitis

D. Hepatitis B infection

E. Hepatitis C infection

32. Microscopic picture of a liver biopsy is shown below. What is the diagnosis?

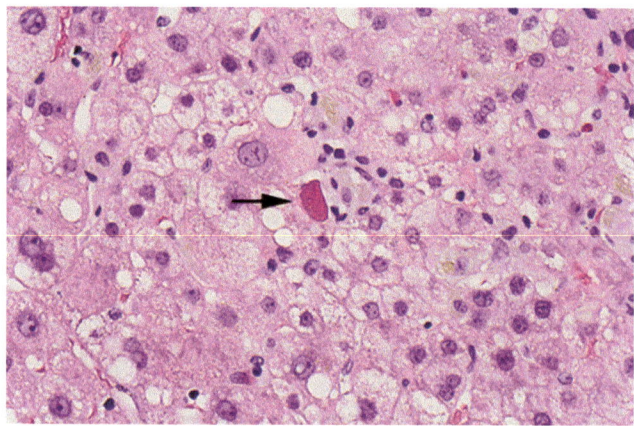

A. Councilman body

B. Concentric fibrosis around bile ducts

C. Segmental stenosis of bile ducts

D. Beaded appearance of bile ducts

E. Mallory body

33. The bile duct neoplasm cholangiocarcinoma is an important complication of which of the following disease?

A. Autoimmune hepatitis

B. Primary sclerosing cholangitis (PSC)

C. Chronic hepatitis C

D. Chronic hepatitis B

E. Primary biliary cirrhosis (PBC)

34. A 3-year-old boy presents with a liver mass. Alpha-fetoprotein (AFP) is elevated in the serum. This tumor is associated with Beckwith–Wiedemann syndrome. What is the diagnosis?

A. Hepatocellular carcinoma

B. Hepatoblastoma

C. Primary hepatic carcinoma

D. Fibrolamellar carcinoma

E. Hepatic adenoma

35. Which serological markers are positive in people who have been vaccinated for Hepatitis B?

A. HBsAg

B. Anti HBs

C. HBcAG

D. Anti HBc

E. Anti-HBe

36. Mallory bodies are characteristic of which of the following condition?
    A. Alcoholic hepatitis
    B. Autoimmune hepatitis
    C. Primary biliary cirrhosis
    D. Wilson disease
    E. Hemochromatosis

37. A 49-year-old woman has multiple nodular lesions ranging from a few millimeters to several centimeters in size in the liver on CT imaging. Biopsy of a mass shows multiple areas of fibrotic lesions. The tumor cells are elongated and cytoplasms are vacuolated. What is the diagnosis?
    A. Leiomyosarcoma
    B. Cholangiocarcinoma
    C. Angiosarcoma
    D. Epithelioid hemangioendothelioma
    E. Adenocarcinoma

38. Which of the following syndrome presents with jaundice of > 20 mg/dL plasma bilirubin and kernicterus?
    A. Budd–Chiari syndrome
    B. Gilbert syndrome
    C. Crigler–Najjar Type 1 syndrome
    D. Crigler–Najjar Type 2 syndrome
    E. Physiological neonatal jaundice

Answers and Explanations

1. Answer: C. Prolonged prothrombin time

   Indicators of liver function are prothrombin time, hypoalbuminemia, and bilirubin. Laboratory findings in cirrhosis are elevated bilirubin, hypoalbuminemia, and elevated prothrombin time (PT). These findings are signs of inadequate liver function resulting in poor prognosis in cirrhotic patients. Partial thromboplastin time (PTT), PT, and INR are tests for identifying and monitoring coagulopathy. A high prothrombin time (PT) signifies serious liver damage and is an important prognostic indicator in patients with cirrhosis.

2. Answer: A. Acetaminophen

   Acetaminophen is safe when taken at therapeutic doses which is usually 4000 mg every day in 24 h.

   Overdose of acetaminophen causes hepatocellular necrosis with inflammation which sometimes can be fatal. Factors which influence hepatotoxicity include chronic alcohol ingestion, malnutrition, older age, genetic polymorphisms and medications that affect CYP2E1 enzyme.

3. Answer: B. Alpha-1 antitrypsin deficiency

   Alpha-1 antitrypsin (AAT) deficiency is a protein-folding disorder because of the deficiency of a serine protease inhibitor in which improper folded AAT pro-

teins aggregate in the hepatocytes. There are hepatic changes due to inflammation and fibrosis. Patients experience hepatomegaly and cirrhosis. There is an increased risk of hepatocellular carcinoma. AAT deficiency leads to alveolar destruction and predisposes patients to panacinar emphysema in adults prior to age 50 years.

4. Answer: C. Liver

   There are different isoenzymes of LDH (LDH-1 to LDH-5). LDH-4 and LDH-5 are found in liver and skeletal muscle. Laboratory findings of LDH-5 greater than LDH-4 indicate that there is liver damage which may include cirrhosis and hepatitis.

5. Answer: A. Primary sclerosing cholangitis (PSC)

   Primary sclerosing cholangitis (PSC) is common in males between 25 and 60 years range. Laboratory diagnosis shows an elevated alkaline phosphatase. There is progressive fibrosis of both intra and extrahepatic bile ducts. The multifocal beading pattern of biliary strictures seen on ERCP is diagnostic. Histologically, liver biopsy shows a mixed inflammatory infiltrate with "onion-skinning" of interlobular bile ducts, and bile ductular proliferation. Majority of patients are associated with ulcerative colitis. There is also an increased incidence of cholangiocarcinoma. Certain HLA haplotypes, HLA-B8, and HLA-DR3 have been associated with PSC. There are no effective pharmacologic treatments, and most patients will need a liver transplant.

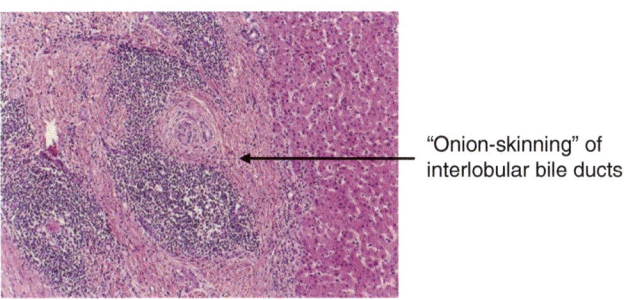

"Onion-skinning" of interlobular bile ducts

6. Answer: B. Metastatic liver disease

   Metastatic liver disease is the most common neoplasm of the liver in adults. It is more common than hepatocellular carcinoma. Common primary sites are colon, breast, lung, pancreas, and ovary. Patients usually present with hepatomegaly. Imaging studies show multiple hypodense masses.

7. Answer: C. Hepatocellular carcinoma

   Hepatocellular carcinoma (HCC) is common in older patients with a history of cirrhosis or infection with Hepatitis B or C. HCC mimics normal liver cells. There may be a trabeculae-cord like pattern or pseudo glands with a single layer of tumor cells and dilated bile canaliculi. Tumor cells are polygonal with eosinophilic cytoplasm. They show mild atypia and a higher nuclear to cytoplasmic ratio. Alpha-fetoprotein is a common marker for HCC and serum values are elevated.

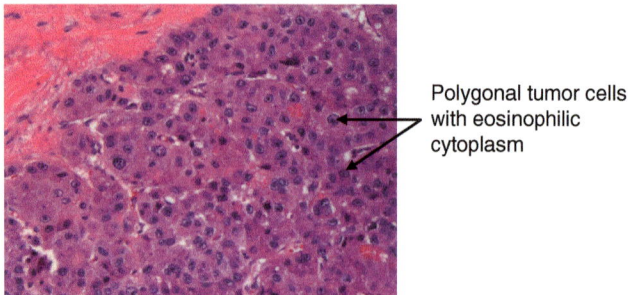

Polygonal tumor cells with eosinophilic cytoplasm

8. Answer: C. Mononuclear inflammatory cells, swollen hepatocytes, and bile plugs in canaliculi

    Viral hepatitis is caused by different hepatotropic. Most common of these viruses are Hepatitis A, Hepatitis B, and Hepatitis C. Common clinical manifestations are nausea, malaise, abdominal pain, and jaundice. The clinical course is usually similar in acute hepatitis caused by different hepatotropic viruses.

9. Answer: C. Primary biliary cholangitis

    Primary biliary cholangitis (PBC) is commonly seen in middle-aged females between the ages of 40 and 60 years. PBC is an autoimmune disease due to autoimmune destruction of the intrahepatic bile ducts and cholestasis. Clinical manifestations include severe pruritus (may be severe at night), hepatosplenomegaly, and xanthomatous lesions in the eyelids or in the skin. Laboratory findings show elevated alkaline phosphatase. 80–90% of the patients have AMA (anti-mitochondrial antibodies) in the serum. Cholangiopancreatography shows bile duct wall thickening, and dilatation of intra- and extrahepatic bile ducts. Primary biliary cholangitis (PBC) is similar to primary biliary cirrhosis (PBC) with common clinical manifestations. Associated autoimmune diseases such as Hashimoto's thyroiditis, Sjogren syndrome, scleroderma, and Raynaud's syndrome may be present. Primary biliary cholangitis (PBC) is a premalignant condition.

10. Answer: A. Liver

    Liver is a common site of metastatic spread after lymph nodes. Most of the metastasis in liver originate from colon, pancreas, stomach, esophagus, breast, lung, gallbladder, uterus, kidney, melanoma, and urinary bladder. Clinically, hepatomegaly is the most common finding besides signs and symptoms attributable to cancer in general and to the primary cancer. Jaundice occurs when the biliary system is invaded or obstructed. Ascites may form a non-specific late event. Unlike in HCC, the liver usually is not cirrhotic, and signs caused by portal hypertension are absent. For diagnosis, there is an increasing list of tumor markers, such as CEA, CA19–9, CA175, AFP. Perhaps CEA is the most frequently tested, and it is useful not only in disease diagnosis but also in the assessment of therapy and progression of disease.

11. Answer: C. Alcoholic fatty liver

    Alcoholic fatty liver is associated with significant drinking history. Laboratory findings show AST:ALT greater than 2:1. In alcoholic fatty liver, there is deposition of fat in hepatocytes, which is particularly seen in centrilobular region. Light microscopy shows macrovesicular steatosis, ballooned hepatocytes, and Mallory bodies. Mallory bodies are damaged cytokeratin filaments and are seen as eosinophilic inclusions within the hepatocytes.

12. Answer: A. Cirrhosis of liver

    Cirrhosis is a chronic disease of the liver in which destruction with the regeneration of liver cells occurs. There is a diffuse increase in fibrous tissue that leads to disorganization of the lobular architecture. Clinically, this leads to portal hypertension and complications depending on the stage of disease. Patients with cirrhosis show triad of parenchymal necrosis, regeneration, and scarring. Infiltration of portal zones with leukocytes, mononuclear cells, or plasma cells may represent inflammation associated with initial injury, a response to continued necrosis, or part of the reparative process. The morphological classification characterizes the gross appearance of the liver (micronodular, macronodular and mixed cirrhosis). Micronodular cirrhosis is characterized by the uniformity of the size of the nodules, virtually all of which are less than 3 mm in diameter. These micronodules lack a normal lobular organization and are surrounded by fibrous tissue. In micronodular cirrhosis, there is variation in nodular size, but most nodules are greater than 3 mm in diameter.

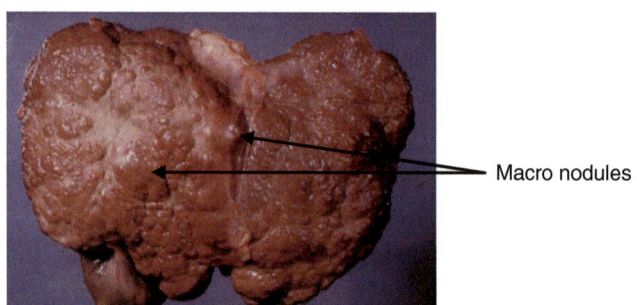

Macro nodules

13. Answer: E. Hepatitis B (HBV) and Hepatitis C (HCV)

    HCC (Hepatocellular carcinoma) is a malignant tumor of the liver. Numerous epidemiological and biological studies have suggested an important role of HBV infection in hepatocarcinogenesis. HCV is transmitted not only by blood transfusion but also by poorly understood routes and causes chronic hepatitis. In due course of time, cirrhosis develops in such patients with significant risk of hepatocellular carcinoma (HCC).

14. Answer: C Hepatitis D (delta agent)

HDV is recognized as a distinct, defective, but highly infectious hepatitis agent. HDV antigen could be identified in the hepatocytes of patients with chronic hepatitis B suggest an intimate linkage of HDV and HBV. Hepatitis D virus (HDV) is a defective, pathogenetic RNA virus, which requires Hepatitis B virus to complete its cycle in human liver cells. It causes symptoms only in hepatitis B positive persons.

15. Answer: A. Acute cholecystitis

The common complication of cholelithiasis is acute cholecystitis (AC). 90–95% of acute cholecystitis is due to cholelithiasis. Acalculous cholecystitis is an acute inflammation without gallstones accounts for 5–10% of the cases. Patients present with fever, nausea, vomiting, and pain in the upper right side of the quadrant. Laboratory findings show leukocytosis and mild elevations in liver function tests. Acalculous cholecystitis is common in critically ill patients. Common causes are sepsis, severe burns, immunosuppression, burns, and trauma. Acute cholecystitis may require emergency surgery.

16. Answer: B. Chronic cholecystitis

Chronic cholecystitis causes thickening of gallbladder due to repeated attacks of acute cholecystitis. Ultrasound shows shrunken, fibrosed gallbladder. Light microscopy shows varying degree of mucosal inflammation, subepithelial and subserosal fibrosis. Rokitansky-sinuses (glandular structures deep in the wall) may be present. Porcelain gallbladder is associated with chronic cholecystitis and may be detected on abdominal imaging as a rim of calcium deposits outlining the bladder. There is an increased risk of gallbladder carcinoma in patients with porcelain bladder.

17. Answer: B. Hepatic adenoma

Liver cell adenoma/hepatic adenoma had been a rare tumor until the introduction of oral contraceptives. It is most common in women in their reproductive years, ages 15–45. Grossly, hepatic adenomas are well demarcated, occasionally encapsulated, yellow and tan. Most of the adenomas have a fairly homogeneous appearance. Histologically, adenomas consist of tumor cells arranged in a cord pattern. The large cells have a pale cytoplasm because of glycogen or fat accumulation. The tumor is found incidentally in 5–10% of the cases. Patients present with acute abdominal pain caused by hemorrhage in about 30–40%. Regression and regressive enlargement of adenomas after withdrawal of oral contraceptives have been reported. Acute abdominal catastrophe can only be treated by emergency surgery.

18. Answer: A. Cholesterolosis

Cholesterolosis is characterized by abnormal accumulation of cholesterol esters and triglycerides in the mucosa and submucosa of the gallbladder. Much of the cholesterol is found in histiocytes, giving them a foamy appearance. Aggregates of these foamy cells are present on the top of mucosal ridges and are visible to the naked eye as yellowish, pinpoint spots or nodules. Many of these nodules are less than 1 mm in diameter. The nodules in about one third of cases are larger and polypoid in appearance. When these spots/nodules are diffusely distributed over the mucosa, they simulate the surface of a strawberry, hence the term strawberry gallbladder. These cholesterol polyps may break off and become a nidus for gallstone formation.

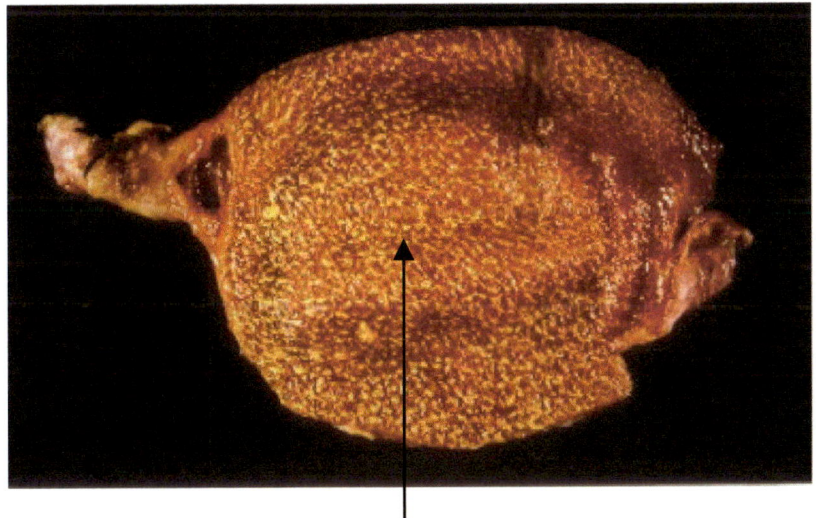

Cholesterolosis

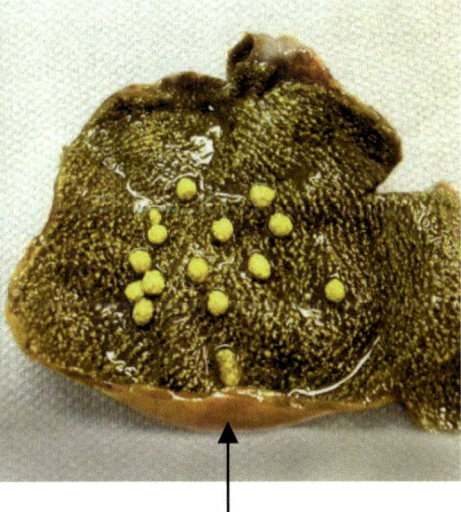

Strawberry gallbladder

19. Answer: B. Cholangiocarcinoma

    Cholangiocarcinoma arises from intra- and extrahepatic bile ducts. Cholangiocarcinoma is a known complication of primary sclerosing cholangitis. Other predisposing diseases which can cause cholangiocarcinoma include fibropolycystic liver disease and infection with liver flukes (*Clonorchis sinensis*). Some other risk factors include the use of anabolic steroids, Caroli's disease, Thorotrast, congenital hepatic fibrosis. On gross examination, there is a tree like mass that grows along the biliary system.

20. Answer: A. Entamoeba histolytica

    The term amoebiasis signifies infection by the protozoan parasite, *Entamoeba histolytica*. Amoeba reaches the liver through the portal blood. Most amoebic abscesses are found in the right lobe of the liver. The right lobe is affected more often than the left lobe because it has a larger volume. The right lobe also receives the venous drainage from the cecum and ascending colon, parts of the bowel commonly affected by amoebiasis. Amoebic liver abscesses are well demarcated lesions. They contain yellow-brown fluid that later retains classic orange-brown anchovy sauce. The fluid consists of necrotic liver tissue mixed with the blood.

21. Answer: A. Cavernous hemangioma

    Cavernous hemangioma is the most common benign mesenchymal tumor of the liver. They are also known as capillary hepatic hemangiomas. This tumor occurs at any age but are they mostly seen in adults. They are usually asymptomatic and are incidental found on imaging. Grossly, hepatic hemangioma is a well-demarcated, reddish tumor ranging in size from a few millimeters to more than 20 cm. Most of the tumors are solitary, but multiple lesions may also be present. Histologically, the tumor is composed of irregular vascular channels lined by endothelial cells surrounded by fibrous stroma of low cellularity. The entire tumor sometimes is replaced by dense, often hyalinized tissue.

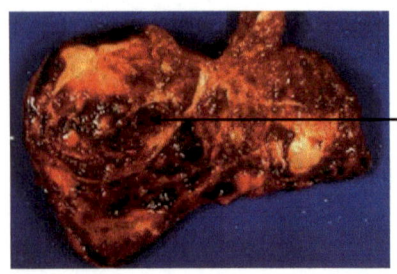

Hepatic hemangioma: areas of focal hemorrhage and fibrosis

22. Answer: C. Adenocarcinoma of gallbladder

    The most common cancer of the biliary tract is the carcinoma of the gallbladder. It is more common in women between sixth and seven decades of life. Gallstones are found in 60–90% of the patients.

Carcinoma of the gallbladder is an infiltrative lesion that eventually involves the whole organ. Histologically, 85% of the carcinoma of gallbladder are adenocarcinomas. The remainder comprises undifferentiated carcinomas, squamous cell carcinoma, and adenoacanthoma. Patient usually present with intermittent pain in the upper abdomen, weight loss, anorexia, nausea, and vomiting. About 50% of the patients present with jaundice and palpable abdominal mass. Carcinoma of the gallbladder is a lethal disease and 5 -year survival rate is 1–3%.

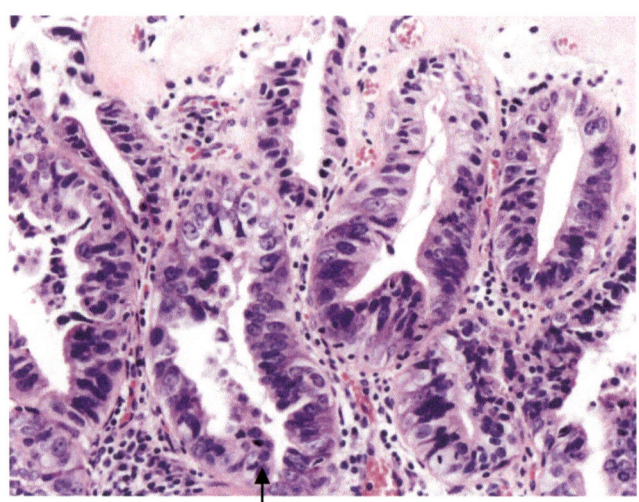

Adenocarcinoma Gallbladder

23. Answer: B. Angiosarcoma of the liver

    Angiosarcoma, the most common malignant mesenchymal tumor of the liver, is derived from endothelial cells. Peak age incidence is in the sixth and seven decades and a male/female ratio of 3:1. Many hepatic angiosarcomas are causatively related to polyvinyl chloride, thorotrast, and arsenic. Other important factors include external radiation, copper, hemochromatosis, steroids, and phenelzine. Grossly, it is various-size hemorrhagic tumor. Histologically, angiosarcoma is characterized by two cell types: spindle-shaped and polyhedral cells. There are spindle shaped tumor cells that show both sinusoidal and solid growths. Liver cords are markedly atrophic.

24. Answer: D. Physiologic jaundice of the newborn

    Transient elevation of plasma bilirubin is a common occurrence during the neonatal period. 97% of the healthy full-term infants manifest hyperbilirubinemia (unconjugated) of more than 1 mg/dL. 5% of newborn infants become jaundiced with hyperbilirubinemia more than 5 mg/dL. This physiological jaundice is multifactorial, resulting from the contributions of accelerated erythrocyte degradation caused by the turnover of fetal red blood cells, relative hepatic immaturity of bilirubin conjugation and increased enterohepatic circulation. Plasma bilirubin returns to normal levels of less than 1 mg/dL within the first 10 days of life in most cases.

25. Answer: A. Portal vein thrombosis

Portal vein thrombosis (PVT) causes an interruption of the normal blood flow in the portal vein (PV), causing portal hypertension. The signs of portal hypertension include esophageal varices and splenic enlargement. Ascites is uncommon. Some of the common causes of PVT are thrombophilic conditions, tumor invasion, and liver cirrhosis.

26. Answer: A. Gilbert syndrome

Gilbert syndrome is an inherited disorder of bilirubin glucuronidation. It is a benign condition. There is a mutation in UGT1A1, in which production of UDP glucuronyl transferase is decreased, the enzymes that mediate the glucuronidation of various compounds. There may be recurrent episodes of jaundice with no apparent disease. It may be triggered by fasting, dehydration, physical exertion, hemolysis, febrile illness, stress, and menses. No specific therapy is required for these patients.

27. Answer: D. Gallbladder adenocarcinoma

Porcelain bladder is a manifestation of chronic gallbladder inflammation in chronic cholecystitis. Majority of patients have associated gallstones. Patients may be asymptomatic or present with right upper quadrant abdominal pain. Findings of porcelain gallbladder are detected incidentally on abdominal imaging. The porcelain gallbladder is used to describe brittle consistency and bluish discoloration of the gallbladder. Gross examination shows a bluish, brittle with thickened gallbladder wall. Histologically, there is a broad continuous band of calcifications in the muscularis. Mucosa shows several punctate calcifications. There is an increased risk of adenocarcinoma in porcelain gallbladder.

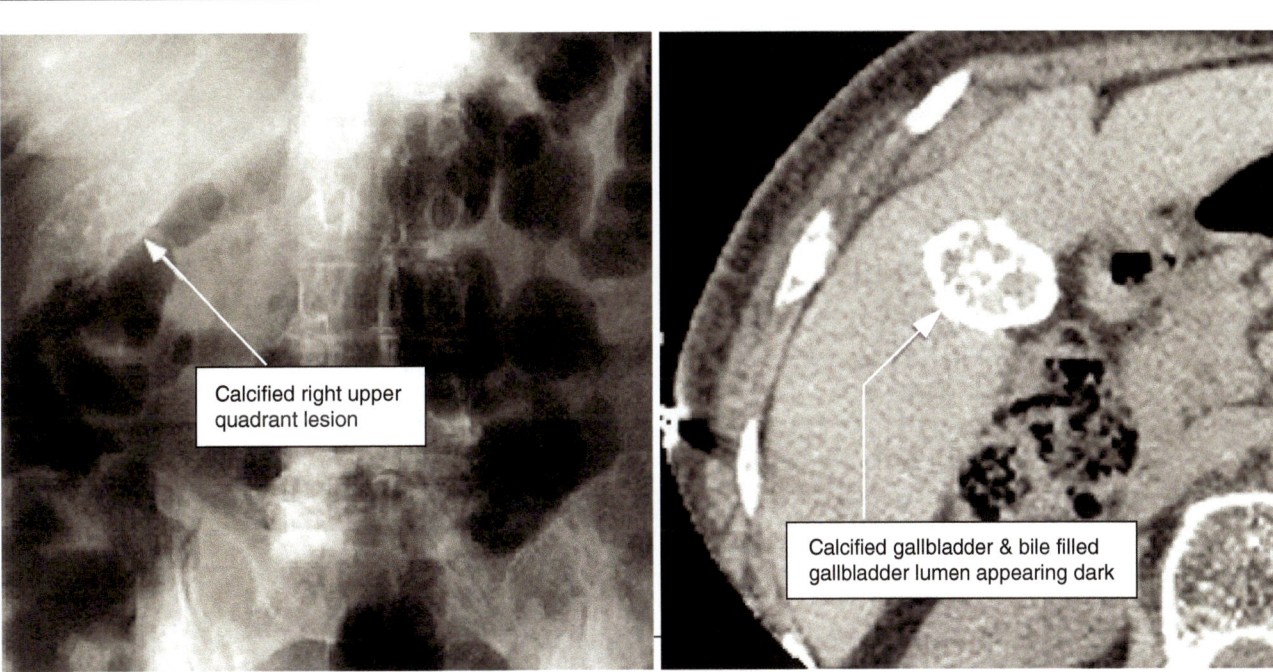

28. Answer: B. Alcoholic hepatitis

Alcoholic hepatitis is a form of toxic liver injury associated chronic excess ethanol consumption. Alcohol-induced liver lesions are fatty liver, alcoholic hepatitis, cirrhosis, and hepatocellular carcinoma. Alcoholic hepatitis represents a serious but often reversible stage in the disease process. Association with some degree of fatty liver and cirrhosis is present in over half the cases. Important features essential for the histologic diagnosis of alcoholic hepatitis include liver cell damage (ballooning degeneration), inflammatory cell infiltration, predominantly polymorphonuclear leukocytes, fibrosis both pericellular, and periventricular (centrilobular). Mallory body formation varies with the severity of the disease. Clinically, there is jaundice. Laboratory findings show serum bilirubin of more than 3 mg/dL and an AST: ALT ratio greater than >1.5 (elevated levels of enzymes not exceeding 400 IU).

29. Answer: D. Budd–Chiari syndrome

Budd–Chiari syndrome arises by thrombotic or nonthrombotic occlusion of hepatic veins and/or the intra-or hepatic suprahepatic inferior vena cava. There is an increase in sinusoidal pressure leading to clinical manifestations of hepatomegaly, ascites and abdominal pain.

Prognosis is poor in untreated patients. Progressive liver failure results in 3 months to 3 years.

30. Answer: D. Fibrolamellar hepatocellular carcinoma

The patient's clinical presentation and imaging results are suggestive for fibrolamellar hepatocellular carcinoma (FLHCC). Fibrolamellar carcinoma is associated with prolonged survival, and occurs in young non-cirrhotic patients. FLHCC demonstrates large polygonal and eosinophilic tumor cells with enlarged nucleoli and nuclei. The tumor cells are separated into cords by intervening parallel layers of prominent fibrous tissue. AFP serum levels are not elevated.

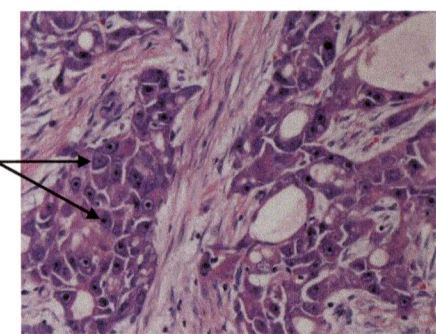

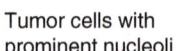
Tumor cells with prominent nucleoli

31. Answer: D. Hepatitis B infection

Intravenous drug use carries a high risk for hepatitis B and C viral infection. Ground glass hepatocytes are found in chronic hepatitis B virus. These hepatocytes have eosinophilic, homogeneous cytoplasm. Ground glass hepatocytes usually surround normal granular hepatocytes. In chronic hepatitis, there is a significant inflammation surrounding portal triad. There is also an increased risk of hepatocellular carcinoma (HCC) with persistent inflammation and HBV viremia.

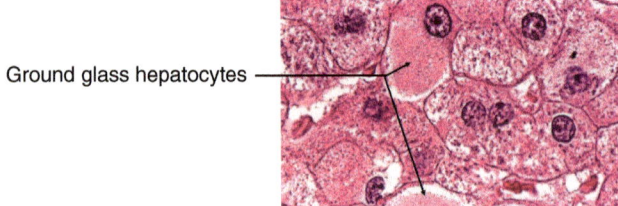
Ground glass hepatocytes

32. Answer: A. Councilman body

Apoptosis is a term used to describe the death of individual cells. In acute liver hepatitis, liver biopsy shows panlobular lymphocytic infiltrate with areas of hepatocyte necrosis. Necrotic hepatocytes present as ballooning hepatocytes. Hepatocytes may also undergo cytotoxic T cell-mediated apoptosis. Apoptotic hepatocytes appear as round, acidophilic bodies and referred to as

Councilman bodies. They are found in various forms of hepatitis including acute viral hepatitis.

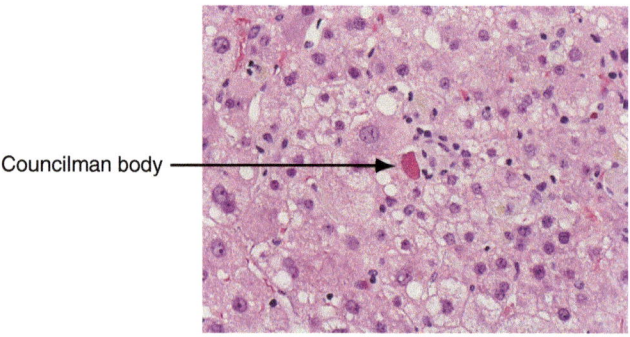
Councilman body

33. Answer: B. Primary sclerosing cholangitis (PSC)

Cholangiocarcinoma is a known complication of long standing primary sclerosing cholangitis. PSC is associated with chronic biliary tract inflammations. PSC in combination with k-ras and c-myc activation plays a key role in the pathogenesis of this cancer.

34. Answer: B. Hepatoblastoma

The most common malignant liver tumor in children is hepatoblastoma. 90% of these tumors occur before the age of 5 years. Incidence in boys is twice that in girls. The associations with Beckwith–Wiedemann syndrome, down syndrome, and familial adenomatous polyposis (FAP) have been demonstrated. Serum AFP is nearly always elevated. Histology shows trabeculae 2–3 cells thick with low nuclear-to-cytoplasmic ratio, small nucleoli, and minimal pleomorphism. The cytoplasm is finely granular and eosinophilic or clear, reflecting variable amounts of glycogen and lipids. This imparts a characteristic light and dark pattern at low magnification. The two subtypes of differentiation are commonly seen; epithelial and mixed epithelial/mesenchymal type. It is usually fatal if not surgically resected.

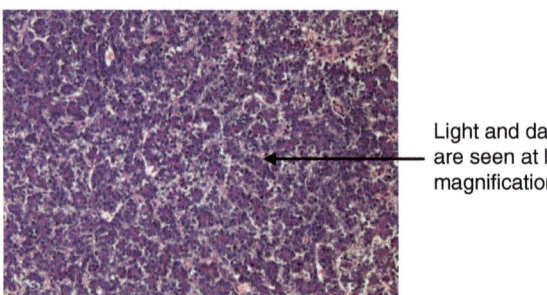
Light and dark areas are seen at low magnification

35. Answer: B. Anti-HBs

Different serological markers are used to identify different phases of HBV infection and to determine whether a person is immune to HBV as a result of vaccination. Human B surface antibody (anti-Hbs) is positive in people who have been successfully vaccinated against

Hepatitis B. HBsAg appears in serum usually between 1 and 10 weeks after exposure to Hepatitis B virus. HBsAg becomes undetectable after 4–6 months. In Chronic HBV infection, HBsAg is positive for more than 6 months. Hepatitis B core antigen (HBcAg) is found in infected hepatocytes. IgM anti-HBc detection is as an indication of acute HBV infection. IgM anti-HBc can be found in serum up to 2 years after acute infection. Permanent immunity is conferred by anti-HBs.

36. Answer: A. Alcoholic hepatitis

Mallory bodies are found in alcoholic hepatitis. Mallory body formation varies with the severity of the disease. Histologically, Mallory's bodies appear as irregular aggregates of purplish red material (as seen with H&E stain), which typically are intracytoplasmic and perinuclear in location. In the centrilobular area, they are characteristic but not pathognomonic of alcoholic hepatitis.

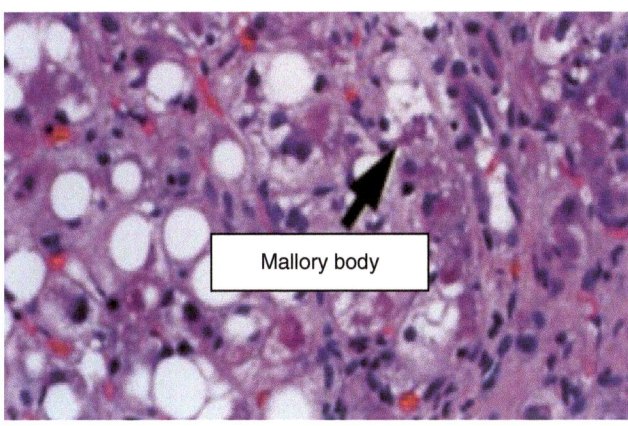

Mallory body

37. Answer: D. Epithelioid hemangioendothelioma

Epithelioid hemangioendothelioma is relatively new disease entity in the liver. The male/female ratio is about 1:2. The mean age is 50 years. The neoplasm shows a myxoid stroma, numerous signet ring type cells, and intracytoplasmic vacuoles. It tends to occlude portal and hepatic vein branches. These tumors can be confused with steatohepatitis or adenocarcinomas. These are positive for D2–40, CD31, and CD34. Sometimes this tumor is mistaken for cholangiocarcinoma or mistaken adenocarcinoma because vacuolated tumor cells look like mucin-producing cancer cells and there is dense fibrosis.

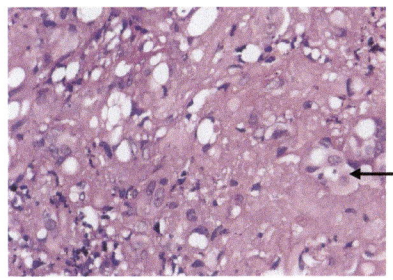

Vacuolated tumor cells look like mucin-producing cancer cells

38. Answer: C. Crigler–Najjar type 1 syndrome

Crigler–Najjar syndrome is subdivided into two entities: type 1 is extremely rare and is characterized by severe with severe neurologic impairment. Type II patients have lower plasma bilirubin concentrations with no neurologic damage. The primary metabolic defect in Crigler–Najjar type 1 syndrome involves the conjugation of bilirubin. Bilirubin-UGT activity in liver biopsy specimen reveals complete absence of bilirubin glucuronide formation. Plasma bilirubin levels generally exceed 20 mg/dL, with all the pigment in the unconjugated form.

Bibliography

1. Harrison MF. The misunderstood coagulopathy of liver disease: a review for the acute setting. West J Emerg Med. 2018;19(5):863–71.
2. Zamzami MA, et al. Amelioration of CCL4-induced hepatotoxicity in rabbits by *Lepidium sativum* seeds. Evid Based Complement Alternat Med. 2019;2019:7234.
3. Mitchell EL, Khan Z. Liver disease in alpha-1 antitrypsin deficiency: current approaches and future directions. Curr Pathobiol Rep. 2017;5(3):243–52.
4. Lactate Dehydrogenase Test. https://www.healthline.com/health/lactate-dehydrogenase-test. Accessed 26 May 2017.
5. Kowdley KV, et al. Primary sclerosing cholangitis in adults: clinical manifestations and diagnosis. Waltham: UptoDate; 2019.
6. Fletcher J, Chun C. What to know about liver metastases. Waltham: The American Cancer Society; 2019.
7. Schwartz JM, et al. Clinical features and diagnosis of hepatocellular carcinoma. Waltham: UptoDate; 2019.
8. Meissner HC. Alphabet soup: differentiating viruses that cause hepatitis. Itasca: AAP Publications; 2018.
9. Kancherla V, et al. Genomic analysis revealed new oncogenic signatures in TP53-mutant hepatocellular carcinoma. Front Genet. 2018;9:2.
10. Torruellas C, French SW, Medici V. Diagnosis of alcoholic liver disease. World J Gastroenterol. 2014;20(33):11684–99.
11. Sharma B, John S. Hepatic cirrhosis. Treasure Island: StatPearls; 2019.
12. Mani SKK, Andrisani O. Hepatitis B virus-associated hepatocellular carcinoma and hepatic cancer stem cells. Genes (Basel). 2018;9(3):137.
13. Axley P, Ahmed Z, Ravi S, Singal AK. Hepatitis C virus and hepatocellular carcinoma: a narrative review. J Clin Transl Hepatol. 2018;6(1):79–84.
14. Mentha N, Clément S, Negro F, Alfaiatea D. A review on hepatitis D: from virology to new therapies. J Adv Res. 2019;17:3–15.
15. Escartin A, et al. Acute cholecystitis in very elderly patients: disease management, outcomes, and risk factors for complications. Surg Res Pract. 2019;2019:9709242.
16. Jones MW, Ferguson T. Chronic cholecystitis. Treasure Island: StatPearls; 2019.
17. Varadarajulu S, et al. Porcelain gallbladder. Waltham: UptoDate; 2019.
18. Healthline. Cholesterolosis of the gallbladder: definition and treatment. San Francisco: Healthline; 2018.
19. Shiao M-S, et al. Emergence of intrahepatic cholangiocarcinoma: how high-throughput technologies expedite the solutions for a rare cancer type. Front Genet. 2018;9:309.
20. Prakash V, Oliver TI. Amebic liver abscess. Treasure Island: StatPearls; 2019.

21. Evans J, Sabih DE. Cavernous hepatic hemangiomas. Treasure Island: StatPearls; 2019.
22. Pandya B, et al. Study of histopathological spectrum of cholecystectomy specimens received in a government hospital. New York: Springer; 2019.
23. American Cancer Society. What is liver cancer? Atlanta: American Cancer Society; 2019.
24. Wong RJ, et al. Pathogenesis and etiology of unconjugated hyperbilirubinemia in the newborn. Waltham: UptoDate; 2019.
25. Mantaka A, et al. Portal vein thrombosis in cirrhosis: diagnosis, natural history, and therapeutic challenges. Ann Gastroenterol. 2018;31(3):315–29.
26. Chandrasekar VT, John S. Gilbert syndrome. Treasure Island: StatPearls; 2019.
27. Wells ML, Venkatesh SK. Congestive hepatopathy. Abdom Radiol (New York). 2018;43(8):2037–51.
28. Axley P, Russ K, Singal AK. Severe alcoholic hepatitis: atypical presentation with markedly elevated alkaline phosphatase. J Clin Transl Hepatol. 2017;5(4):414–5.
29. Roy PK, Anand BS. Budd–Chiari Syndrome. New York: Springer; 2018.
30. Samji NS, Anand BS. Viral hepatitis. Treasure Island: StatPearls; 2017.
31. Peters MG. Hepatitis B virus infection: what is current and new. Top Antivir Med. 2019;26(4):112–6.
32. Krishna M. Patterns of necrosis in liver disease. Clin Liver Dis. 2017;10(2):53.

Pancreas

13

Multiple Choice Questions

1. Which of the following is the most common islet cell tumor of the pancreas?
   A. Gastrinoma
   B. Alpha cell tumor
   C. Beta cell tumor
   D. Vipoma
   E. Somatostatinoma

2. Which of the following is NOT a feature of type 1 diabetes mellitus?
   A. Decrease in the number and size of islets
   B. Mild acinar atrophy
   C. Pheochromocytoma
   D. Amyloid deposits in islets
   E. Insulitis

3. A middle-aged man presents to the emergency department with stabbing epigastric abdominal pain radiating to the back. Laboratory findings show elevation of serum amylase and lipase. What is the diagnosis?
   A. Acute cholecystitis
   B. Perforated peptic ulcer
   C. Acute pancreatitis
   D. Occlusion of mesenteric vessels with bowel infarction
   E. Acute peritonitis

4. Migratory thrombophlebitis is associated with which one of the following diseases?
   A. Diabetes mellitus
   B. Cholangitis
   C. Acute pancreatitis
   D. Chronic relapsing pancreatitis
   E. Pancreatic carcinoma

5. A 55-year-old male presents with abdominal pain. He does not consume alcohol. There is a family history of pancreatic cancer. Endoscopic retrograde cholangiopancreatography (ERCP) shows normal appearing pancreatic duct. Biopsy shows papillary formation with tall columnar mucinous cells with mild, focal nuclear abnormalities including nuclear crowding, hyperchromatism, and pseudostratification. What is the diagnosis?
   A. Pancreatic adenocarcinoma
   B. Squamous metaplasia of the pancreas
   C. Pancreatic intraepithelial neoplasia (PanIN)
   D. Intraductal papillary mucinous neoplasm
   E. Chronic pancreatitis

6. Which of the following disease is associated with HLA DR 3 & 4?
   A. Type 1-Juvenile onset diabetes mellitus
   B. Type 2-adult onset diabetes mellitus
   C. Diabetes insipidus
   D. Syndrome of inappropriate antidiuretic hormone
   E. Zollinger–Ellison syndrome

7. Hyperglycemia, anion gap metabolic acidosis, increased blood ketone levels, leukocytosis are seen in which of the following disease?
   A. Diabetes insipidus
   B. Syndrome of inappropriate antidiuretic hormone
   C. Acute pancreatitis
   D. Lactic acidosis
   E. Diabetic ketoacidosis

8. What is true about insulinoma?
   A. β cell tumor
   B. G cell tumor
   C. α cell tumor
   D. δ cell tumor
   E. It is type of Vipoma

9. A middle-aged patient comes to the emergency department with symptoms of hyperglycemia, anemia, skin rash and confusion. What is the diagnosis?
   A. Insulinoma
   B. Gastrinoma
   C. Glucagonoma
   D. Somatostatinoma
   E. Vipoma

V. K. Kohli et al., *Comprehensive Multiple-Choice Questions in Pathology*, https://doi.org/10.1007/978-3-031-08767-7_13

10. A 48-year-old woman presents with a 4 cm mass in the body of the pancreas. Histological examinations shows features of microcystic adenoma of the pancreas. This lesion is associated with which syndrome?
    A. Neurofibromatosis, type 2
    B. Cowden syndrome
    C. Gorlin syndrome
    D. Von Hippe–Lindau syndrome
    E. Tuberous sclerosis

11. Autoimmune insulitis with progressive beta cell loss is the most common cause of which disease?
    A. Type 2 diabetes mellitus
    B. Diabetes insipidus
    C. Carcinoid syndrome
    D. Zollinger–Ellison syndrome
    E. Type 1 diabetes mellitus

12. A 5-year-old child presents with steatorrhea, failure to thrive, bulky, foul smelling oily stool. There is also history of recurrent pneumonia. What is the diagnosis?
    A. Primary ciliary dyskinesia
    B. Cystic fibrosis
    C. Shwachman diamond syndrome
    D. Severe combined immunodeficiency
    E. Alpha1 antitrypsin deficiency

13. A male patient aged 75 years with a history of smoking, presents with symptoms of abdominal pain, obstructive jaundice. CT scan of abdomen shows a small mass in the head of the pancreas. What is the diagnosis?
    A. Chronic pancreatitis
    B. Lymphoma
    C. Pancreatic carcinoma
    D. Colonic neuroendocrine carcinoma
    E. Duodenal adenocarcinoma

14. Pancreatic islet amyloid deposition is seen in which of the following medical condition?
    A. Type 1 diabetes mellitus
    B. Diabetes insipidus
    C. Carcinoid syndrome
    D. Type 2 diabetes mellitus
    E. Zollinger–Ellison syndrome

15. Pancreatic pseudocysts are the potential complication of which of the following condition involving the pancreas?
    A. Acute pancreatitis
    B. Pancreatic adenocarcinoma
    C. Pancreatic abscess
    D. Insulinoma of pancreas
    E. Gastrinoma of pancreas

16. Hyperparathyroidism (e.g., hypercalcemia, constipation, kidney stones), pituitary tumors, and pancreatic endocrine tumors (e.g., gastrinoma) are seen in which of the following condition?
    A. Multiple endocrine neoplasia type 2A
    B. Multiple endocrine neoplasia type 2B
    C. Von Hippel–Lindau disease
    D. Vipomas
    E. Multiple endocrine neoplasia type 1

17. A 40-year-old man presents with watery diarrhea, mid epigastric pain for the last 1 month. Upper endoscopy shows distal duodenal ulcerations. Laboratory findings show elevated basal serum gastrin levels. What is the diagnosis?
    A. Antral G cell hyperplasia
    B. Retained antrum syndrome
    C. Autoimmune gastritis
    D. Zollinger–Ellison syndrome
    E. Enterochromaffin cell tumor

18. Recurrent intractable peptic ulcer disease suggests an underlying:
    A. Acinar cell carcinoma
    B. Adenocarcinoma of the pancreas
    C. Pancreatoblastoma
    D. Poorly differentiated neuroendocrine carcinoma
    E. Pancreatic neuroendocrine neoplasms (NENs)

19. Which of the following is correct regarding Hemoglobin A1c (HbA1c)?
    A. Measures average blood sugar for the past 1 month
    B. Measures average blood sugar for the past 3 months
    C. Measures average blood sugar for the past 6 months
    D. Measures average blood sugar for the past 12 months
    E. Hemoglobin A1c has no relation with diabetes mellitus

20. Relatively reduced insulin secretion and peripheral insulin resistance are the pathogenesis of which of the following medical condition?
    A. Adult onset diabetes mellitus
    B. Diabetes insipidus
    C. Syndrome of inappropriate antidiuretic hormone
    D. Juvenile onset diabetes mellitus
    E. Zollinger–Ellison syndrome

21. A middle-aged man history of consuming regular alcohol presents with epigastric pain, chronic diarrhea and weight loss. Abdominal X-ray is done which shows epigastric calcifications. What is the diagnosis?
    A. Autoimmune pancreatitis
    B. Pancreatic endocrine tumors
    C. Lymphoma
    D. Pancreatic adenocarcinoma
    E. Chronic alcoholic pancreatitis

22. A 2-year-old male child is drought to the pediatrician office for abdominal pain, vomiting, and yellow skin. On physical examination, the child is jaundiced and his abdomen is tender to palpation. Laboratory studies reveal elevated alpha-fetoprotein (AFP). What is the diagnosis?
    A. Pancreatoblastoma
    B. Hepatocellular carcinoma
    C. Pancreatic intraepithelial neoplasia
    D. Acinar cell carcinoma
    E. Pancreatic cystadenoma

Answers and Explanations

1. Answer: C. Beta cell tumor

   Beta cell tumors are the most common islet tumors of the pancreas. When functioning, they are also referred as insulinoma because they secrete insulin. Common clinical manifestation is fasting hypoglycemia. Insulinomas are usually benign and solitary. High serum insulin concentrations are present during an episode of hypoglycemia. Light microscopy shows the presence of amyloid in fibrovascular stroma adjacent to tumor cells.

2. Answer: D. Amyloid deposition in islets

   Type 1 diabetes mellitus (T1DM) is caused by the destruction of beta cells of the pancreas, resulting in insulin deficiency. Common signs and symptoms are polyuria, polydipsia, weight loss, and lethargy. Diabetic ketoacidosis may be the first presentation of T1DM. Amyloid deposition is usually seen in type 2 diabetes mellitus and not seen in type 1.

3. Answer: C. Acute pancreatitis

   Patients of acute pancreatitis usually present with an acute onset of severe epigastric pain, often radiating to back, fever, nausea, and vomiting. There is an abdominal tenderness to palpation. Laboratory findings show elevation in serum amylase or lipase three times or greater than the upper normal range. Common causes of acute pancreatitis are gall bladder stones and alcohol abuse. Pancreatitis due to alcohol abuse is indistinguishable from pancreatitis due to other causes.

4. Answer: E. Pancreatic carcinoma

   Migratory thrombophlebitis (i.e., Trousseau sign) may be the first presentation of pancreatic cancer. Majority of pancreatic cancers arise from the exocrine component of the pancreas.

5. Answer: C. Pancreatic intraepithelial neoplasia (PanIN)

   The patient has an incidental pancreatic mass identified on imaging. PanIN lesions generally involve the smaller pancreatic ducts, and represent the progression through a series of grades to the development of invasive pancreatic adenocarcinoma. They are classified as PanIN IA, IB, II, and III. Multiple genetic abnormalities are associated with increasing PanIN grades, including activation of K-ras oncogene, positive MUC1 expression, inactivation of tumor suppressor genes p16 and p53.

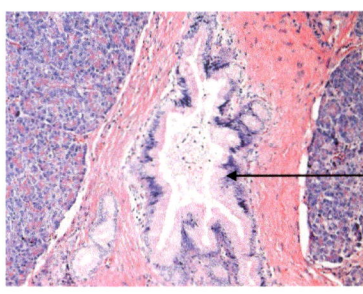

Papillary formation with tall columnar mucinous cells

6. Answer: A. Type I—Juvenile onset diabetes mellitus

   The HLA complex on chromosome 6 is the strongest genetic risk and accounts for approximately 40–50% of type 1 diabetes. The genetic determinants are polymorphisms of class II HLA genes which encode DQ and DR. The DR-DQ haplotypes conferring the highest risk are DR3 and DR4.

7. Answer: E. Diabetic ketoacidosis

   Diabetic ketoacidosis (DKA) is a condition that affects patients with type1 diabetes mellitus due to absolute insulin deficiency. Laboratory findings show hyperglycemia (blood glucose >200 mg/dL), increased blood ketones, anion gap metabolic acidosis. Venous pH is usually <7.3 with serum bicarbonate <15 mEq/L, and the presence of ketonuria. Diabetic ketoacidosis (DKA) is one the commonest causes of hospitalization leading to mortality, and morbidity in patients with type 1 diabetes mellitus.

8. Answer: A. β cell tumor

   Insulinoma is the most common type of islet cell tumor. This tumor produces insulin. Insulinomas are β cell tumors and are the most common cause of hypoglycemia resulting from endogenous hyperinsulinism. Approximately 90–95% of insulinomas are benign, and complete resection is the long-term cure with total resolution of preoperative symptoms.

9. Answer: C. Glucagonoma

   Glucagonoma is an α-islet cell tumor of pancreas. Common clinical manifestations are necrotizing migratory erythema (NME), diabetes mellitus, weight loss, and normocytic normochromic anemia. There may be depression and tendency to develop deep vein thrombosis. It is more common in women and is located in the distal portion of the pancreas. Glucagonoma has both trabecular and diffuse pattern of growth.

10. Answer: D. Von Hippel–Lindau syndrome

    A serous cystadenoma is a benign cystic neoplasm, generally located in the body or tail of the pancreas. It is mainly found in elderly. The multiloculated pattern, termed microcystic cystadenoma, is the most common. While most lesions arise sporadically, it is associated with Von Hippel–Lindau syndrome. Grossly, microcystic adenoma shows a sponge like appearance with a central stellate scar. Histologically, the lining cells demonstrate clearing due to glycogen.

11. Answer: E. Type I diabetes mellitus

    Diabetes type 1 is also known as insulin dependent diabetes. Peak age of onset is between 10 and 14 years. Progeny of affected individuals have 10% higher incidence. It is an autoimmune phenomenon in which insulin producing islets cells (beta cells) are destroyed by T cells of the immune system. CD4 and C8 cells infiltrate and also cause beta cell destruction. Autoantibodies (anti-islet cell, anti-insulin, and anti-insulin receptor) are found. There are one or more environmental triggering events which cause critical B cell mass and subclinical beta cell dysfunction. This process takes months and years before clinical type 1 diabetes mellitus develops.

12. Answer: B. Cystic fibrosis

Clinical features of cystic fibrosis (CF) in pancreatic disease are due to exocrine pancreatic insufficiency and cystic fibrosis related diabetes. In cystic fibrosis, there is a mutation in transmembrane conductance regulator (CFTR) protein. Dysfunctional CFTR causes thick, viscous secretions in the pancreas and lungs. Common manifestation is pancreatic insufficiency (PI). Insufficiency of the exocrine pancreas is present from birth in majority of patients. Defective pancreatic secretion, pancreatic duct obstruction, and distension due to viscous mucus and inflammation leads to fibrosis. Because of pancreatic insufficiency, patients are unable to absorb fat soluble vitamins. Patients present with steatorrhea, failure to thrive, frequent, bulky, foul smelling oily stools. The most important diagnostic test is sweat chloride testing. Approximately 25%of the cases develop cystic fibrosis related diabetes (CFRD) by 20 years of age.

13. Answer: C. Pancreatic carcinoma

Pancreatic adenocarcinoma occurs after the age of 50 years and median age at diagnosis in both sexes is after 65 years. Head of pancreas is the common site of pancreatic adenocarcinoma. Besides head, it can occur in the body and tail. Patients usually present with symptoms of anorexia, nausea, fatigue. Tumors of the head of pancreas produce obstructive jaundice due to the compression of common bile duct. Pancreatic cancers of the body present with mid-epigastric pain with radiation of pain to the back due to invasion of the nerves around the pancreas. Patients can also present with clinical jaundice and palpable gallbladder (Courvoisier sign). Physical examination can show hepatomegaly and ascites. Laboratory investigations show elevated bilirubin, dark urine, and pale stools. Imaging modalities including CT help in the diagnosis. CA19–9 antigen is an important tumor marker. Tobacco smoking is the most important risk factor. Other recognized risk factors are obesity, high alcohol consumption, chronic pancreatitis, diabetes, family history of pancreatic cancer. 5–10% are hereditary in nature. Common hereditary risk factors are hereditary pancreatitis, multiple endocrine neoplasia, hereditary nonpolyposis rectal cancer (HNPCC), familial adenomatous polyposis (FAP), Gardner syndrome, and Peutz–Jeghers syndrome. Majority of pancreatic cancers are adenocarcinomas of the ductal epithelium. Pancreatic carcinoma is a fatal disease and median survival time is 4–6 months.

14. Answer: D. Type 2 diabetes mellitus

Islet amyloid polypeptide (amylin) is deposited in insulin secretory granules in the beta cells of the pancreas. Amylin causes the inhibition of endogenous insulin secretion. Amylin may be involved in the pathogenesis of adult onset diabetes mellitus. Relative insulin deficiency and insulin resistance are key factors in type 2 diabetes. The most important risk factors are weight gain and decreased physical activity. Adult onset diabetes (type 2 diabetes mellitus) is a multifactorial disease with a lower incidence of autoantibodies than type 1.

15. Answer: A. Acute pancreatitis

The most common cystic lesions of the pancreas are pancreatic pseudocysts. They are the potential complications of pancreatitis. This event usually takes 4–6 weeks following the episode of acute pancreatitis. Besides acute and chronic pancreatitis, other causes may include pancreatic trauma and iatrogenic (post partial gastrectomy). In acute pancreatitis, proteolytic enzymes cause disruption of pancreatic duct structure and leakage of pancreatic juice into peripancreatic space. There is a severe inflammatory reaction which leads to encapsulation of the cysts by fibrosed granulation tissue. Radiologically, they are seen as fluid filled oval or round collections with a thick wall. The pseudocyst is commonly located in lesser sac, posterior to the stomach. They are not lined by epithelium. Pancreatic pseudocysts may regress on its own or interventions are required in selected cases.

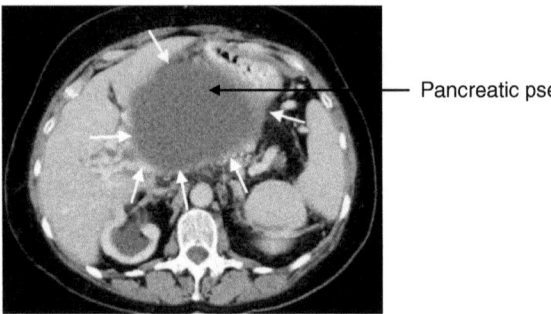

Pancreatic pseudocyst

16. Answer: E. Multiple endocrine neoplasia type 1

Multiple endocrine neoplasia type 1 (also called MEN1) is a rare heritable disorder. Tumors are usually found in parathyroid gland, anterior pituitary, and pancreatic islet cells. Enteropancreatic neuroendocrine tumors with malignant potential may be the primary life threatening manifestation of MEN1 as there is a treatment for hyperparathyroidism and pituitary disease. The most common manifestation of multiple endocrine neoplasia (MEN1) is multiple parathyroid tumors displaying almost 100% by age 40–50 years. The most common site of tumors (gastrinomas) is duodenum.

17. Answer: D. Zollinger–Ellison syndrome

Patient's high gastrin levels and distal duodenal ulcers on endoscopy are indicative of Zollinger–Ellison syndrome (ZES). Secretion of gastrin by duodenal or pancreatic neuroendocrine tumors causes Zollinger–Ellison syndrome. Zollinger–Ellison syndrome is common in men between the ages of 20 and 50. Chronic diarrhea results due to excess gastric acid which impairs intestinal epithelial cells and inactivation of pancreatic enzymes. Gastrin stimulates gastric acid secretion resulting in heartburn and development of peptic ulcers. Zollinger–Ellison syndrome is caused by gastrinomas located in pancreas, duodenum, and upper jejunum.

18. Answer: E. Pancreatic neuroendocrine neoplasms (NENs)

There are numerous pancreatic neuroendocrine neoplasms (NENs). Well differentiated endocrine tumors are gastrinoma, insulinoma, glucagonoma, somatostatinoma, and vipoma. Gastrinoma produces unregulated hypergastrinemia and Zollinger–Ellison syndrome. There is elevated serum gastrin levels and massive gastric acid hypersecretion leading to peptic ulcerations. Ulcers are frequently multiple.

19. Answer: B. Measures average blood sugar for the past 3 months

Hemoglobin A1c (HbA1c) is a type of hemoglobin bound to glucose. HbA1c is produced by nonenzymatic glycosylation of the N-terminal of the hemoglobin molecule. Hemoglobin A1c (HbA1c) provides the average blood sugar levels over the time of 3 months (lifespan of circulating red blood cells) and reflect how well diabetes is controlled. Higher blood glucose levels over the time of 3 months give increase in values of HbA1c. It is an important and essential test for patients with diabetes mellitus.

20. Answer: A. Adult onset diabetes mellitus

In type 2 diabetes mellitus, there is a combination of relatively reduced insulin secretion, peripheral insulin resistance, and excessive or inappropriate glucagon secretion. Majority of patients are asymptomatic. Patients may present polyuria, polydipsia, polyphagia, and weight loss. There may be lower extremity paresthesias and blurred vision. Obesity and decreased physical activity increase the risk of diabetes mellitus. There are some conditions which may accompany type 2 diabetes which include hypertension, high LDL, and low serum HDL concentrations.

21. Answer: E. Chronic alcoholic pancreatitis

Chronic alcoholic pancreatitis occurs in patients with regular history of alcohol use. Patients present with epigastric pain, weight loss, and chronic diarrhea. Pancreatic exocrine insufficiency results in malabsorption with chronic diarrhea. Abdominal imaging may show epigastric calcifications.

22. Answer: A. Pancreatoblastoma

Pancreatoblastoma occurs most frequently in males during infancy and childhood. It may be associated with Beckwith–Wiedemann syndrome or familial adenomatous polyposis. Histologically, it is a cellular tumor composed of sheets/nests of acini and squamoid corpuscles. Tumors exhibit mixed differentiation by immunohistochemical positivity for keratin, EMA, CEA, neuron-specific enolase, synaptophysin, lipase, alpha-1-antitrypsin, and chymotrypsin.

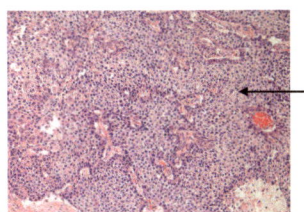

Tumor composed of sheets/nests of acini and squamoid corpuscles

Bibliography

1. Chen J-S, et al. Venous thromboembolism in Asian patients with pancreatic cancer following palliative chemotherapy: low incidence but a negative prognosticator for those with early onset. Cancers. 2018;10(12):501.
2. Qiu W, et al. Utility of chromogranin a, pancreatic polypeptide, glucagon and gastrin in the diagnosis and follow-up of pancreatic neuroendocrine tumours in multiple endocrine neoplasia type 1 patients. Clin Endocrinol. 2016;85(3):400–7.
3. Vege SS, et al. Clinical manifestations and diagnosis of acute pancreatitis. Waltham: UptoDate; 2019.
4. Dragovich T, Espat NJ. Pancreatic cancer. Treasure Island: StatPearls; 2019.
5. Adigun R, Basit H, Murray J. Necrosis, cell (liquefactive, coagulative, caseous, fat, fibrinoid, and gangrenous). Treasure Island: StatPearls Publishing; 2019.
6. Müller D, Telieps T, Eugster A, Weinzierl C, Jolink M, Ziegler AG, Bonifacio E. Novel minor HLA DR associated antigens in type 1 diabetes. Clin Immunol. 2018;194:87–91.
7. Henquin JC, Nenquin M, Guiot Y, Rahier J, Sempoux C. Human Insulinomas show distinct patterns of insulin secretion in vitro. Diabetes. 2015;64(10):3543–53.
8. Ali ZA, Radhakrishnan N. Insulinoma. Treasure Island: StatPearls; 2018.
9. Bonheur JL, Anand BS. Gastrinoma. Treasure Island: StatPearls; 2019.
10. Mohan JF, Kohler RH, Hill JA, Weissleder R, Mathis D, Benoista C. Imaging the emergence and natural progression of spontaneous autoimmune diabetes. Proc Natl Acad Sci USA. 2017;114(37):E7776–85.
11. Bhavsar AR, Khardori R. Diabetic retinopathy. New York: Springer; 2019.
12. McGuigan A, Kelly P, Turkington RC, Jones C, Coleman HG, McCain RS. Pancreatic cancer: a review of clinical diagnosis,

epidemiology, treatment and outcomes. World J Gastroenterol. 2018;24(43):4846–61.

13. Akter R, Cao P, Noor H, Ridgway Z, Tu LH, Wang H, Wong AG, Zhang X, Abedini A, Schmidt AM, Raleigh DP. Islet amyloid polypeptide: structure, function, and pathophysiology. J Diabetes Res. 2016;2016:8269.

14. Kamilaris CDC, Stratakis CA. Multiple endocrine neoplasia type 1 (MEN1): an update and the significance of early genetic and clinical diagnosis. Front Endocrinol. 2019;10:399.

15. Hui C, Radbel JM. Diabetes insipidus. Treasure Island: StatPearls Publishing; 2019.

16. PDQ Adult Treatment Editorial Board. Pancreatic neuroendocrine tumors (islet cell tumors) treatment (PDQ®) (health professional version). Rockville: National Cancer Institute; 2019.

17. MacGill M, Weatherspoon D. Everything you need to know about the A1C test. Waltham: UptoDate; 2019.

18. Khardori R, Griffing GT. Type 2 diabetes mellitus. Treasure Island: StatPearls; 2019.

19. Song X, Zheng S, Yang G, Xiong G, Cao Z, Feng M, Zhang T, Zhao Y. Glucagonoma and the glucagonoma syndrome. Oncol Lett. 2018;15(3):2749–55.

Kidney

14

Multiple Choice Questions

1. H&E microscopic picture of a 68-year-old man suffering from a chronic medical condition is shown below. What is the diagnosis?

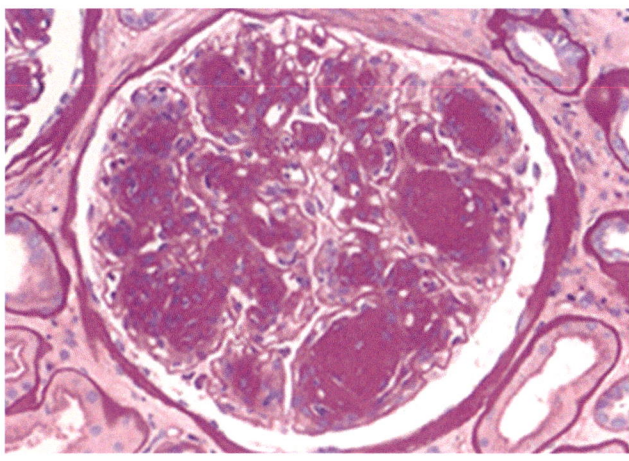

   A. IgA nephropathy
   B. Lupus glomerulonephritis
   C. Membranoproliferative glomerulonephritis (MPGN)
   D. Diabetic nephropathy
   E. Amyloidosis

2. A 6-year-old boy is brought to the pediatrician office due to puffy face. Physical examination shows marked periorbital edema and pitting edema of both feet. Urinalysis show 4+ proteinuria. Laboratory findings show decreased serum albumin and increased cholesterol. The most likely cause of child's disease is:
   A. Membranous nephropathy
   B. Minimal change disease
   C. Poststreptococcal disease
   D. IgA Nephropathy
   E. Goodpasture's syndrome

3. An important factor for chronic pyelonephritis is:
   A. Obstruction
   B. Vesico-ureteral reflux
   C. Pelvi-ureteric junction obstruction
   D. Catheter induced
   E. Hypertension

4. Paraneoplastic syndromes of RCC such as polycythemia, hypertension, hyperparathyroidism are sometimes the earliest manifestation of renal cell carcinoma. What is the cause of polycythemia?
   A. Renin secretion
   B. Parathyroid-like substance
   C. Excess erythropoietin production
   D. Hypercalcemia
   E. Myeloproliferative disorders

5. Which of the following condition presents with characteristic triad of microangiopathic hemolytic anemia, thrombocytopenia, and acute kidney injury?
   A. Hemolytic uremic syndrome
   B. Systemic vasculitis
   C. Henoch–Schonlein purpura
   D. Thrombotic thrombocytopenic purpura
   E. Disseminated intravascular coagulation

6. A 51-year-old man is brought to the emergency department with symptoms of severe headaches, vomiting, and visual disturbances. Physical examination shows blood pressure 220/150 mmHg. Which of the following renal pathology will be present in this patient?
   A. Hyaline arteriolosclerosis
   B. Hyperplastic arteriolosclerosis
   C. Tubulointerstitial nephritis
   D. Papillary necrosis
   E. Chronic glomerulonephritis

V. K. Kohli et al., *Comprehensive Multiple-Choice Questions in Pathology*, https://doi.org/10.1007/978-3-031-08767-7_14

7. A 59-year-old male patient present with long standing hypertension. Physical examination shows blood pressure of 160/95 mmHg. Ultrasound examination shows small sized kidneys. Which of the following renal lesions is characteristic of this long standing hypertension?
   A. Hyaline arteriosclerosis
   B. Fibrinoid necrosis
   C. Hyperplastic arteriosclerosis
   D. Rapidly progressive glomerulonephritis
   E. Acute tubular necrosis

8. Which is the following is additional finding in Von Hippel–Lindau syndrome in addition to renal cell carcinoma?
   A. Renal amyloidosis
   B. Renal calculi
   C. Renal cysts
   D. Renal carcinoid tumors
   E. Renal oncocytoma

9. A 4-year-old child presents as a large abdominal mass. What is the diagnosis?
   A. Renal cell carcinoma
   B. Wilms tumor
   C. Neuroblastoma
   D. Renal sarcomas
   E. Transitional cell carcinoma

10. Which of the following condition is a common cause of recurrent kidney stones, hypercalcemia, and hypophosphatemia?
    A. Hyperparathyroidism
    B. Hyperthyroidism
    C. Hypothyroidism
    D. Gout
    E. Vitamin D deficiency

11. Which inheritance is found in polycystic kidney disease (PKD) in children?
    A. Autosomal recessive
    B. Autosomal dominance
    C. X-linked dominant
    D. X-linked recessive
    E. Mutations in genes on the X chromosome

12. Which of the following glomerulonephritis shows tram-track appearance?
    A. Membranoproliferative glomerulonephritis (MPGN)
    B. Rapidly progressive glomerulonephritis (RPGN)
    C. Minimal change disease
    D. Lupus nephritis
    E. Membranous glomerulonephritis

13. Gross presentation of a kidney tumor is shown below. What is the diagnosis?

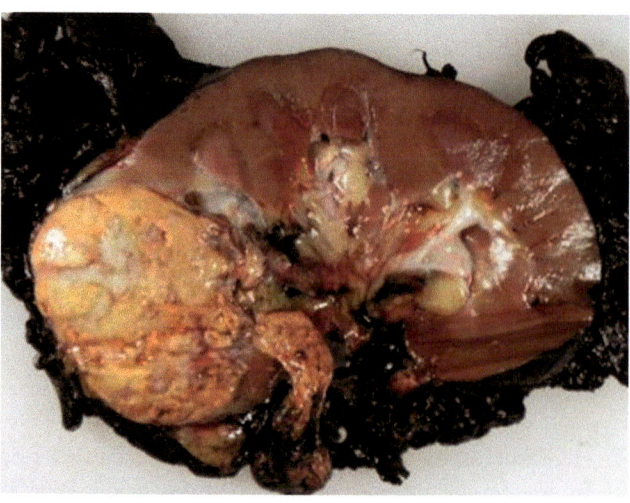

   A. Adenoma
   B. Hypernephroma
   C. Clear cell tubulopapillary carcinoma
   D. Collecting duct carcinoma
   E. Papillary oncocytoma

14. A 49-year-old man presents with hematuria and hypertension. Laboratory findings show blood urea nitrogen of 45 mg/dL and serum creatinine of 5.8 mg/dL. Kidney biopsy is done and light microscopy shows hypercellular glomeruli, crescent formation in Bowman's space. What is the diagnosis?
    A. Rapidly progressive glomerulonephritis (RPGN)
    B. Lupus nephritis
    C. IgA nephropathy (Berger's disease)
    D. Membranous nephropathy
    E. Nephrotic syndrome

15. Unilateral small smooth kidney is seen in:
    A. Reflux nephropathy
    B. Lobar infarction
    C. Renal artery stenosis
    D. Chronic glomerulonephritis
    E. Membranous glomerulopathy

16. Which of the following organism causes recurrent urinary infections leading to staghorn calculus in the renal pelvis?
    A. Klebsiella infection
    B. Escherichia infection
    C. Enterococcus faecalis
    D. Staphylococcus saprophyticus
    E. Streptococcus pyogenes

17. Subendothelial electron-dense deposits within the glomerulus is seen in:
   A. MPGN type I
   B. Crescentic glomerulonephritis
   C. Dense deposit disease
   D. IgA nephropathy
   E. Minimal change disease

18. A 10-year-old male child presents with pink color urine. Physical examination shows edema, hypertension. Laboratory findings showed proteinuria, red blood cell casts, and hypocomplementemia. Immunofluorescence shows diffuse granular pattern in the mesangium and glomerular capillary walls. Dome shaped subepithelial deposits are seen by electron microscope. What is the diagnosis?
   A. Focal segmental glomerulosclerosis
   B. Membranoproliferative glomerulonephritis
   C. Membranous glomerulonephritis
   D. Minimal change disease
   E. Poststreptococcal glomerulonephritis

19. Finnish type of congenital nephrotic syndrome is caused by defects in the following protein:
   A. Alpha actinin
   B. CD2 activated protein
   C. Nephrin
   D. ACTN4
   E. Myosin-9

20. H&E microscopic picture of renal pathology is shown below. What is the diagnosis?

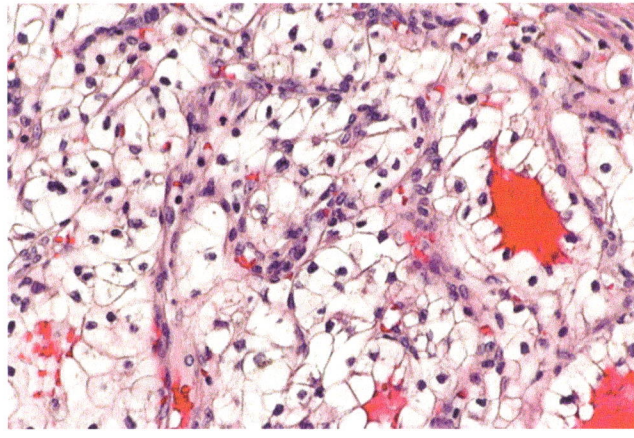

   A. Adenoma
   B. Clear cell tubulopapillary carcinoma
   C. Collecting duct carcinoma
   D. Clear cell renal cell carcinoma
   E. Papillary oncocytoma

21. A 47-year-old male presents with decrease in urine output. The patient was prescribed injectable aminoglycosides for a severe ear infection. Lab findings show BUN 65 mg/dL and serum creatinine of 2 mg/dL. Which of the following conditions is most likely to account for his findings?
   A. Acute tubular necrosis
   B. Rapidly progressive glomerulonephritis
   C. Papillary necrosis
   D. Malignant nephrosclerosis
   E. Goodpasture syndrome

22. A 27-year-old IV drug abuser is brought to the hospital with symptoms of chills and fever. Laboratory findings show elevated BUN and serum creatinine. Urinalysis reveals microscopic hematuria, granular, and cellular casts. He later died and an autopsy is performed. The most likely diagnosis is:
   A. IgA nephropathy
   B. Viral hepatitis B
   C. Goodpasture's syndrome
   D. Diffuse glomerulonephritis secondary to infectious endocarditis
   E. AIDS

23. A 32-year-old heroin addict develops nephrotic syndrome. Renal biopsy shows focal deposition of hyaline masses in portions of affected glomeruli and increased mesangial matrix on light microscopy. The most likely diagnosis is:
   A. Postinfectious glomerulonephritis
   B. Rapidly progressive glomerulonephritis
   C. Membranoproliferative glomerulonephritis
   D. Berger's disease
   E. Focal segmental glomerulosclerosis

24. A 30-year-old male presents with sore throat and pink/brown urine. Kidney biopsy showed mesangial proliferation, immunofluorescence shows mesangial deposits of IgA. What is the diagnosis?
   A. Membranoproliferative glomerulonephritis (MPGN)
   B. lupus nephritis
   C. IgA nephropathy (Berger's disease)
   D. Membranous nephropathy
   E. Nephrotic syndrome

25. A 45-year-old man with rheumatoid arthritis presents with nephrotic range proteinuria, severe edema. Laboratory findings show elevated BUN and serum creatinine. What is the diagnosis?
   A. Membranous glomerulonephritis
   B. Renal amyloidosis
   C. Rapidly progressive glomerulonephritis
   D. Acute tubular necrosis
   E. Chronic glomerulonephritis

26. A 25-year-old female presents with skin rashes, arthralgia, and arthritis of knee joints. Laboratory findings show anemia, elevated BUN, and serum creatinine. Urinalysis shows proteinuria and red blood cells. Which of the following condition is most likely to account for her findings?

A. Lupus nephritis
B. Chronic pyelonephritis
C. Amyloidosis
D. Renal papillary necrosis
E. Acute tubular necrosis

27. What is the most common cause of nephrotic syndrome in adults?
    A. Focal segmental glomerulosclerosis
    B. Acute pyelonephritis
    C. Minimal change disease
    D. Chronic glomerulonephritis
    E. Membranous glomerulonephritis

28. Immunofluorescence microscopic picture showing linear deposits along the glomerular basement membrane, is shown below. What is the diagnosis?

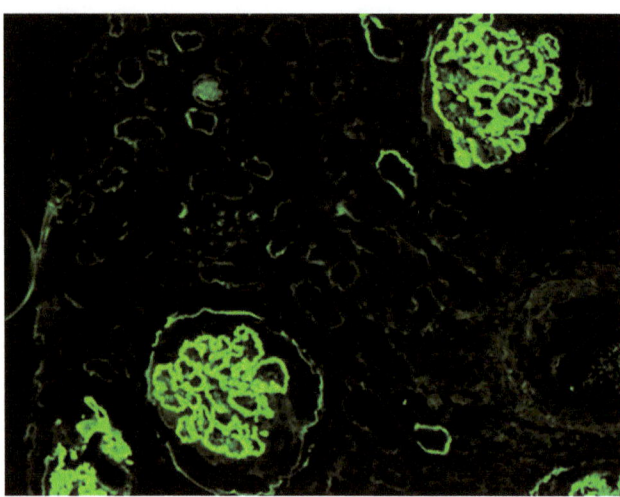

A. Rapidly progressive glomerulonephritis
B. Poststreptococcal glomerulonephritis
C. Membranoproliferative glomerulonephritis
D. Goodpasture syndrome
E. Membranous glomerulonephritis

29. A 5-year-old child is brought by his mother to pediatrician office with symptoms of pink urine, hearing and vision problems. Urinalysis shows red blood cells. The most probable diagnosis is:
    A. IgA nephropathy
    B. Alport syndrome
    C. Epstein syndrome
    D. Thin GBM disease
    E. Medullary cystic disease

Answers and Explanations

1. Answer: D. Diabetic nephropathy

   Diabetic nephropathy, either type 1 or type 2 can cause diabetic nephropathy. A classification of type 1 and type 2 diabetic kidney disease is developed by research committee of Renal Pathology Society. Class III is nodular glomerulosclerosis. Thickening of the glomerular basement membrane is the initial abnormality. Other glomerular changes include mesangial expansion, which can be diffuse or nodular. Nodular glomerulosclerosis leads to the formation of Kimmelstiel–Wilson nodules. In class III, there is at least 1 KW nodule observed on biopsy.

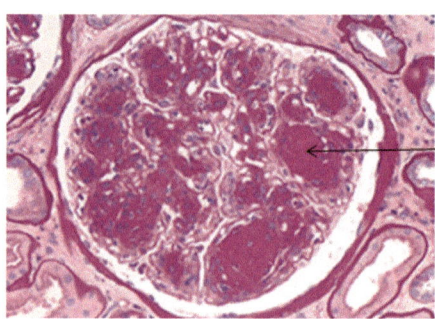

Kimmelstiel-Wilson nodule

2. Answer: B. Minimal change disease

   Minimal change disease is a common cause of nephrotic syndrome in children. It is usually seen in between 2 and 3 years. It presents suddenly after an upper respiratory infection. The proteinuria is termed "selective" because primarily albumin (low-molecular weight) is lost. Renal function is normally maintained. Key findings in nephrotic syndrome include proteinuria (more than 3.5 g/24 h). There is also hypoalbuminemia (plasma albumin level less than 3 g/dL), edema, and hyperlipidemia. Urinalysis shows 4 + proteinuria. Two mechanisms including underfilling and overfilling contribute to the pathogenesis of edema. Light microscopy shows no obvious morphologic changes in the glomeruli. Definitive diagnosis of minimal change disease can only be made by electron microscopy which shows the effacement of visceral epithelial processes.

Fusion of the epithelial foot processes

GBM

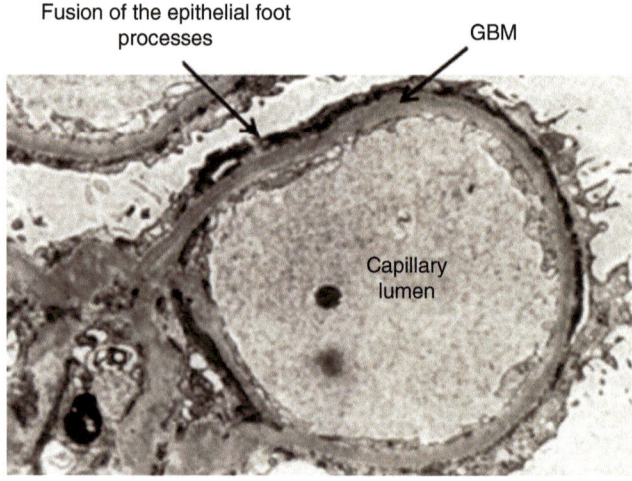

Capillary lumen

3. Answer: B. Vesico-ureteral reflux

In vesico-ureteral reflux (VUR), urine goes back to the ureter and kidneys because normal flip-valve mechanism does not work. The flip valve is present where the ureter joins with the bladder and allows one-way flow of urine to the bladder from the ureters. VUR leads to renal scarring. Most of the scars are present in the upper and lower poles of the kidneys. There is an increased risk of chronic pyelonephritis in patients with vesicoureteral reflux (VUR). Ultrasonography shows dilated calyces and cortical atrophy in both kidneys in the upper and lower lobes.

4. Answer: C. Excess erythropoietin production

This patient of RCC with an elevated erythropoietin is the cause of erythrocytosis due to excessive erythropoietin production. Paraneoplastic syndromes such as polycythemia from excess erythropoietin, hypertension due to renin secretion, and hyperparathyroidism due to secretion of parathormone like substances are often the earliest manifestation of renal cell carcinoma.

5. Answer: A. Hemolytic uremic syndrome

Hemolytic uremic syndrome (HUS) occurs following intestinal infection caused by *Escherichia coli* O157:H7 which produces Shiga-like toxins. Shiga toxin (verotoxin) injures the endothelium of glomerular capillaries. It leads to the formation of microthrombi. Platelet consumption causes thrombocytopenia. Patients present with diarrhea (often bloody), abdominal pain, cramping, vomiting, and fever. In HUS, there is microangiopathic hemolytic anemia and thrombocytopenia. It also causes acute kidney injury (oliguria, hematuria, increased creatinine). Microangiopathic hemolytic anemia occurs due to the damage of erythrocytes into schistocytes.

6. Answer: B. Hyperplastic arteriolosclerosis

Malignant hypertension is a severe, rapid increase in blood pressure usually more than 240/120 mmHg. It is usually seen in a younger age group (35–50 years) and associated with organ damage. Clinically, it is characterized by chest pain, dyspnea, angina, and headache. Physical examination shows papilledema, evidence of left ventricular hypertrophy, and retinal hemorrhages. Grossly, kidneys show small petechial hemorrhages on the cortical surface giving a flea-bitten appearance. Histologically, there is eosinophilic material in the interlobular arteries and arterioles which represent fibrinoid necrosis of the vessel walls. It is characterized by thickening of the arteriolar wall due to the concentric proliferation of smooth muscle cells, giving the arterioles an "onion skin" appearance. These changes represent an adaptive response of arterioles to severe malignant hypertension.

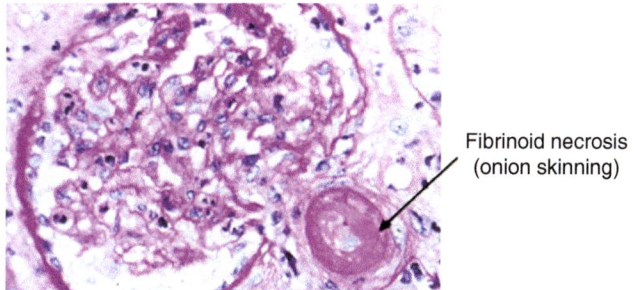

Fibrinoid necrosis (onion skinning)

7. Answer: A. Hyaline arteriosclerosis

Benign nephrosclerosis is seen in patients who have moderate hypertension. Patients may have varying proteinuria with renal insufficiency. Gross examination shows small kidneys with fine granularity of the surface. Cortex is thinned. On microscopic examination, there is an accumulation of hyaline within the walls of arterioles which is characteristic of hyaline arteriosclerosis. There is also intimal hyperplasia leading to narrowing of the lumen along with reduplication of internal elastic lamina.

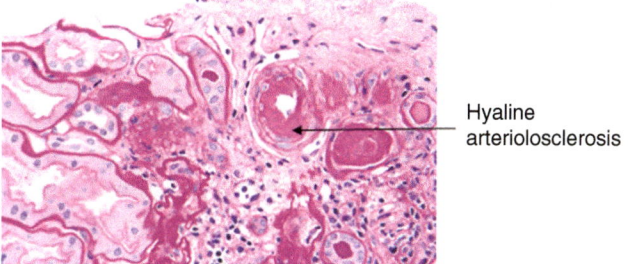

Hyaline arteriolosclerosis

8. Answer: C. Renal cysts

Von Hippel–Lindau syndrome is an autosomal disorder characterized by retinal and CNS hemangioblastomas. Approximately, 50% of VHL syndromes develop renal cell carcinoma. VHL gene is found on chromosome 3p25.3. This syndrome is also associated with pheochromocytoma, renal cysts in the kidneys. Renal cysts are at higher risk for developing renal cell carcinoma. Kidney cysts are closed sacs filled with fluid.

9. Answer: B. Wilms tumor

Wilms tumor is commonly seen below 10 years old. Patients present with a firm mass in the abdomen. Histologically, there is an admixture of blastema, epithelium, and stroma. Blastemal elements are sheets of uniform small blue cells. Anaplasia may be focal or diffuse. Cells have large, hyperchromatic nuclei with frequent mitosis. Epithelial cells may be present in a variety of patterns forming abortive glomeruli or tubules, supported by fibrovascular stroma. Wilms tumor is associated with a variety of syndromes including Wilms-aniridia-genital anomaly retardation (WAGR), Beckwith–Wiedemann syndrome, and Denys–Drash syndrome (BWS).

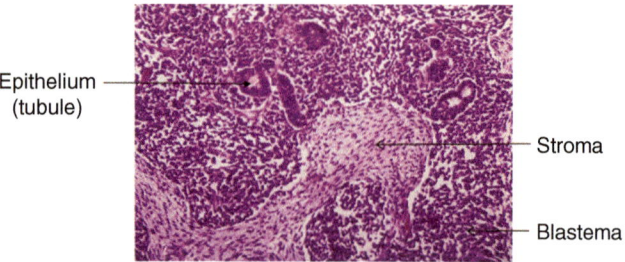

Epithelium (tubule)

Stroma

Blastema

10. Answer: A. Hyperparathyroidism

Types of stones in kidney are calcium stones, struvite (staghorn) or uric acid. The most common of the kidney stones are calcium stones. Staghorn calculi are composed of magnesium ammonium phosphate. Hypercalcemia and hypophosphatemia are caused by primary hyperparathyroidism which can result in the formation of renal stones.

11. Answer: A. Autosomal recessive

Polycystic kidney disease in children is a rare disorder. It presents at birth or during the first year of life. The common presentation is bilateral flank masses. Kidneys are grossly enlarged and may occupy almost the complete abdominal cavity. Cortex and medulla show many small cysts. Cysts are formed by dilated collecting ducts and are lined by a flattened cuboidal epithelium. Several hepatic cysts may also be present along with this disorder.

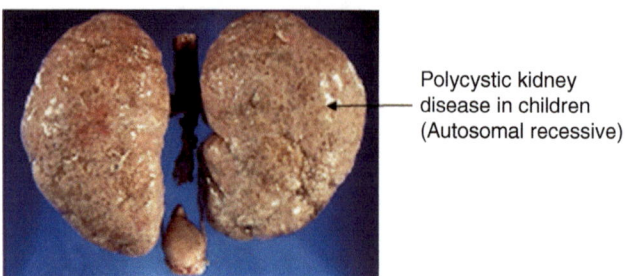

Polycystic kidney disease in children (Autosomal recessive)

12. Answer: A. Membranoproliferative glomerulonephritis (MPGN)

Membranoproliferative glomerulonephritis occurs mostly in children and young adults. Most of the patients are between the ages of 5 and 30. It is characterized by basement membrane thickening, endothelial, and mesangial cell proliferation. Light microscopy shows diffuse glomerular enlargement with lobular appearance, secondary to mesangial hypercellularity, and increased mesangial matrix. There is duplication of the glomerular basement membrane giving it a tram-track or double-contour appearance. Tram-track appearance is seen on PAS and silver stains.

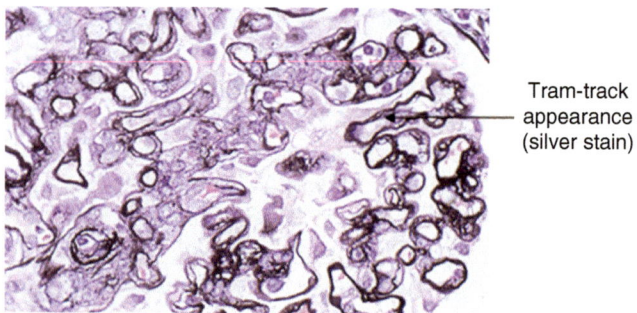

Tram-track appearance (silver stain)

13. Answer: B. Hypernephroma

Hypernephroma (clear cell renal cell carcinoma) is a spherical, yellow tumor on gross examination. On cut section, RCC is golden yellow in color due to high lipid content. There is a variegated appearance due to the presence of areas of hemorrhage, necrosis, and calcifications. RCC may invade perinephric fat and renal vein. On histology, clear renal cell carcinoma may show cuboidal or polygonal cells with clear cytoplasm. Renal cell carcinoma can cause hematuria and hypertension.

14. Answer: A. Rapidly progressive glomerulonephritis (RPGN)

Rapidly progressive glomerulonephritis (RPGN) presents with rapid and progressive loss of renal function. The glomerular injury is due to anti-GBM antibodies, immune complex deposition or no evidence of immune mechanisms (pauci-immune type). Light microscopy depends on the underlying cause. Proliferation of endothelial and mesangial cells occurs. It may show crescent formation due to epithelial parietal cell proliferation and abnormal deposition of fibrin. Crescents are diagnostic of rapidly progressive glomerulonephritis (RPGN). Proteinuria, hematuria, azotemia, and anemia are constant findings. Immunofluorescence microscopy shows linear deposits of IgG in RPGN due to anti-GBM disease and granular immune deposits in immune complex-mediated cases. Diagnosis of specific subtype is made by serum analysis of anti-GBM antibodies, antinuclear antibodies, and antineutrophil cytoplasmic antibodies (ANCA). ANCA is virtually always present in pauci-immune GN.

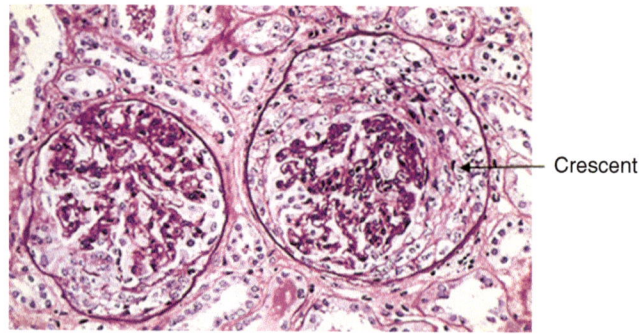

Crescent

15. Answer: C. Renal artery stenosis

Atherosclerosis is a major cause of the unilateral renal stenosis. It accounts for 70% of the cases. Besides atherosclerosis, fibromuscular dysplasia is the other lesion which can cause unilateral renal artery stenosis. Fibromuscular dysplasia is responsible for 10–30% of the cases. Stenosis of renal artery leads to hyperplasia of the juxtaglomerular apparatus and increase renin secretion. It is a rare cause of hypertension which is potentially curable with surgical treatment. The kidney is shrunken to less than normal size due to restricted blood supply on ultrasonography.

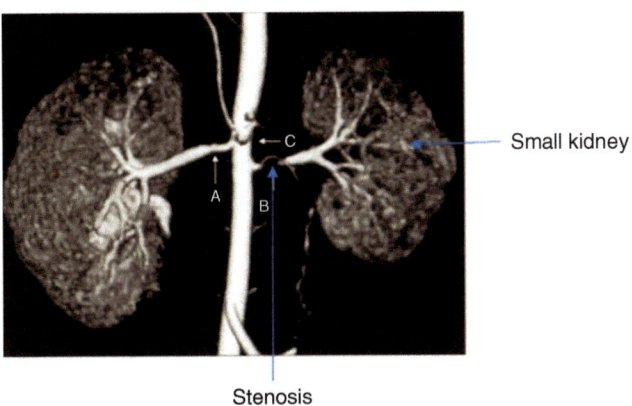

Stenosis

16. Answer: A: Klebsiella infection

Staghorn kidney stone is a large renal stone when it creates a cast of renal pelvis and calyceal system. They are caused by urease-positive organisms such as proteus, Klebsiella and occur in patients with persistent alkaline urine from urinary tract infections. Staghorn calculi are composed of struvite. Struvite is a magnesium ammonium phosphate.

17. Answer: A. MPGN type I

There are three subtypes of MPGN. By electronic microscopy, numerous deposits in subendothelial and mesangial areas are seen in MPGN type I. Dense deposit disease is seen in MPGN type II. In MPGN type III, subepithelial and subendothelial deposits are noted.

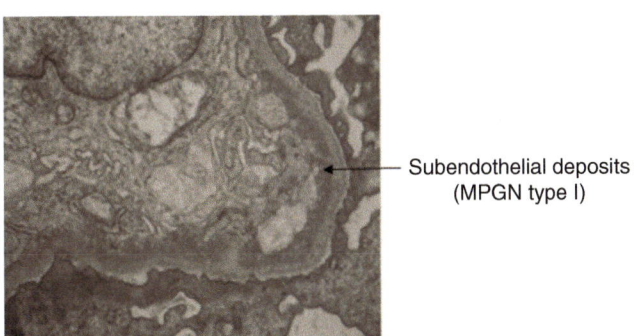

Subendothelial deposits (MPGN type I)

18. Answer: E: Poststreptococcal glomerulonephritis

Postinfectious glomerulonephritis occurs within 1–4 weeks of an upper respiratory tract or skin infection with nephritogenic strains of β hemolytic group A streptococci. Age of the patient is an important factor in prognosis. Most children recover completely, but in adults, 15–50% of cases progress to irreversible renal damage. Common clinical features include facial edema, hematuria, mild proteinuria, and hypertension. Urinalysis shows red cell casts, hematuria, and proteinuria. Laboratory findings show elevated BUN, decreased C3, and increased antistreptolysin O (ASO) titer. Light microscopy shows large, hypercellular glomeruli with neutrophils. There is obliteration of the capillary spaces due to mesangial and endothelial cells proliferation. Immunofluorescence shows lumpy-bumpy deposits of C3 and IgG. EM shows electron-dense deposits (humps) on the epithelial side of the basement membrane.

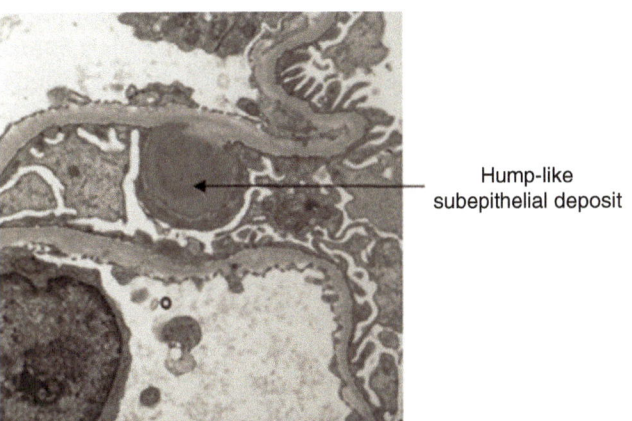

Hump-like subepithelial deposit

19. Answer: C. Nephrin

Congenital nephrotic syndrome is caused by nephrin gene (NPHS1) mutations. It is a rare disease inherited as an autosomal recessive trait. There is proteinuria, hypoproteinemia, and edema soon after birth. Light microscopy shows unremarkable glomeruli and microcystic dilatation of proximal tubules. Nephrin is a cell surface protein of podocytes.

20. Answer: D. Clear cell renal cell carcinoma

Renal cell carcinoma (Hypernephroma) presents in sixth and seventh decades. Risk factors include cigarette smoking and cadmium exposure and Von-Hippel–Lindau disease (inherited). Classical triad of hematuria, flank pain, and palpable abdominal mass occurs in less than 10% of cases. Metastasis is often the presenting symptom. Microscopic examination shows a clear cell pattern (classic), accounts for 70–80% of the cases, papillary pattern (10–15% of RCC) and chromophobe pattern (5% of RCC). Clear cell pattern shows cells with a clear or empty appearance and eccentric nuclei. There is branching, "chicken-wire" like vasculature.

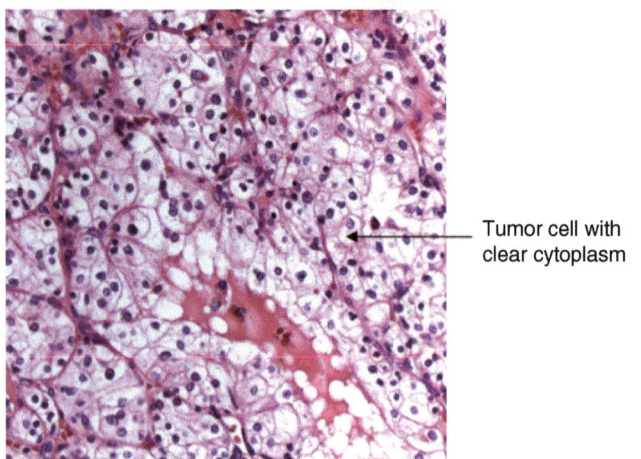

Tumor cell with clear cytoplasm

21. Answer: A. Acute tubular necrosis

In acute kidney necrosis (acute tubular injury), proximal tubular epithelium is damaged by ischemia or toxins. Common nephrotoxins such as drugs (aminoglycosides), heavy metals, and X-ray contrast media are associated with acute tubular necrosis. Common presentation is oliguria, anuria and elevated BUN and serum creatinine. On light microscopy, the tubular epithelial cells become flattened and loose surface microvilli. Individual cell undergoes necrosis with detachment from their basement membranes along with sloughing of cells into tubular lumens. The interstitium becomes edematous with the presence of inflammatory cells. The process resolves in 1–2 weeks with a normal urinary output.

22. Answer: D. Diffuse glomerulonephritis secondary to infectious endocarditis

Intravenous drug abusers are prone to develop infective endocarditis. Infective endocarditis can cause glomerulonephritis due to immune complex deposition in the glomerular capillary wall resulting in acute renal insufficiency. There are subendothelial and subepithelial deposits along with capillary wall thickenings. Light microscopy shows hypercellularity. Staphylococcus and streptococci are the most common pathogens.

23. Answer: E. Focal segmental glomerulosclerosis

Focal segmental glomerulosclerosis (FSGS) accounts for 5–10% of nephrotic syndrome in children and 35% in adults. There is an association with IV drug abuse (heroin abuse), HIV infection, morbid obesity, systemic diseases (SLE, sickle cell disease). Light microscopy shows sclerosis and hyalinosis of some tufts in a glomerulus sparing the others. Immunofluorescence shows IgM and C3 in sclerotic areas. EM shows diffuse efface-

ment of foot processes. Immune deposits are present in the sclerotic areas of glomerulus.

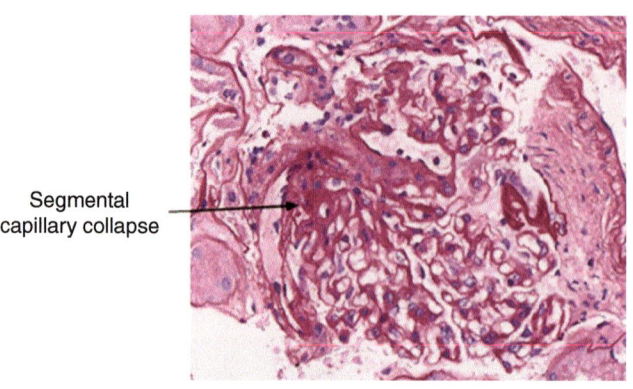

Segmental capillary collapse

24. Answer: C. IgA nephropathy (Berger's disease)

IgA nephropathy is common in males between aged between 15 and 30 years. Most patients have asymptomatic hematuria and proteinuria. Some have recurrent gross hematuria following an upper respiratory infection or viral gastroenteritis. Light microscopy shows a variety of histologies ranging from mesangial hypercellularity to focal GN to diffuse GN. Serum complements are normal. Immunofluorescence shows granular mesangial deposits of IgA. Electron microscopy shows deposits in mesangial matrix.

25. Answer: B: Renal amyloidosis

Nonselective proteinuria with nephrotic syndrome is the most common presentation of renal amyloidosis. Amyloid A (AA) amyloidosis is common in patients with chronic inflammatory diseases. On light microscopy, amyloid is seen as acellular pale amorphous eosinophilic material. Amyloid gives apple-green birefringence with congo red stain. Protein structure of amyloid comprises beta-pleated sheet and accounts for this phenomenon. Electron microscopy shows nonbranching fibrillary deposits.

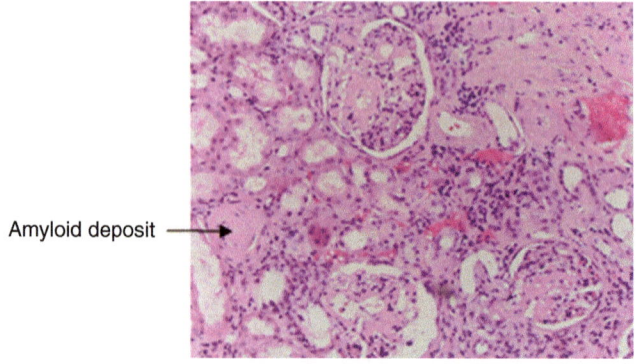

Amyloid deposit

26. Answer: A. Lupus nephritis

In systemic lupus erythematosus (SLE), there is multisystem involvement. It is an autoimmune disease.

There can be skin rashes, arthralgias and arthritis, serosal surface inflammation, anemia, renal, and CNS involvement. Renal involvement in systemic lupus erythematosus is the most common cause of morbidity and mortality. Lupus nephritis usually presents with proteinuria and hematuria. In lupus nephritis, there is a deposition of DNA/anti-DNA immune complexes within the glomeruli. There are six histological types (class 1–class VI).

27. Answer: E. Membranous glomerulonephritis

Membranous nephropathy (MN) accounts for 30–40% of nephrotic syndrome in adults. Idiopathic membranous nephropathy patients show phospholipase A2 antibodies (PLA2R). Other cases are associated with systemic diseases (SLE, sarcoidosis, malignancies), infections (hepatitis B, syphilis), toxins (gold, bismuth, mercury), and drugs (NSAID, penicillamine, captopril). Clinical manifestations range from proteinuria to nephrotic syndrome. Light microscopy shows capillary walls appear thickened and mesangial hypercellularity. The characteristic findings that allows the diagnosis in most of the cases are the perpendicular projections (spikes), seen with silver stain.

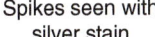

Spikes seen with silver stain

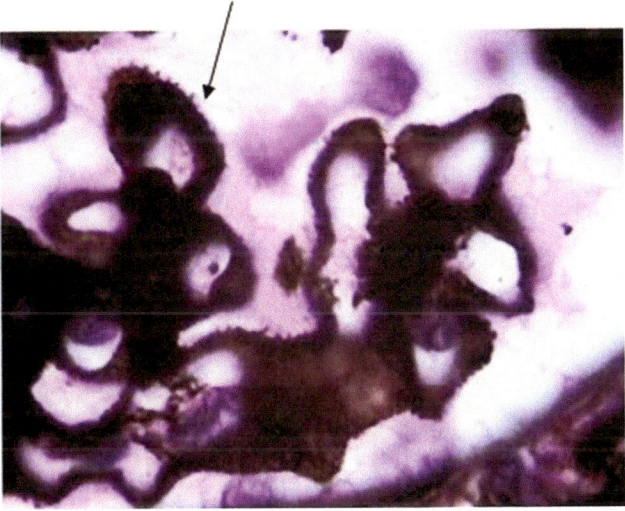

28. Answer: D. Goodpasture syndrome

Immunofluorescence shows linear deposits of IgG in Goodpasture syndrome. Most common clinical manifestation of Goodpasture syndrome is combination of glomerulonephritis and pulmonary hemorrhages of varying severity. An upper respiratory tract infection may precede the onset of Goodpasture syndrome. Hemoptysis usually precedes renal disease by several months. Antibodies are directed against glomerular and pulmonary basement membranes. Common features of this syndrome are features of nephritic syndrome, and hemoptysis.

29. Answer: B. Alport syndrome

Inheritance of Alport syndrome is X-linked or autosomal. Nephritis is associated with nerve deafness, lens dislocation and cataracts. There is a mutation in type IV collagen genes encoding alpha-5 chain. Light microscopy shows basement membrane thickening and alternating with thinning. There are prominent tubular foam cells.

Bibliography

1. Tervaert TWC, et al. Pathologic classification of diabetic nephropathy. JASN. 2010;21(4):556–63.
2. Niaudet P, et al. Etiology, clinical manifestations, and diagnosis of nephrotic syndrome in children. Waltham: UptoDate; 2019.
3. Fogo AB, et al. AJKD atlas of renal pathology: chronic pyelonephritis. Am J Kidney Dis. 2016;68(4):e23–5.
4. Mandal SK, et al. Renal cell carcinoma with paraneoplastic leucocytosis. J Cancer Res Ther. 2015;11(3):660.
5. Chugh A, Bakris GL. Microalbuminuria: what is it? Why is it important? What should be done about it? An update. J Clin Hypertens (Greenwich). 2007;9(3):196–200.
6. Hopkins C, Brenner BE. What is the pathologic hallmark of a malignant hypertensive emergency? Treasure Island: StatPearlsg; 2018.
7. Fervenza FC, Batuman V. Nephrosclerosis. Chicago: American Medical Association; 2018.
8. Varshney N, et al. A review of Von Hippel–Lindau syndrome. J Kidney Cancer VHL. 2017;4(3):20–9.
9. Chintagumpala M, et al. Presentation, diagnosis, and staging of Wilms tumor. Alameda: American Cancer Society; 2019.
10. Stöppler MC. Medical definition of chronic glomerulonephritis. Treasure Island: StatPearls; 2018.
11. Early BC. Early and severe polycystic kidney disease and related ciliopathies: an emerging field of interest. Nephron. 2019;141:50–60.
12. Fervenza FC, et al. Clinical presentation, classification, and causes of membranoproliferative glomerulonephritis. Waltham: UptoDate; 2019.
13. Appel GB, et al. Overview of the classification and treatment of rapidly progressive (crescentic) glomerulonephritis. Waltham: UptoDate; 2019.
14. Bokhari MR, Bokhari SRA. Renal artery stenosis. Treasure Island: StatPearls; 2019.
15. Powell C, Schwartz BF. Papillary necrosis. Waltham: UptoDate; 2017.
16. Cohen EP, Batuman V. Nephrotic syndrome. Treasure Island: StatPearls; 2019.
17. Jalanko H. Congenital nephrotic syndrome. Pediatr Nephrol. 2009;24(11):2121–8.
18. Cohen RJ, Cheng L. Pathology of clear cell renal cell carcinoma. Treasure Island: StatPearls; 2019.
19. Atkins MB, et al. Epidemiology, pathology, and pathogenesis of renal cell carcinoma. Waltham: UptoDate; 2019.
20. Cornec-Le Gall E, Alam A, Perrone RD. Autosomal dominant polycystic kidney disease. Seminar. 2019;393(10174):919–35.
21. Pusey CD, et al. Pathogenesis and diagnosis of anti-GBM antibody (Goodpasture's) disease. Waltham: UptoDate; 2019.
22. Appel GB, Kaplan AA, Glassock RJ, Fervenza FC, Lam AQ. Overview of the classification and treatment of rapidly

progressive (crescentic) glomerulonephritis. Baltimore: Wolters Kluwer; 2019.

23. Bertelli R, Bonanni A, Caridi G, Canepa A, Ghiggeri GM. Molecular and cellular mechanisms for proteinuria in minimal change disease. Front Med (Lausanne). 2018;5:170.

24. Krishna CK, et al. Primary membranous nephropathy: comprehensive review and historical perspective. Postgrad Med J. 2019;95(1119):23–31.

25. McAdoo SP, Pusey CD. Anti-glomerular basement membrane disease. CJASN. 2017;12(7):1162–72.

Male Genital Tract

15

Multiple Choice Questions

1. What is the best definition of Balanitis?
   A. Inflammation of the glans penis
   B. Ulcer of the glans penis
   C. Infection of the glans penis
   D. Abnormality of the glans penis
   E. Abnormality in the curvature of the penis

2. A 32-year-old man comes to the physician with a solid mass in his left testis. Ultrasound reveals partially necrotic mass. Patient has elevated alpha-fetoprotein (AFP) and human chorionic gonadotropin (hCG). Which of the following is the diagnosis?
   A. Leydig cell tumor
   B. Yolk sac tumor
   C. Granulosa cell tumor
   D. Nonseminomatous germ cell tumor
   E. Sertoli cell tumor

3. A 44-year-old male patient presents with symptoms of hematuria to his urologist. Cystoscopy is done which reveals a small tumor like lesion with gritty appearance. What is the diagnosis?
   A. Squamous cell carcinoma of the bladder
   B. Interstitial cystitis
   C. Eosinophilic cystitis
   D. Radiation cystitis
   E. Schistosomiasis-related cystitis

4. A 2-year-old boy was brought by his mother with a mass in the left testis. Serum level of alpha-fetoprotein (AFP) is elevated. What is the diagnosis?
   A. Seminoma
   B. Yolk sac tumor
   C. Granulosa cell tumor
   D. Teratoma
   E. Sertoli cell tumor

5. A 30-year-old man with a large bulky mass comes to the physician office. Biopsy is done. Microscopic findings show polygonal germ cells with clear cytoplasm and round nuclei. Tumor cells are arranged in lobules, separated by fibrous septae. What is the diagnosis?
   A. Seminoma
   B. Leydig cell tumor
   C. Granulosa cell tumor
   D. Choriocarcinoma
   E. Sertoli cell tumor

6. A 19-year-old boy comes to the physician office with a swollen, red scrotum on the right side. There is pain and tenderness in the testicle. There is also painful urination along with urgency and frequency. What is the diagnosis?
   A. Epididymitis
   B. Testicular torsion
   C. Inguinal hernia
   D. Testicular cancer
   E. Testicular tumor

7. A 40-year-old man comes to the physician office with complaints of painless testicular mass, bilateral breast enlargement. Immunohisto-chemical stain is positive for inhibin and Ki-67. What is the diagnosis?
   A. Seminoma
   B. Yolk sac tumor
   C. Granulosa cell tumor
   D. Leydig cell tumor
   E. Sertoli cell tumor

8. A 45-year-old man presents with painless slowly enlarging testicular mass. He has also features of precocious masculinization. What is the diagnosis?
   A. Seminoma
   B. Yolk sac tumor
   C. Granulosa cell tumor
   D. Leydig cell tumor
   E. Sertoli cell tumor

9. Sclerosing adenosis, a pseudo neoplastic lesion in the prostate gland that can mimic prostate cancer is most likely to occur in which zone:

V. K. Kohli et al., *Comprehensive Multiple-Choice Questions in Pathology*, https://doi.org/10.1007/978-3-031-08767-7_15

A. Central zone
B. Peripheral zone
C. Anterior fibromuscular zone
D. Transition zone
E. None of the above

10. A 69-year-old male presents with obstructive urinary systems. Transurethral resection biopsy of the prostate is done. Microscopic findings show marked proliferation of round, smaller and crowded glands. What is the diagnosis?
    A. Benign prostatic hyperplasia (BPH)
    B. Prostatic adenocarcinoma
    C. Acute bacterial prostatitis and prostatic abscess
    D. Invasive squamous cell carcinoma
    E. Invasive urothelial carcinoma

11. Which one of the following is NOT used as a tumor marker in testicular tumors?
    A. Beta human chorionic gonadotropin (ß-hCG)
    B. Carcinoembryonic antigen (CEA)
    C. Alpha-fetoprotein (AFP)
    D. Lactate dehydrogenase (LDH)
    E. Placental alkaline phosphatase (PLAP)

12. A 40-year-old male patient with symptoms of polyuria, dysuria, hematuria, and abdominal pain. Cystoscopy done which shows a distensible bladder with ulceration and areas of pinpoint petechiae and ulceration. What is the diagnosis?
    A. Interstitial cystitis
    B. Schistosomal cystitis
    C. Eosinophilic cystitis
    D. Tuberculous cystitis
    E. Follicular cystitis

13. A 65-year-old male patient presents with urinary problems. He complains of frequent or urgent need to urinate, increased frequency of urination at night, difficulty starting urination, weak urine stream, dribbling at the end of urination, inability to completely empty the bladder. What is the diagnosis?
    A. Prostate cancer
    B. Cystitis
    C. Prostatitis
    D. Carcinoma of the bladder
    E. Benign prostatic hyperplasia

14. A 30-year-old male comes to the physician office with small, flesh-colored/gray swellings in genital area. He also complained of itching and discomfort in genital area. Physical examination shows several warts close together taking a cauliflower like shape. What is the diagnosis?
    A. Molluscum contagiosum
    B. Condyloma lata
    C. Condyloma acuminatum

D. Familial benign pemphigus
E. Keratosis follicularis

15. Which of the following conditions in penis is associated with human papillomavirus infection?
    A. Epididymitis
    B. Squamous cell carcinoma of penis
    C. Orchitis
    D. Varicocele
    E. Peyronie's disease

16. Which of the following primary testicular neoplasm are NOT considered to be a teratoma?
    A. Yolk sac tumors
    B. Embryonal carcinomas
    C. Choriocarcinomas
    D. Diffuse embryoma
    E. Teratomas

17. A 20-year-old man comes to the physician's office for a regular checkup. On physical examination, no testis is palpable in the left scrotum. Which of the following complications this patient can have in the future?
    A. Carcinoma
    B. Varicocele
    C. Tuberculosis
    D. Prostatitis
    E. Gynecomastia

18. A 38-year-old man comes to the physician office with painless swelling of the left scrotum for the last 11 months. He also complains of discomfort, and feeling of heaviness in the left scrotum. Physical examination shows swollen scrotum and the transillumination test result is positive. What is the diagnosis?
    A. Spermatocele
    B. Varicocele
    C. Hematocele
    D. Hydrocele
    E. Testicular tumor

19. A 15-year-old teenager presents with symptoms of inability to urinate and empty the bladder properly. He also complaints of redness, soreness, and swelling on foreskin. Physical examination shows narrowing of the opening of the foreskin and it cannot be retracted. What is the diagnosis?
    A. Epispadias
    B. Hypospadias
    C. Phimosis
    D. Balanitis
    E. Cellulitis

20. Embryonal carcinomas are germ cell tumors of the testis. Which of the following staining profile is typical immunophenotype for embryonal carcinomas?
    A. PLAP(+); CK(+); EMA(−); CD30(+)
    B. PLAP(+); CK (+); EMA (+); CD30 (+)

C. PLAP(−); CK(−); EMA (+); CD30(−)

D. PLAP(−); CK (+); EMA (−); CD30(+)

E. PLAP(+); CK (+); EMA (−); CD 30(−)

21. Which statement best defines epispadias?

   A. Urethra ends in an opening on the upper aspect of the penis

   B. Opening on the urethra on the underside of penis

   C. It is an abnormality at the external urethral meatus

   D. It is an abnormality in the shaft of the penis

   E. It is an abnormality in the dorsal nerve and blood vessels of the penis

22. A 9-year-old male patient is brought by his mother to the pediatrician office with symptoms of right testicular pain. Physical examination shows an extra testicular tumour scrotal mass. Imaging studies demonstrate a 2.5 × 2.0 cm spermatic cord mass. A right radical orchiectomy is done. Microscopic picture shows malignant cells with rhabdoid differentiation. What is the diagnosis?

   A. Non-Hodgkin lymphoma

   B. Rhabdomyosarcoma

   C. Liposarcoma

   D. Hibernoma

   E. Adenomatoid tumor

Answers and Explanations

1. Answer: A. Inflammation of the glans penis

   Balanitis is an inflammation of the glans penis. Common causes are poor hygiene and lack of circumcision. When there is also inflammation of the foreskin of the glans penis, it is called balanoposthitis. Patients usually present with pain and pruritus on the glans and the foreskin.

2. Answer: D. Nonseminomatous germ cell tumor

   Nonseminomatous germ cell tumors are more aggressive and may present with widespread metastasis. Beta-hCG tumor marker is elevated in nonseminomatous germ cell tumors. Yolk sac tumor produces alpha-fetoprotein (AFP) in men.

3. Answer: E. Schistosomiasis-related cystitis

   Patient of Schistosomiasis-related cystitis almost always present as hematuria. Early changes are ulcer and numerous eosinophils with noncalcified schistosoma eggs. Chronic changes can be difficult to diagnose due to extensive fibrosis. Schistosomiasis-related cystitis is prone to develop squamous cell carcinoma of the bladder.

4. Answer: B. Yolk sac tumor

   There are two common types of germ cell tumors that occur in infants and children. Yolk sac tumors account for about 60% of germ cell tumors. Patients of yolk sac tumors commonly present as painless bulky masses. There is elevated serum alpha fetoprotein in the serum.

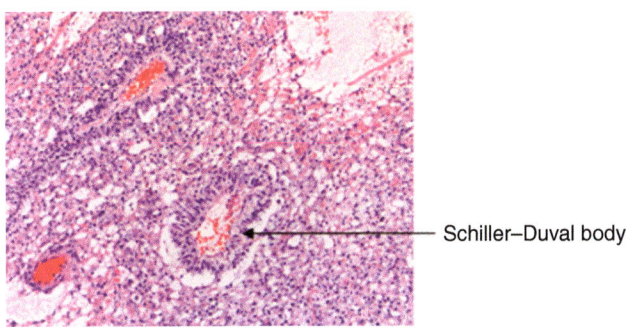
Schiller–Duval body

5. Answer: A. Seminoma

   Testicular seminomas commonly present as painless mass. It is the most common malignant tumor of the testis and mean age at presentation is 40 years. Light microscopy shows the tumor is composed of monotonous cells. Tumor cells have pale cytoplasm with large nuclei and intervening thin fibrous septa. In seminomas, immunostains, PLAP, vimentin, ferritin, PAS, and ACE are positive. There is elevated serum beta-hCG in approximately 15–20% of seminomas.

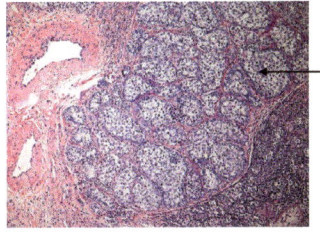
Monotonous tumor cells with large nuclei and intervening thin fibrous septa

6. Answer: A. Epididymitis

   Infection or inflammation of the epididymis testis is defined as epididymitis. The commonest organism causing acute epididymitis below the age of 35 years is *Neisseria gonorrhoeae* and *Chlamydia trachomatis*. *Escherichia coli* and pseudomonas are common organisms causing epididymitis in an older men. Patients present with scrotal pain and testicular torsion.

7. Answer: D. Leydig cell tumor

   Leydig cell tumors are called sex cord stromal tumors. Patients present between the second and sixth decades of life. They may produce androgens and estrogens. Common clinical manifestations are painless testicular mass, gynecomastia in adults, and precocious puberty in children. Majority of the tumors have an excellent prognosis and approximately 10% may undergo malignant transformation.

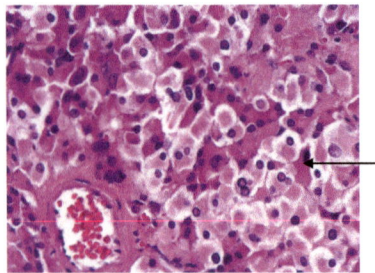

Large uniform tumor cells with distinct cell borders

8. Answer: E. Sertoli cell tumor

Sertoli cell tumors are rare tumors. These tumors present with the symptoms of precocious puberty and gynecomastia by releasing sex hormones. Leydig cell tumors and granulosa cell tumors also belong to sex cord stromal tumors.

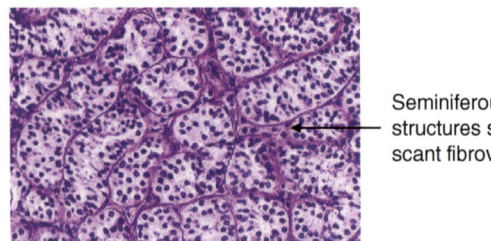

Seminiferous-like tubular structures separated by a scant fibrovascular stroma

9. Answer: D. Transition zone

Sclerosing adenosis of the prostate is most likely to occur in the transition zone. It is a pseudoneoplastic lesion and can mimic prostate carcinoma. It can be found in some 1–5% of prostatectomy specimens.

10. Answer: B. Prostatic adenocarcinoma

In prostatic adenocarcinoma crowded glandular proliferation of round glands are seen. Benign glands tend to be larger and have a fluffy appearance while glands in prostatic adenocarcinoma are more crowded, smaller, and usually have an infiltrative configuration. Cytological features include round nuclei and prominent nucleoli. Immunohistochemistry usually confirms the diagnosis of prostatic adenocarcinoma. Immunohistochemistry commonly used is a PIN4 triple cocktail comprising of two brown strains (p63 and high molecular weight cytokeratin) along with alpha-methylacyl-CoA racemase (AMACR or P5045) protein. Basal cells which are seen in benign prostatic glands are not seen in prostatic adenocarcinoma.

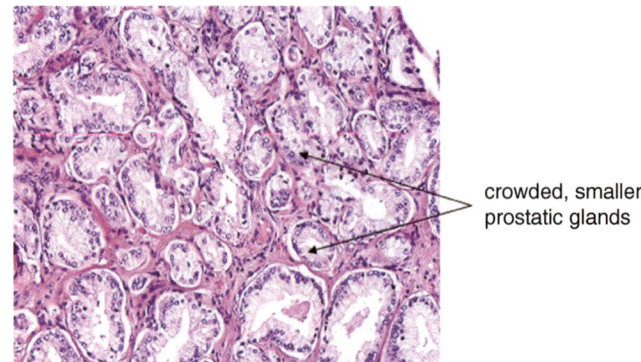

crowded, smaller prostatic glands

11. Answer: B. Carcinoembryonic antigen (CEA)

Testicular cancer patients usually present with firm, painless testicular mass. Risk factor includes cryptorchidism testicular dysgenesis and family history. Diagnosis is usually meet by ultrasonography and tumor marker studies. Radical orchiectomy is the treatment and also helps in diagnosing the type of testicular cancer.

Common testicular marker includes alpha-fetoprotein (AFP), beta human chorionic gonadotropin (ß-hCG), and lactate dehydrogenase (LDH).

12. Answer: A. Interstitial cystitis

Interstitial cystitis is a painful chronic inflammation of the bladder. Patients usually present with symptoms of dysuria, hematuria, and severe abdominal pain. Cystoscopy helps in the diagnosis and shows a distensible bladder with multiple areas of pinpoint petechiae and ulceration. It is a diagnosis of exclusion.

13. Answer: E. Benign prostatic hyperplasia

Benign prostatic hyperplasia is commonly seen in males more than 50 years of age. It usually occurs due to cellular proliferation at the periurethral central zone. Patients present with urinary symptoms including frequency, urgency, dribbling of urine, nocturia (increase frequency during the night). Other associated symptoms may be sensation of incomplete voiding, incontinence, and often urinary tract infections. Digital rectal examination (DRE) shows firm, smooth, and uniform enlargement of the prostate. Ultrasonography may show a diffuse and enlarged prostate. Prostate specific antigen (PSA) is elevated but is typically < 10 ng/mL. Grossly, the prostate is enlarged with well demarcated nodules usually in the transition and periurethral zones. Light microscopy shows proliferating glands and fibromuscular stroma. The glands are lined by double layered epithelium (inner columnar and outer cuboidal). The lumen of the glands show laminated proteinaceous material (corpora amylacea).

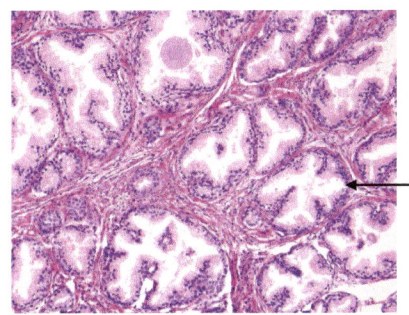

Proliferating glands and fibromuscular stroma

14. Answer: C. Condyloma acuminatum

Condyloma acuminatum is warty, cauliflower like growth. They are usually found in the anogenital region (penis, groin, perineum, perianal skin, and/or suprapubic skin). Human papillomavirus, serotypes 6 and 11 commonly cause condyloma acuminatum.

15. Answer: B. Squamous cell carcinoma of penis

Squamous cell carcinoma of penis is associated with human papillomavirus (HPV) infection, serotypes 16 and 18. There is an increased incidence in uncircumcised males. Precursors are Bowen's disease and bowenoid papulosis, erythroplasia of Queyrat, and Lichen sclerosus (also called balanitis xerotica obliterans).

16. Answer: D. Diffuse embryoma

Diffuse embryoma of the testis is a newly recognized form of mixed germ cell tumor. Diffuse embryoma is a mixed germ cell tumor with features of embryonal carcinoma and yolk sac tumor. Dermoid cyst, carcinoid tumor, and primitive neuroectodermal tumors (PNET) are considered to be a variant of teratoma.

17. Answer: A. Carcinoma

Cryptorchidism is a condition in which one or both of the testes has not moved into its proper position into the scrotum before birth. Usually, one testicle is affected but in about 10% of the cases, both testes fail to descend into the scrotum. Common complications of cryptorchidism are infertility and carcinoma of testes.

18. Answer: D. Hydrocele

Hydrocele is presence of fluid within the tunica vaginalis. It is more common in children but can also occur in adult patients. Some common causes which lead to the formation of hydrocele include infections, inflammation. Injuries to the testis and tumors of the testis may also lead to the formation of hydrocele.

19. Answer: C. Phimosis

Phimosis is a congenital narrowing of the opening of the foreskin and inability to retract the foreskin. Patients usually present with frequent urinary tract infections, hematuria, and a weakened urinary stream. They also have symptoms of inability to retract the foreskin routine cleaning or bathing and painful erections.

20. Answer: A. PLAP(+); CK(+); EMA(−); CD30(+)

Embryonal carcinomas are germ cell tumors which are positive for pan cytokeratin (CK), negative for epithelial membrane antigen (EMA), and positive for CD30 and placental alkaline phosphatase (PLAP). When epithelial tumors that are CK positive but completely negative for EMA, the possibility of germ cell tumors should be considered.

21. Answer: A. Urethra ends in an opening on the upper aspect of the penis

In epispadias, there is urethral opening on the dorsal surface of the penis. Epispadias cause backward flow of urine leading to kidney problems (reflux nephropathy and hydronephrosis). There may be frequent urinary tract infections.

22. Answer: B. Rhabdomyosarcoma

Rhabdomyosarcoma (RMS) is a primitive sarcoma. Light microscopy picture shows presence of malignant cells with rhabdoid differentiation. RMS can be classified as favorable or unfavorable. Favorable rhabdomyosarcoma (RMS) are well-differentiated. Tumors cells may be spindle cell type, botryoid, and the majority are embryonal rhabdomyosarcoma (RMS). In unfavorable rhabdomyosarcoma (RMS), tumor cells are poorly differentiated with numerous monotonous round cells. Anaplasia is usually present and alveolar features may be seen. Approximately, 20% of rhabdomyosarcoma (RMS) cases are classified as unfavorable. The embryonal subtypes are the commonest rhabdomyosarcoma (RMS) tumors and demonstrate round cell morphology with poorly to moderately differentiation.

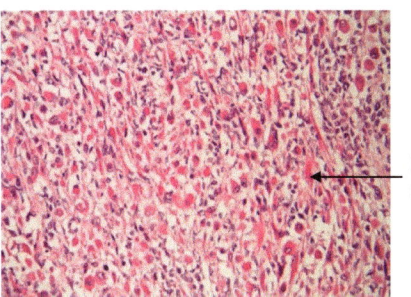

Malignant cells with rhabdoid differentiation

Bibliography

1. Wray AA, Khetarpal S. Balanitis. Treasure Island: StatPearls; 2019.
2. Saltzman AF, Cost NG. Adolescent and young adult testicular germ cell tumors: special considerations. Adv Urol. 2018;2018:2375176.
3. Steele GS. Clinical manifestations, diagnosis, and staging of testicular germ cell tumors. Waltham: UptoDate; 2019.
4. Janugade H, Monteiro J, Gouda S. Pure yolk sac tumour, postpubertal type, arising from cryptorchid testes. BMJ Case Rep CP. 2019;12(7):e229541.

5. Marko J, Wolfman DJ, Aubin AL, Sesterhenn IA. Testicular semi-noma and its mimics: from the radiologic pathology archives. Radiographics. 2017;37(4):1085.

6. Liu T, Wang Y, Zhou R, Li H, Cheng H, Zhang J. The update of prostatic ductal adenocarcinoma. Chin J Cancer Res. 2016;28(1):50–7.

7. Milose JC, et al. Role of biochemical markers in testicular cancer: diagnosis, staging, and surveillance. Open Access J Urol. 2012;4:1–8.

8. Kidd LC, et al. Relationship between human papillomavirus and penile cancer—implications for prevention and treatment. Transl Androl Urol. 2017;6(5):791–802.

9. Campobasso D, et al. Synchronous bilateral testis cancer: clinical and oncological management. Contemp Oncol (Pozn). 2017;21(1):70–6.

Female Genital Tract

16

Multiple Choice Questions

1. Which of the following is the most common ovarian cancer and shows psammoma bodies on microscopic examination?
   A. Granulosa cell tumor
   B. Serous cystadenocarcinoma
   C. Dysgerminoma
   D. Granulosa cell tumor
   E. Yolk sac tumor

2. Which are the following human papilloma virus (HPV) is NOT a high risk for cervical carcinoma?
   A. HPV 16
   B. HPV 18
   C. HPV 31
   D. HPV 33
   E. HPV 6

3. Cervical intraepithelial neoplasia (CIN) occurs commonly at which site?
   A. At the squamocolumnar junction of the cervix
   B. In the cervix
   C. In the vulva
   D. At the squamous junction of the cervix
   E. At the columnar junction of the cervix

4. What is the microscopic finding of chronic endometritis?
   A. Lymphocytes and neutrophils in the endometrium
   B. Plasma cells in the endometrium
   C. Monocytes in the endometrium
   D. Macrophages in the endometrium
   E. Eosinophils in the endometrium

5. A 35-year-old female come to the physician office with symptoms of cyclical pelvic pain which occurs at time of menstruation. What is the diagnosis?
   A. Endometriosis
   B. Appendicitis
   C. Diverticulitis

   D. Ectopic pregnancy
   E. Pelvic inflammatory disease

6. What are the laboratory findings in polycystic ovarian disease (Stein-Leventhal syndrome)?
   A. Elevated luteinizing hormone (LH) and low follicle stimulating hormone (FSH)
   B. Decreased luteinizing hormone (LH)
   C. Increased follicle stimulating hormone (FSH)
   D. Decreased testosterone
   E. Decreased luteinizing hormone (LH) and elevated follicle stimulating hormone (FSH)

7. Which is the most common benign ovarian tumor?
   A. Cystadenoma
   B. Teratoma
   C. Dysgerminoma
   D. Yolk sac tumor
   E. Granulosa cell tumor

8. Immature teratoma is graded by:
   A. Amount of mature tissue
   B. Amount of immature neuroepithelium
   C. Amount of immature cartilage
   D. Amount of bone and well-formed teeth
   E. Amount of immature tissue types

9. What is the percentage of the teratoma which develops malignant transformation; usually squamous cell carcinoma (SCC)?
   A. 5%
   B. 10%
   C. 15%
   D. 20%
   E. 2%

10. A female in her early 20s presented to her physician with complaints of right lower quadrant pain for approximately 2 weeks and adnexal mass. Laboratory values may include elevated beta lactate dehydrogenase (LDH). What is the diagnosis?
    A. Serous cystadenocarcinoma

V. K. Kohli et al., *Comprehensive Multiple-Choice Questions in Pathology*, https://doi.org/10.1007/978-3-031-08767-7_16

B. Dysgerminoma

C. Mucinous cystadenocarcinoma

D. Endodermal sinus tumor

E. Granulosa cell tumor

11. Which of the following is correct regarding Meigs' syndrome?

A. Ovarian fibroma and ascites

B. Ovarian fibroma and pleural effusion

C. Ovarian fibroma, ascites and pleural effusion

D. It is an androgen producing tumor

E. It produces β-HCG

12. Call-Exner bodies are found in which tumor?

A. Teratoma

B. Dysgerminoma

C. Granulosa cell tumor

D. Sertoli-Leydig cell tumor (androblastoma)

E. Cystadenocarcinoma

13. A uterine mass is found in a 52-year-old woman. Gross examination shows 10 cm, yellow-tan mural lesion. Microscopic examination shows coagulative tumor necrosis, mitotic count >10/10 HPF. What is the diagnosis?

A. Leiomyosarcoma

B. Adnexal tumor

C. Leiomyoma

D. Carcinosarcoma

E. Adenosarcoma

14. Which of the following is the correct answer for the molar karyotype of hydatidiform mole?

A. 69, XXY

B. 46, XX

C. 69, XXX

D. 46, XY

E. 69, XYY

15. A 25-year-old woman has a spontaneous abortion at 16 weeks. The male fetus is deformed and nonviable. The placenta is also small. It shows grape-like villi among morphologically normal villi. What is the diagnosis?

A. Partial hydatidiform mole

B. Complete hydatidiform mole

C. Invasive hydatidiform mole

D. Choriocarcinoma

E. Turner syndrome

16. A 38-year-old female presents with irregular vaginal bleeding and pelvic pain. Pelvic ultrasound reveals a pelvic mass. Endometrial biopsy reveals enlarged, non-spindled pleomorphic cells with large nuclei and no mitotic figures. What is the diagnosis?

A. Leiomyosarcoma

B. Adenomatoid tumor

C. Adenomyoma

D. Adnexal tumor

E. Uterine epithelioid leiomyoma

17. A 32-year-old woman presents with vaginal bleeding, shortness of breath, hemoptysis and chest pain. Chest X-ray shows multiple infiltrates of various shapes in both lungs. Serum level of human chorionic gonadotropin (hCG) is elevated. What is the diagnosis?

A. Seminoma

B. Yolk sac tumor

C. Granulosa cell tumor

D. Leydig cell tumor

E. Choriocarcinoma

18. A 58-year-old markedly obese, single, diabetic nulliparous woman presents with vaginal bleeding. A pap smear is done which shows cells that are consistent with endometrial adenocarcinoma. Which of the following disease can progress to endometrial carcinoma?

A. Adenomyosis

B. Human papillomavirus infection

C. Endometrial hyperplasia

D. Leiomyoma

E. Chronic endometritis

19. The epithelial lining of fallopian tube is:

A. Squamous

B. Cuboid

C. Ciliated columnar

D. Pseudostratified columnar

E. Transitional

20. A 25-year-old woman in her fifth month of pregnancy complains of vaginal bleeding and no fetal movement. Physical examination reveals a larger uterus than expected for her duration of pregnancy. During the examination, she spontaneously passes some grape-like tissue. Which of the following is the most likely complication?

A. Granulosa cell tumor

B. Invasive mole

C. Polycystic ovaries

D. Serous cystadenocarcinoma

E. Increased risk for breast carcinoma

21. Microscopic picture of an ovarian lesion is shown below. What is the most likely diagnosis?

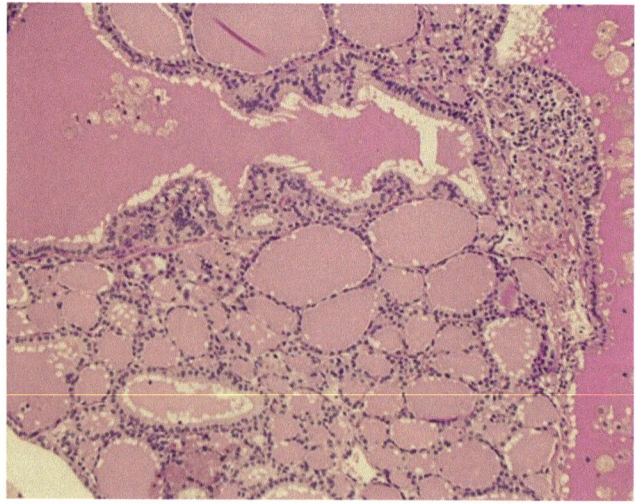

A. Brenner tumor

B. Struma ovarii

C. Thecoma

D. Serous cystadenoma

E. Choriocarcinoma

22. A 49-year-old woman presents to her primary care physician with a recent history of a malodorous bloody discharge following intercourse. Her last PAP smear was done 12 years ago. What would be the most likely diagnosis?

A. Endometriosis

B. Cervicitis

C. Vaginitis

D. Pelvic inflammatory disease

E. Squamous cell carcinoma of cervix

23. A 30-year-old woman shows ASC-H (atypical squamous cells-favor high grade). What is the most appropriate follow up for this patient?

A. Repeat pap smear in 6 months

B. Repeat pap smear in 1 year

C. Hysterectomy

D. Loop electrocautery excision procedure

E. Colposcopy

24. An 8-year-old girl has intermittent lower abdominal pain and fever for 3 weeks. On physical examination, lower abdomen tenderness is noted. Ultrasonography (US) showed a huge pelvic tumor with cystic mass. Biopsy of the tumor is done. Microscopic picture shows solid, tubular and focal papillary patterns with Schiller–Duval bodies. What is the diagnosis?

A. Embryonal carcinoma

B. Choriocarcinoma

C. Yolk sac tumor

D. Teratoma

E. Dysgerminoma

25. Gross specimen of the ovary of 19-year-old female is shown below. What is the diagnosis?

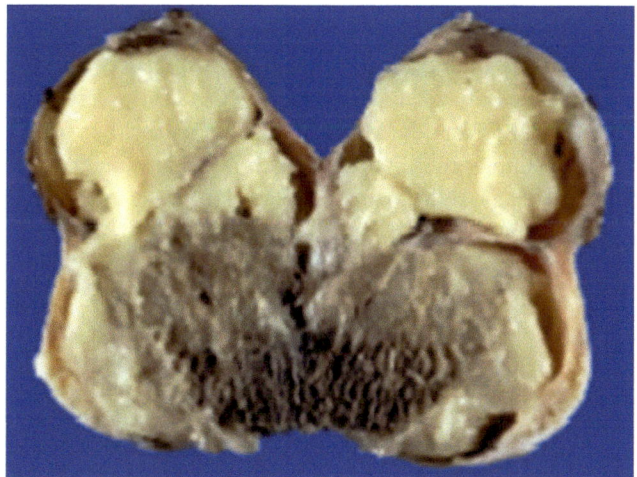

A. Cystadenoma

B. Cystadenocarcinoma

C. Mature cystic teratoma of ovary

D. Dysgerminoma

E. Ovarian fibroma

26. A middle-aged woman complaints of menorrhagia and dysmenorrhea. Patient has a uniformly enlarged uterus with normal-appearing endometrial tissue on biopsy. What is the diagnosis?

A. Leiomyoma

B. Adenomyosis

C. Pelvic adhesive disease

D. Uterine cancer

E. Chronic endometritis

Answers and Explanations

1. Answer: B. Serous cystadenocarcinoma

    Serous cystadenocarcinoma is the most common ovarian carcinoma. It usually pursues a rapidly malignant course with extensive peritoneal implantation and ascites. One of the hallmarks of the serous cystadenocarcinoma is the formation of psammoma bodies. They are bilateral in approximately two-thirds of all cases.

2. Answer: E. HPV 6

    Low-risk types of HPV (types 6, 11) are rarely identified in high grade lesions. High-grade lesions including carcinomas are infected with HPV types 16, 18, 31, 33, 35.

3. Answer: A. At the squamocolumnar junction of the cervix

    Majority of cervical cancers develop at the transformation zone. It is a small region of metaplastic squamous epithelium at the squamocolumnar junction between endocervix and ectocervix. The strongest risk factor for cervical intraepithelial neoplasia (cervical dysplasia) and carcinoma is persistent infection with human papilloma virus (HPV) type 16 or 18.

4. Answer: B. Plasma cells in the endometrium

    Chronic endometritis shows increased number of plasma cells, which is characteristic of this condition. While an etiology is diagnosed sometimes, most cases are non-specific. Chronic endometritis has potential adverse effects on fertility.

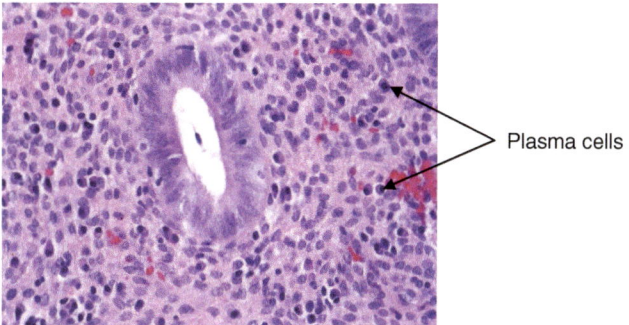

Plasma cells

5. Answer: A. Endometriosis

Endometriosis refers to the presence of endometrial glands and stroma outside the uterus in places such as peritoneum, ovaries, and ligaments. Bleeding and shedding of extra uterine endometrium causes blood collections in the ectopic locations resulting in inflammation and adhesions. Patients usually present with chronic pelvic pain, dysmenorrheal (painful menses), painful intercourse, and pain during urination and bowel movements. Endometriosis often causes infertility. Common risk factors are prolonged menses, nulliparity, and early menarche.

6. Answer: A. Elevated luteinizing hormone (LH) and low follicle stimulating hormone (FSH)

Polycystic ovaries are usually bilateral and show a mixture of follicular cysts and cystic follicles without evidence of ovulation. Polycystic ovarian syndrome presents with clinical evidence of hyperandrogenism. If prolonged, the surface can be become fibrotic. In addition to the cystic follicles, there is both a follicular and stromal hyperthecosis. Follicular stimulating hormone (FSH) levels are low. Luteinizing hormone (LH) level is elevated. The LH to FSH ratio is usually greater than 3.

7. Answer: A. Cystadenoma

Benign serous tumors of the ovary are common and accounts for about 50–70% of all ovarian serous tumors. They can occur at any age, but are common between the fourth and fifth decades of life and may occasionally be bilateral. Serous cystadenomas are unilocular, but may be multilocular ranging in size from 5 to 20 cm. Cystadenomas appear grossly as cystic structures with a smooth, glistening lining, and occasional tiny papillary projections. Microscopically, they are characterized by papillae lined by single layer of columnar epithelium.

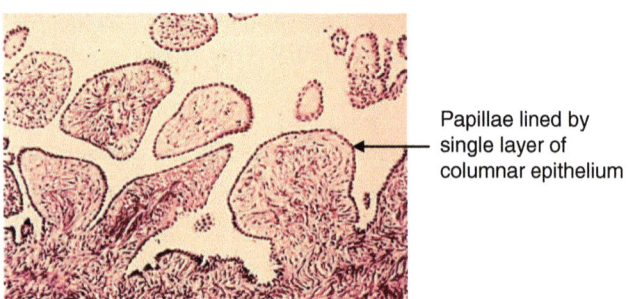

Papillae lined by single layer of columnar epithelium

8. Answer: B. Amount of immature neuroepithelium

An ovarian immature teratoma's histological grade is based upon amount of immature neuroepithelium. Mature teratoma has a better prognosis than an immature teratoma.

9. Answer: E. 2%

Teratomas are subdivided into immature, mature, and monodermal subtypes. Immature teratomas are charac-

terized by the presence of embryonal type of tissue. The most significant embryonal tissue is neuroectodermal. Most immature teratomas are predominantly solid. Mature cystic teratoma occurs most commonly during the reproductive years. Mature teratomas are usually cystic (dermoid cyst), almost always contain abundant hair and keratinous debris. Bone and well-formed teeth may be identified. Malignant transformation occurs in about 2% of cases, especially in older women. The most common malignant tumor is squamous cell carcinoma.

10. Answer: B. Dysgerminoma

Dysgerminoma is the ovarian counterpart of testicular seminoma. It is composed of a uniform population of germ cells that show morphological and histochemical similarity to primordial germ cells. Dysgerminoma is unilateral and occurs in patients under the age of 30. The tumors are solid with a smooth surface. Histologically, the tumor consists of large aggregates of uniform cells surrounded by delicate strands of connective tissue containing lymphocytes. Most dysgerminomas are related to elevated serum lactic dehydrogenase (LDH, sometimes used as a tumor marker). Dysgerminiomas are positive for OCT4 (nuclear positivity) and CD117 (membranous positivity).

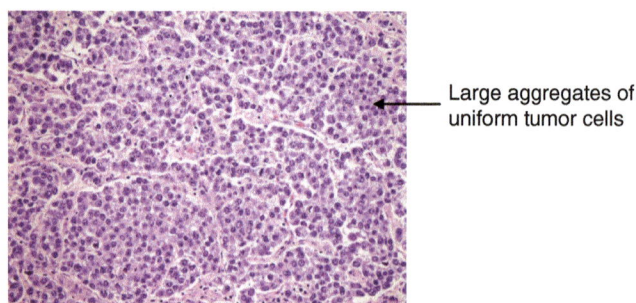

Large aggregates of uniform tumor cells

11. Answer: C. Ovarian fibroma, ascites and pleural effusion

Metastatic carcinomas to the ovary are usually bilateral and multicentric. They may be solid or cystic. The Classic Krukenberg tumor is a metastatic carcinoma typically from the stomach that has signet ring mucin-containing cells infiltrating stroma. This tumor has a triad of solid ovarian tumor, ascites, and pleural effusion.

12. Answer: C. Granulosa cell tumor

Adult granulosa cell tumors account for 95% of all granulosa cell tumors. Histologically, granulosa cells are cuboidal in shape, and form rosette like structures (Call-Exner bodies) with grooved, pale, and round nuclei (coffee bean nuclei). Granulosa cells grow in several varieties of patterns: macrofollicular, microfollicular, insular, trabecular, and diffuse or sarcomatoid. These patterns are often mixed in the same neoplasm. Granulosa cell tumors are of low malignant potential and can recur. A subtype of granulosa cell tumors that occurs in younger patients are called juvenile granulosa cell tumor. These tumors have better prognosis. Adult granulosa cell tumor present with amenorrhea, menometrorrhagia, or post-menopausal bleeding. Juvenile tumors may present with sexual precocity.

13. Answer: A. Leiomyosarcoma

The median age of women with leiomyosarcoma is 50–55 years. Grossly, these tumors are 10 cm on average and usually there is only one mass/lesion. Microscopic examination shows tumor necrosis, severe cellular atypia, and high mitotic activity (>10/HPF). Nuclear atypia on low power examination is also an important feature.

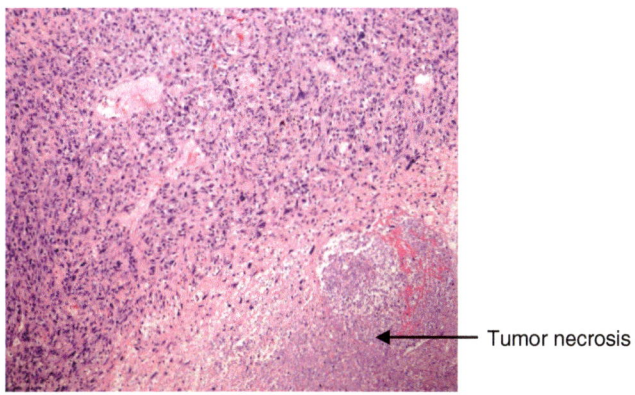

Tumor necrosis

14. Answer: B. 46, XX

Hydatidiform moles are divided into complete and partial moles and represent an abnormal placenta characterized by marked enlargement of chorionic villi due to central stromal edema. Complete mole is a more common type and the most common genotype responsible for complete molar pregnancies is 46, XX. Complete mole does not contain a fetus and cause an abnormal elevation of β-human chorionic gonadotropin.

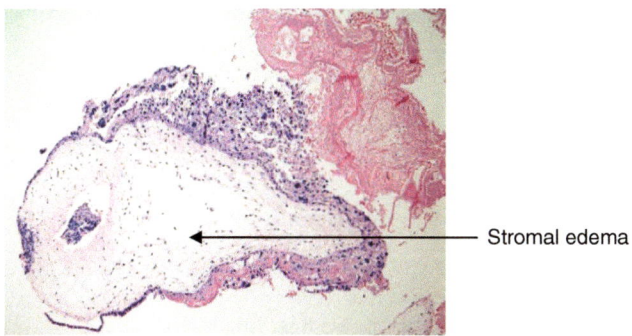

Stromal edema

15. Answer: A. Partial hydatidiform mole

There are two common types of hydatidiform moles. Partial hydatidiform mole results from triploidy. A par-

tial mole has deformed, nonviable fetus because maternal chromosomes are present. Complete mole is the more common type and does not contain a fetus. In partial moles, the karyotype is usually 69 XXY.

16. Answer: E. Uterine epithelioid leiomyoma

Uterine epithelioid leiomyoma is a benign uterine smooth muscle tumor. Endometrial biopsy shows enlarged, non-spindled pleomorphic cells with large, atypical appearing nuclei. There are no mitotic figures or necrosis.

17. Answer: E. Choriocarcinoma

Choriocarcinoma is a trophoblastic epithelial malignancy deriving from normal or abnormal pregnancy. Choriocarcinoma frequently arises within a complete hydatidiform mole. There is an elevated HCG level. Grossly, it has fleshy areas of both ischemic necrosis and hemorrhage. Histologically, choriocarcinoma is composed of cytotrophoblast cells and syncytiotrophoblasts. Cytotrophoblast cells are smaller cells and syncytiotrophoblasts are the larger, multinucleated cells with eosinophilic cytoplasm. It rapidly penetrates myometrium with early vascular and lymphatic invasion. Choriocarcinoma commonly metastasizes hematogenously. The most common metastatic sites are lung, pelvis, vagina, liver, and brain. Immunohistochemically, it is positive for cytokeratin, hCG, human placental lactogen (hPL), and placental alkaline phosphatase (PLAP).

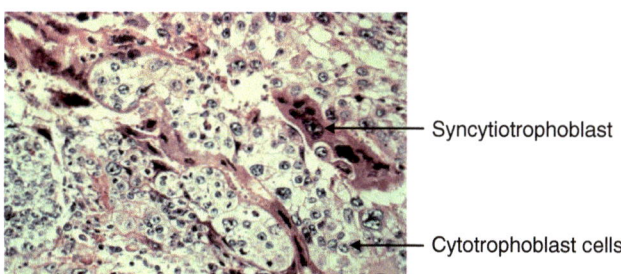

Syncytiotrophoblast

Cytotrophoblast cells

18. Answer: C. Endometrial hyperplasia

Endometrial hyperplasia is disordered glandular and stromal growth. It is important because of its relationship to endometrial carcinoma, i.e. a continuum of atypical changes lead eventually to endometrial carcinoma. Hyperplasia usually occurs in the peri-menopausal state or post-menopausal and is associated with abnormal bleeding. Risk factors include obesity, diabetes, and nulliparity.

19. Answer: C. Ciliated columnar

Histologically, there are three layers in the uterine tubes: mucosa, muscularis, and serosa. The fallopian tube is lined by ciliated columnar epithelium. Ciliated cells help in the transport of the embryo.

20. Answer: B. Invasive mole

    Gestational trophoblastic neoplasia occurs due to abnormal proliferation of trophoblastic tissue. Common histologic types are invasive mole and choriocarcinoma. There is an elevated level of HCG in an invasive mole and choriocarcinoma. Invasive mole is common after a molar pregnancy. There may be edematous chorionic villi with trophoblastic proliferation invading the myometrium. Invasive mole (chorioadenoma destruens) is a cellular mole that may perforate the uterus leading to significant morbidity and even death.

21. Answer: B. Struma ovarii

    Although some thyroid tissue can be identified in a benign teratoma, a significant portion of the lesion must have thyroid tissue to be deemed struma ovarii. Majority of these lesions are benign. Sometimes, they could present with hyperfunctioning thyroid tissue or malignancy like papillary thyroid carcinoma.

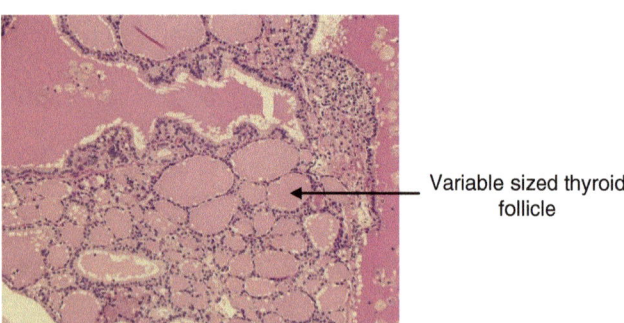

Variable sized thyroid follicle

22. Answer: E. Squamous cell carcinoma of cervix

    Virtually, all high-grade lesions including carcinomas are infected with high risk types of HPV 16, 18, 31, 33, 35. HPV DNA is detected in >90% of carcinomas and squamous intraepithelial lesions (SILs). E6 and E7 genes of HPV have oncogenic properties. E6 binds p53 promoting its degradation. Squamous cell carcinoma of the cervix is the most common histologic types of cervical cancer. Patients usually present with abnormal vaginal bleeding or postcoital bleeding. The diagnosis of carcinoma of the cervix is established by biopsy. Adenocarcinoma accounts for 5–15% of cervical cancers and arise from endocervical glandular epithelium. Extent of invasion is a valuable prognostic indicator.

23. Answer: E. Colposcopy

    The recommended next step for women with a diagnosis of ASC-H is colposcopy. ASC-H means the woman has atypical squamous cells with the possibility of her having high grade squamous intraepithelial lesion (HSIL).

24. Answer: C. Yolk sac tumor

    The yolk sac (endodermal sinus) tumor recapitulates the embryonic development of the yolk sac. Yolk sac tumors occur most commonly in childhood and adolescence and are the second most common malignant tumor of the ovary. The tumor is soft and friable with areas of hemorrhage and necrosis. The tumors are almost unilateral. A variety of histologic patterns are seen, but the most frequent type is reticular or microcystic pattern. This pattern is characterized by a loose meshwork of spaces and channels lined by mitotically active cells. There are characteristic Schiller–Duval bodies that have a central vessel and lined by primitive tumor cells. Other histologic patterns are polyvesicular vitelline pattern, hepatoid pattern, and endometrioid-like pattern. Clinically, yolk cell tumors are aggressive neoplasms, often presenting as an advanced stage. Alpha fetoprotein (AFP) is elevated in YST and is a useful serum marker in monitoring treatment.

25. Answer: C. Mature cystic teratoma of ovary

    Teratomas are germ-cell tumors that contain all the three germ cell layers: ectoderm, endoderm, and mesoderm. Teratomas account for about 20% of ovarian tumors and usually arise in the first two decades of life. They are also called dermoid cysts. They often present with cysts containing mature tissues. The most common mature tissues are skin, hair, and teeth. Histologically, teratomas consist of various tissues, such as cartilage, glandular tissue, and keratinizing squamous epithelium. Teratomas are usually benign, and surgical excision is curative.

26. Answer: B. Adenomyosis

    Adenomyosis refers to the presence of endometrial glands and stroma within the myometrium. This results in hypertrophy and hyperplasia of the surrounding myometrium causing globular enlargement of the uterus. Common symptoms are heavy menstrual bleeding and painful menses. Endometriosis is presence of endometrial glands and stroma outside the uterus. Some common sites are ovaries and uterine ligaments.

Bibliography

1. Burd EM. Human papillomavirus and cervical cancer. Clin Microbiol Rev. 2003;16(1):1–17.
2. Deng H, et al. HPV16-immortalized cells from human transformation zone and endocervix are more dysplastic than ectocervical cells in organotypic culture. Sci Rep. 2018;8(1):15402.
3. Maeda K, et al. A case of ovarian clear cell carcinoma arising from ovarian mature cystic teratoma. J Ovarian Res. 2018;11:74.
4. Tsai W-C, Chang F-W, Chang J-L, Chao H-M. Meigs' syndrome in an elderly woman with short of breath. J Med Sci. 2015;35(3):125–7.

5. Inada Y, et al. Rapidly growing juvenile granulosa cell tumor of the ovary arising in adult: a case report and review of the literature. J Ovarian Res. 2018;11(1):100.

6. Kubeček O, et al. The pathogenesis, diagnosis, and management of metastatic tumors to the ovary: a comprehensive review. Clin Exp Metastasis. 2017;34(5):295–307.

7. Ghassemzadeh S, Kang M. Hydatidiform mole, vol. 4. Treasure Island, FL: StatPearls; 2019.

8. Kwan GWM, Koo C-K. Peripartum respiratory failure with bilateral pulmonary infiltrates on chest X-ray. Case Rep Oncol. 2009;2(2):133–9.

9. El Hasbani G, et al. Uterine choriocarcinoma diagnosed 11 years after menopause: a case report. Case Rep Womens Health. 2018;20:e00076.

10. Maggiore ULR, et al. Bladder endometriosis: a systematic review of pathogenesis, diagnosis, treatment, impact on fertility, and risk of malignant transformation. Eur Urol. 2017;71(5):790–807.

11. Baergen RN. Gestational trophoblastic disease: pathology. Waltham: UpToDate; 2019.

12. Frumovitz M. Invasive cervical cancer: epidemiology, risk factors, clinical manifestations and diagnosis. Baltimore: Wolters Kluwer; 2019.

13. Chen LH, Yip K-C, Wu H-J, Yong S-B. Yolk sac tumor in an eight-year-old girl: a case report and literature review. Front Pediatr. 2019;7:169.

14. Chad AH, Sonoda Y. Cystic teratoma. Baltimore: Wolters Kluwer; 2018.

15. Elizabeth AS, Barbieri RL, Levine D, Eckler K. Uterine adenomyosis. Baltimore: Wolters Kluwer; 2019.

Breast

17

Multiple Choice Questions

1. The distinction between phyllodes tumor and fibroadenoma is based on?
   A. Proliferating epithelial elements
   B. Tumor size
   C. Age of the patient
   D. Stromal cellularity
   E. Mucinous change

2. Which of the following breast pathology has 4–5 times increased risk of breast cancer?
   A. Apocrine metaplasia
   B. Sclerosing adenosis
   C. Usual ductal hyperplasia
   D. Intraductal papilloma
   E. Atypical ductal hyperplasia

3. The most likely cause of a 1-cm mass in the upper outer quadrant of the breast of a 65-year-old woman is?
   A. Fibrocystic disease
   B. Acute mastitis
   C. Fibroadenoma
   D. Carcinoma
   E. Paget disease of the breast

4. A 42-year-old woman noticed lumps in both breasts. Fine needle aspiration of both breasts reveals additional foci of similar cells. What is the diagnosis?
   A. Medullary carcinoma
   B. Metaplastic carcinoma
   C. Papillary carcinoma
   D. Lobular carcinoma in situ (LCIS)
   E. Infiltrating ductal carcinoma

5. A 33-year-old woman presents with bloody nipple discharge from her left breast. Core needle biopsy of the breast is done and microscopic examination shows papillae with a delicate fibrovascular core. What is the diagnosis?
   A. Fibroadenoma
   B. Fibrocystic changes
   C. Intraductal papilloma
   D. Lobular carcinoma
   E. Carcinoma of the breast

6. A 52-year-old woman presents with a large, massive size mass distanding the right breast. Core biopsy of the breast is done. Microscopic examination shows an increased cellularity, stromal overgrowth. What is the diagnosis?
   A. Phyllodes tumor
   B. Fibroadenoma
   C. Medullary carcinoma
   D. Fibrocystic changes
   E. Lobular carcinoma

7. Which of the following benign breast lesions does NOT have a myoepithelial lining?
   A. Fibroadenoma
   B. Microglandular adenosis
   C. Tubular adenoma
   D. Ductal ectasia
   E. Lipoma

8. A 61-year-old woman presents with red warm edematous skin of the right breast with a diffuse erythema and edema. There is also an orange red thickened skin. What is the diagnosis?
   A. Paget disease of the breast
   B. Inflammatory carcinoma of the breast
   C. Fat necrosis
   D. Apocrine metaplasia
   E. Medullary carcinoma

9. A 52-year-old woman presents with ulceration, oozing, crusting and fissuring of the nipple and areola. On examination, there is redness, flaky, and scaly skin on the nipple with an inverted nipple. What is the diagnosis?
   A. Paget disease of the nipple
   B. Medullary carcinoma
   C. Inflammatory carcinoma
   D. Infiltrating ductal carcinoma
   E. Ductal carcinoma in situ

© The Author(s), under exclusive license to Springer Nature Switzerland AG 2022
V. K. Kohli et al., *Comprehensive Multiple-Choice Questions in Pathology*, https://doi.org/10.1007/978-3-031-08767-7_17

10. Which is the most important prognostic factor for determining outcomes in invasive breast carcinoma?
    A. Age of the patient
    B. Axillary lymph node status
    C. Distance of resection margin to the tumor location in the breast
    D. Estrogen/progesterone receptor (ER/PR) status of Invasive carcinoma
    E. Radiation therapy to the breast and axillary lymph nodes

11. A 55-year-old woman has a screening mammogram. The mammographic findings show microcalcifications. An excisional biopsy show pleomorphic cells with central necrosis, central calcification, and stromal fibrosis. What is the diagnosis?
    A. Apocrine metaplasia
    B. Fat necrosis
    C. Ductal carcinoma in situ (DCIS)
    D. Inflammatory carcinoma
    E. Fibrocystic changes

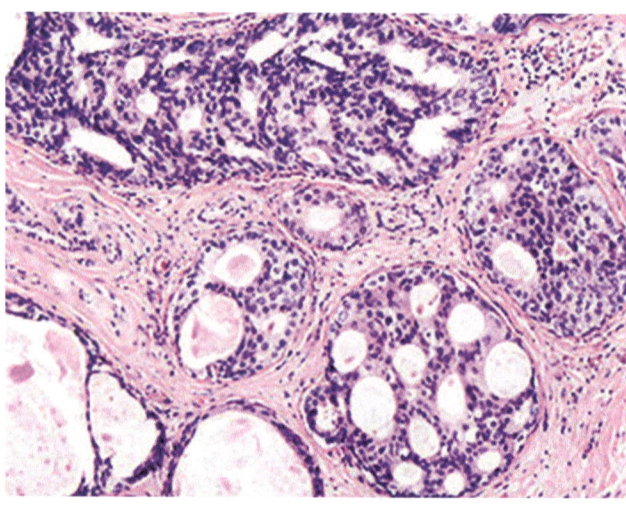

12. HER-2/NEU receptor gene mutation is seen in which of the following breast disease?
    A. Fibroadenoma
    B. Breast cancer
    C. Apocrine metaplasia
    D. Sclerosing adenosis
    E. Fibrocystic breast changes

13. A 24-year-old woman finds a 2 cm mass in the upper outer quadrant of her left breast while taking a shower. She comes to family practice clinic for evaluation. Examination reveals that the mass is nontender, smooth, round, and freely mobile. What is the most likely diagnosis?
    A. Infiltrating ductal carcinoma
    B. Fibroadenoma
    C. Fibrocystic change

D. Infiltrating ductal carcinoma, comedo type
    E. Lobular carcinoma in situ

14. A 55-year-old female presents with a breast lump. Microscopic picture is composed of two cells population. What is the diagnosis?
    A. Infiltrating carcinoma of the breast
    B. Ductal carcinoma in situ
    C. Adenoid cystic carcinoma of the breast
    D. Inflammatory carcinoma of the breast
    E. Lobular carcinoma of the breast

15. Which of the following elements in fibrocystic change is having increased risk of breast cancer?
    A. Cyst formation
    B. Epithelial hyperplasia
    C. Apocrine metaplasia
    D. Sclerosing adenosis
    E. Papillomas

16. A 29-year-old diabetic female patient presents for evaluation of a painful breast mass. On physical examination, there is small, tender nodule in the left breast. Imaging studies show an ill-defined mass with calcifications. Biopsy shows dense fibrosis, lobular atrophy, and aggregates of lymphocytes. What is the diagnosis?
    A. Fat necrosis
    B. Granulomatous mastitis
    C. Duct ectasia
    D. Lymphocytic mastitis
    E. Fibroadenoma

17. A 54-year-old female presents with breast lump. Excisional biopsy is done which shows tumor cells in single lines (Indian filing). What is the diagnosis?
    A. Infiltrating ductal carcinoma of the breast
    B. Infiltrating lobular carcinoma of the breast
    C. Ductal carcinoma in situ
    D. Inflammatory carcinoma of the breast
    E. Tubular carcinoma

18. Which of the following breast carcinoma is estrogen receptor negative by immunohistochemistry?
    A. Medullary carcinoma
    B. Ductal carcinoma, low grade
    C. Lobular carcinoma in situ (LCIS)
    D. Colloid carcinoma
    E. Tubular carcinoma

19. Which of the following is NOT a risk factor for breast cancer?
    A. Age
    B. Age at menarche
    C. Overweight
    D. Race
    E. Second degree relatives with breast cancer

20. A 30-year-old female presents for evaluation of a breast mass. On physical examination, there is a small nontender nodule in the right breast. Imaging studies reveal

ill-defined mass with calcifications. Biopsy is performed and shows foamy histiocytes and multinucleated giant cells. What is the diagnosis?

A. Atypical ductal hyperplasia
B. Fat necrosis of the breast
C. Infiltrating carcinoma of the breast
D. Ductal carcinoma in situ
E. Usual epithelial hyperplasia

21. What is the most common organism which causes acute mastitis?
A. Staphylococcus aureus
B. Pseudomonas aeruginosa
C. Escherichia coli
D. Streptococcus pyogenes
E. Proteus vulgaris

22. Fibrocystic changes most often involve which quadrant of the breast?
A. Upper outer quadrant
B. Upper inner quadrant
C. Lower outer quadrant
D. Lower inner quadrant
E. Upper inner and lower inner quadrants

Answers and Explanations

1. Answer: D. Stromal cellularity

    Fibroadenoma and phyllodes tumors are the most common biphasic tumors, in which there are combinations of proliferating epithelial and stromal elements. The most reliable distinguishing feature is stromal cellularity.

2. Answer: E. Atypical ductal hyperplasia

    Atypical ductal hyperplasia is a form of proliferative breast disease. The common histological findings in fibrocystic changes are cyst formation (micro/macro, blue domed), apocrine metaplasia, fibrosis, and adenosis. Histologically, atypical ductal hyperplasia shows filling and distention of the involved ducts by monotonous epithelial cells. It may also form cribriform-like secondary lumens or micropapillary formations. In atypical ductal hyperplasia, the risk of breast cancer rises to 4–5 times that of the general population. This risk relates to both breasts.

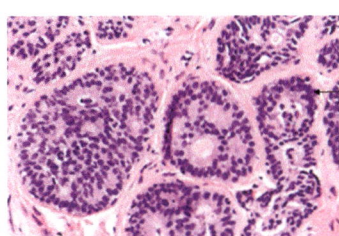

Low-grade nuclear atypia and monotonous cell proliferation

3. Answer: D. Carcinoma

    In many of the patients, tumors of the breast are found in the upper outer quadrant. Breast tumors are usually found at stages II or III. Some malignant carcinomas are infiltrating ductal carcinoma and medullary carcinoma.

4. Answer: D. Lobular carcinoma in situ (LCIS)

    Lobular carcinoma in situ (LCIS) is common in premenopausal women. It is always an incidental finding. Careful observations of the contralateral breast is required if LCIS is confirmed in one breast. In light microscopy, lobules and acini are filled and distended by the proliferation of uniform population of monotonous cells. These cells are arranged in sheets with scant cytoplasm and small round nuclei lacking nucleoli. There is a loss of E-cadherin expression. Cells are often positive for mucin, keratin, EMA and occasionally 5–100. LCIS is frequently multicentric (70% of cases), and often bilateral (30–40% of cases). The rick of subsequent breast cancer (ductal or lobular) is increased by eight to ten times compared to the general population.

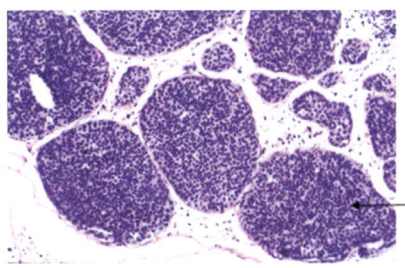

Expansion of lobule by monomorphic cells

5. Answer: C. Intraductal papilloma

    Papillomas are generally solitary. It is located in the subareolar region and arises in the lactiferous sinus or major ducts. The presenting symptom is serious or bloody nipple discharge. Light microscopy shows papillae with a delicate fibrovascular core. Epithelial cells line the luminal aspect of the papillae. There is a distinct layer of myoepithelial cells beneath it. Solitary papillomas are not in a large risk for invasive breast carcinoma.

6. Answer: A. Phyllodes tumor

    Phyllodes tumor occurs at an older age, 15–20 years older than patients with fibroadenoma. Gross appearance shows a large cystic and solid mass. Cut surface shows clefted cauliflower such as appearance, firm, and rubbery. Histologically, the tumor consists of leaf like processes that are protruding into cystic spaces. Stromal and epithelial hyperplasia is seen. Stromal hypercellularity is most pronounced in the peri-epithelial location. Treatment is excision of the tumor with wide margins or by mastectomy as recurrences develop in about 30% of the cases. Metastasis is usually blood borne and seen with a stromal element.

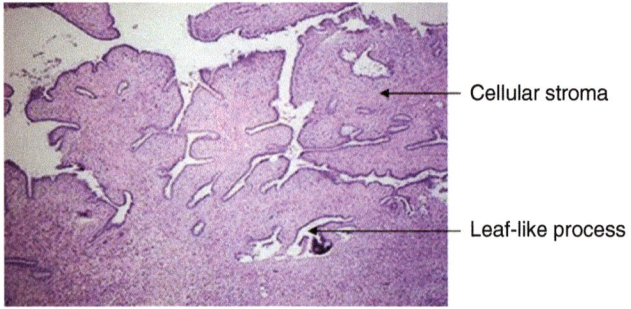

Cellular stroma

Leaf-like process

7. Answer: B. Microglandular adenosis

Microglandular adenosis is a benign tumor of the breast. It lacks the two layer lining (epithelial–myoepithelial) typical of benign lesions. It consists of tubules containing PAS-positive material. There is a negative staining for myoepithelial markers confirming this diagnosis.

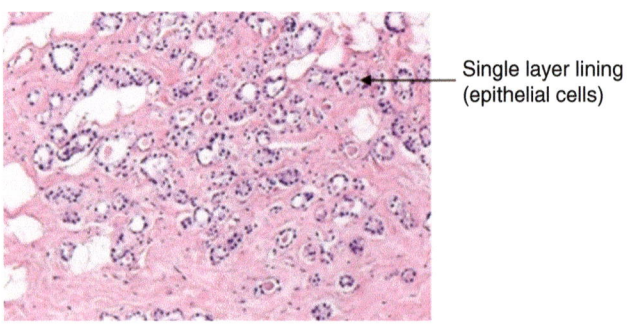

Single layer lining (epithelial cells)

8. Answer: B. Inflammatory carcinoma of the breast

Inflamed breast and skin edema- peau d'orange is seen in Inflammatory carcinoma of the breast. There is an underlying invasive ductal carcinoma with an extensive dermal angiolymphatic invasion.

9. Answer: A. Paget disease of the nipple

Paget disease is a specialized form of ductal carcinoma. Initially, it causes reddening of the nipple and areola. Pruritus is common. Lesion has an eczematous change with eventual erosion and ulceration. Light microscopy shows large paget cells with abundant cytoplasm and large nuclei with nucleoli, singly or in clusters in the surface epithelium of the nipple, areola, or both. There is an underlying carcinoma in 95% of the cases.

10. Answer: B. Axillary lymph node status

Outcome of the invasive carcinoma of breast depends on axillary lymph node status. It is the most important prognostic factor. The second most important prognostic factor after lymph node status is the tumor size. Other prognostic factors include tumor grade, receptor status, lymphovascular invasion, expression of oncogenes, and loss of expression of tumor suppressor genes. The mar-

gins and radiation predict local control, but they do not predict distant metastasis.

11. Answer: C. Ductal carcinoma in situ (DCIS)

Ductal carcinoma in situ (DCIS) is detected by calcifications with the advent of screening mammography. Light microscopy shows pleomorphic cells with central necrosis, central calcification, and stromal fibrosis. Comedo DCIS is more aggressive than noncomedo type DCIS. DCIS is a precursor to invasive ductal carcinoma. Low grade ductal carcinoma in situ is usually positive for estrogen (ER) and progesterone (PR) receptors while high grade DCIS is usually not. Compared to high grade DCIS, low grade DCIS has a low proliferative index and fewer stromal vessels.

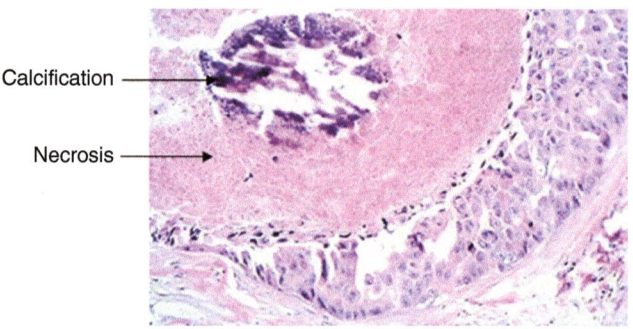

Calcification

Necrosis

12. Answer: B. Breast cancer

Human epidermal growth factor (HER2) gene mutation causes abnormal increase of HER2 on the breast cells. If the HER2 gene is mutated, this will cause an irregular increase in the amount of HER2 proteins on the cell surface. It promotes cell growth which may lead to cancer. About 20% of breast cancers are HER2-positive.

13. Answer: B. Fibroadenoma

Fibroadenoma is the most common benign breast tumor (third most common breast lesion after fibrocystic changes and carcinoma). Peak incidence is between 20 and 35 years and occurs most often in women of childbearing age. On gross examination, it is sharply encapsulated and demarcated from the adjacent parenchyma. Cut surface is firm and white. Histologically, fibroadenomas are composed of loose variably cellular fibrous stroma and glands or ducts lined by benign epithelium. When the granular pattern appears more prominent with open tubular spaces, it is termed a pericanalicular pattern. The intracanalicular growth pattern is more common. In intracanalicular pattern, the glandular epithelium is compressed into cleft-like irregular structures. The two patterns do coexist but one pattern often dominates. The stroma is hypercellular and may show myxoid changes. Malignant transformation occurs in 0.1% of cases.

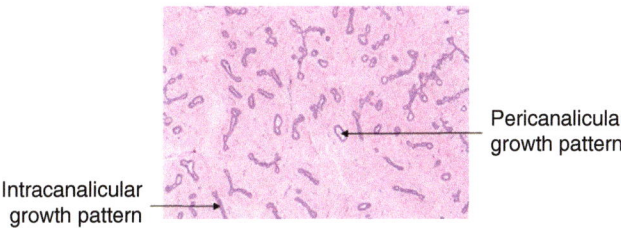

Intracanalicular growth pattern

Pericanalicular growth pattern

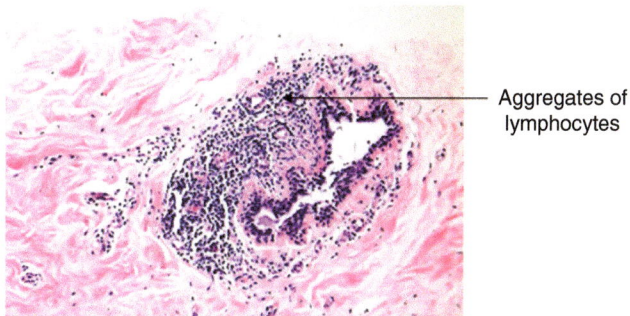

Aggregates of lymphocytes

14. Answer: C. Adenoid cystic carcinoma of the breast

Adenoid cystic carcinoma of the breast (ACC) accounts for < 0.1% of breast tumors. Light microscopy shows features similar to adenoid cystic carcinoma of the salivary gland showing luminal and basal cells. It is a triple negative tumor. Prognosis is excellent and never metastasizes to the axillary lymph nodes.

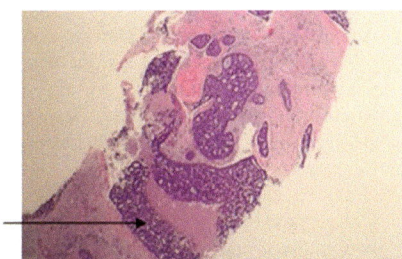

Luminal and basal cells

15. Answer: B. Epithelial hyperplasia

Proliferative breast disease without atypia is an incidental finding in breast biopsies. It includes epithelial hyperplasia, sclerosing adenosis, radial scar, papilloma. Epithelial hyperplasia is correlated with the risk of breast cancer development. Epithelial hyperplasia refers to an increased number of ductal epithelial cells layers.

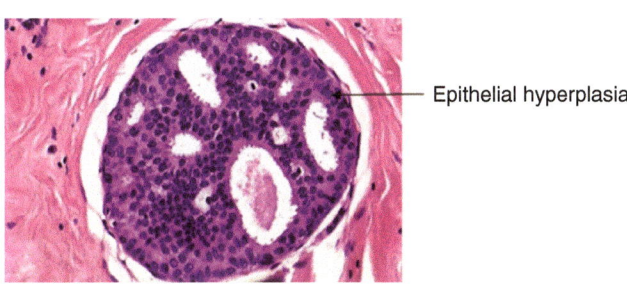

Epithelial hyperplasia

16. Answer: D. Lymphocytic mastitis

Lymphocytic mastitis is an inflammatory condition. It affects young-to-middle aged women. It is usually associated with type 1 diabetes or other autoimmune conditions. The patients usually present with a painful breast lump or nodule. Histologically, there is dense fibrosis, lobular atrophy, and aggregates of lymphocytes seen in a perivascular and perilobular distribution. Circulating autoantibodies associated with HLA-DR3, -DR4, and -DR5 are commonly present in lymphocytic mastitis, supporting autoimmune origin.

17. Answer: B. Infiltrating lobular carcinoma of the breast

Infiltrating lobular carcinoma represents around 10% of all invasive breast cancer. This carcinoma is often bilateral and multicentric. It has propensity to infiltrate surrounding tissue in a diffuse manner. Histologically, carcinoma is composed of cells arranged in single lines (Indian filing), which is characteristic of this carcinoma. There is high frequency of metastatic spread. Mutations and lack of expression of the E-cadherin gene is commonly seen. There are several variants of this carcinoma. They include solid, alveolar, tubulolobular, and pleomorphic.

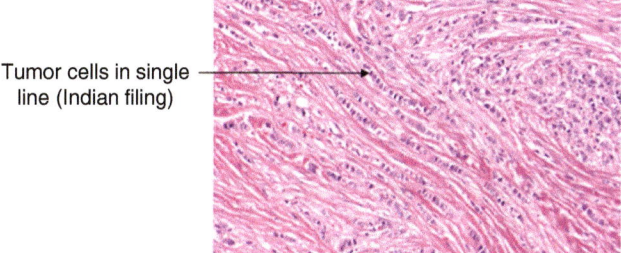

Tumor cells in single line (Indian filing)

18. Answer: A. Medullary carcinoma

Breast tumors show positivity in about 80% of cases and PR-positivity in 65% of cases. Medullary carcinoma and apocrine carcinoma are usually estrogen receptor negative. Lobular, tubular, colloid, and ductal carcinoma of low grade are almost always estrogen receptor positive. ER/PR-positive tumors respond to hormone therapy. The mean age of medullary carcinoma is 50 years and accounts for about 7% of breast carcinomas. On gross examination, medullary carcinoma shows soft gray-white masses with well circumscribed margins. Light microscopy shows round tumor cells with abundant cytoplasm. Nuclei are round vesicular with one or more prominent nucleoli. Mitotic figures are common. In patients carrying the BRCA1 gene, it accounts for 13% of the patients.

19. Answer: E. Second degree relatives with breast cancer

There are several factors that can increase breast cancer. They include increasing age, family history (BRCA1 and BRCA2 genes, Li–Fraumeni Syndrome, Cowden disease) and proliferative breast disease. Other factors are a long duration of reproductive life (first menstrual period before age 12, first birth age at the age 30), nulliparity and late menopause (after age 50) and race (overall incidence is lower in blacks). Possible risk factors also include estrogen replacement therapy, high doses of radiation, high fat diet, alcohol, too little exercise.

20. Answer: B. Fat necrosis of the breast

Fat necrosis is usually seen at the trauma or radiation implants. It can sometimes mimic carcinoma. Histologically, there are areas of necrotic fat surrounded by lymphocytes, foamy histiocytes, and multinucleated giant cells.

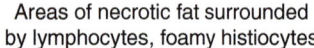
Areas of necrotic fat surrounded by lymphocytes, foamy histiocytes

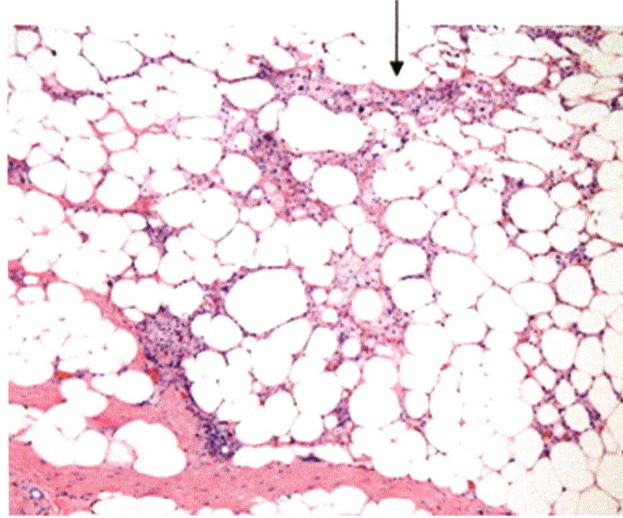

21. Answer: A. Staphylococcus aureus

Acute mastitis is generally unilateral and occurs in early weeks of nursing. *Staphylococcus aureus* is the most common pathogen causing acute mastitis followed by streptococci. Postabscess may lead to fibrosis and may form an area of increased consistency and skin or nipple contraction.

22. Answer: A. Upper outer quadrant

Fibrocystic changes of the breast are a complex of morphologic changes. They are common with the greatest prevalence between 25 and 45 years. They are usually bilateral, but may be asymmetrical. The key morphologic changes are cystic changes, apocrine metaplasia, stromal fibrosis, and adenosis. Common symptoms are pain, tenderness. Physical examination usually shows a nodular texture of the breasts. Fibrocystic changes most often involve the upper outer quadrant.

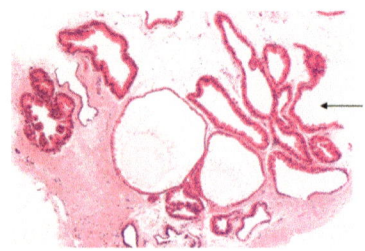
Fibrocystic changes of the breast (cystic changes, apocrine metaplasia, stromal fibrosis and adenosis)

Bibliography

1. Adani-Ifè A, et al. Very late recurrence of diethylstilbestrol—related clear cell carcinoma of the cervix: a case report. Gynecol Oncol Res Pract. 2015;2:3.
2. Koppiker CB, et al. Extreme oncoplastic surgery for multifocal/multicentric and locally advanced breast cancer. Int J Breast Cancer. 2019;2019:4262589.
3. Ginter PS, D'Alfonso TM. Current concepts in diagnosis, molecular features, and management of lobular carcinoma in situ of the breast with a discussion of morphologic variants. Arch Pathol Lab Med. 2017;141(12):1668–78.
4. Han S-H, et al. Benign intraductal papilloma without atypia on core needle biopsy has a low rate of upgrading to malignancy after excision. J Breast Cancer. 2018;21(1):80–6.
5. Fletcher J, Ranchod Y. What's to know about phyllodes tumors? Baltimore: Wolters Kluwer; 2019.
6. Opdahl S, et al. Joint effects of nulliparity and other breast cancer risk factors. Br J Cancer. 2011;105(5):731–6.
7. Eske J, Ranchod Y. What to know about medullary breast carcinoma. Baltimore: Wolters Kluwer; 2019.
8. Taghian A, et al. Inflammatory breast cancer: clinical features and treatment. Baltimore: Wolters Kluwer; 2018.
9. Gaurav A, et al. Practical consensus recommendations for Paget's disease in breast cancer. S Asian J Cancer. 2018;7(2):83–6.
10. Cui X, et al. Preoperative prediction of axillary lymph node metastasis in breast cancer using radiomics features of DCE-MRI. Sci Rep. 2019;9(1):1–9.
11. Parikh U, Chhor CM, Mercado CL. Ductal carcinoma in situ: the whole truth. Am J Roentgenol. 2018;210(2):246–55.
12. Connell CM, Doherty GJ. Activating HER2 mutations as emerging targets in multiple solid cancers. ESMO Open. 2017;2:e000279.
13. Ajmal M, Van Fossen K. Breast fibroadenoma. Treasure Island, FL: StatPearls; 2018.
14. Thomas DN, Asarian A, Xiao P. Adenoid cystic carcinoma of the breast. J Surg Case Rep. 2019;2019:355.
15. Wen HY, Brogi E. Lobular carcinoma in situ. Surg Pathol Clin. 2018;11(1):123–45.
16. Abdelmessieh P, Lee MC. Breast cancer histology. London: Cancer Research Institute; 2018.
17. McCart Reed AE, et al. Invasive lobular carcinoma of the breast: morphology, biomarkers and omics. Breast Cancer Res. 2015;17(1):12.

18. Al-Balas M, et al. Granular cell tumour of the breast: a rare presentation of a breast mass in an elderly female with a subsequent breast cancer diagnosis. SAGE Open Med Case Rep. 2019;7:1154.

19. Kim M, et al. Microinvasive carcinoma versus ductal carcinoma in situ: a comparison of clinicopathological features and clinical outcomes. J Breast Cancer. 2018;21(2):197–205.

20. Myers DJ, Walls AL. Atypical breast hyperplasia. Treasure Island, FL: StatPearls; 2019.

21. Boakes E, Johnson N, Kadoglou N. Breast infection: a review of diagnosis and management practices. Eur J Breast Health. 2018;14(3):136–43.

22. Thomas L, Khetrapal A. Fibrocystic breast disease causes and treatments. Baltimore: Wolters Kluwer; 2019.

Endocrine System

18

Multiple Choice Questions

1. The most common cause of Addison's disease is:
   A. Autoimmune adrenalitis
   B. Meningococcal septicemia
   C. Malignancy
   D. Tuberculosis
   E. Adrenal cortical adenoma
2. Spontaneous regression of tumor is seen is:
   A. Follicular adenoma of thyroid
   B. Neuroblastoma
   C. Acute monocytic leukemia
   D. Hepatoblastoma
   E. Pheochromocytoma
3. Which is the best confirmatory diagnosis for Cushing disease?
   A. Adrenocorticotropic hormone (ACTH) level
   B. Vitamin D and calcium level
   C. High dose dexamethasone suppression
   D. Metyrapone stimulation test
   E. Low dose dexamethasone suppression
4. A 40-year-old woman presents with round moon face dorsal buffalo hump, hypertension, and weight gain. There is also truncal obesity. What is the diagnosis?
   A. Sipple's syndrome
   B. Cushing's syndrome
   C. Addison disease
   D. Conn's syndrome
   E. Cushing disease
5. A 39-year-old female presents with headaches, bitemporal hemianopsia, menstrual irregularities, and infertility. What is the diagnosis?
   A. Adrenal cortical adenoma
   B. Adrenal cortical hyperplasia
   C. Pheochromocytoma
   D. Pituitary adenoma
   E. Addison's disease

6. MEN2A syndrome is associated with which of the following conditions?
   A. Medullary thyroid cancer (MTC) and parathyroid tumors
   B. Medullary thyroid cancer, pheochromocytoma, and primary hyperparathyroidism
   C. Parathyroid tumors, and pheochromocytoma
   D. Pheochromocytoma, and primary hyperparathyroidism
   E. Medullary thyroid cancer and pheochromocytoma
7. Diagram of a female patient aged 35 years is shown below. What is the diagnosis?

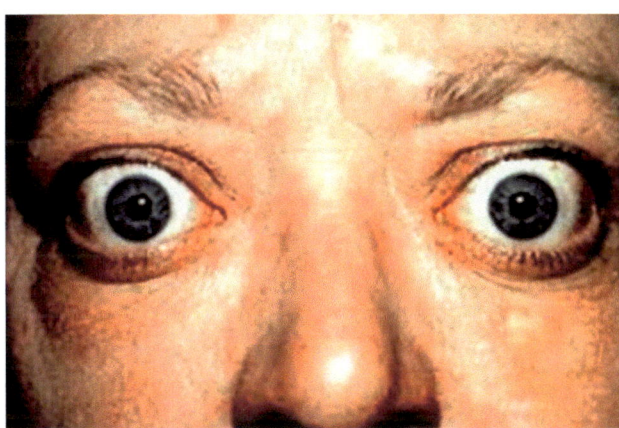

   A. Hypothyroidism
   B. Graves' disease
   C. Toxic nodular goiter
   D. Painless and postpartum thyroiditis
   E. Gestational hyperthyroidism
8. A 16-year-old girl develops cold intolerance, progressive weakness and myxedema for the last 7 years. Serum TSH is 10 mU/mL. The most likely cause is
   A. Graves' disease
   B. De Qurvain's thyroiditis

© The Author(s), under exclusive license to Springer Nature Switzerland AG 2022
V. K. Kohli et al., *Comprehensive Multiple-Choice Questions in Pathology*, https://doi.org/10.1007/978-3-031-08767-7_18

C. Hashimoto's thyroiditis
D. Endemic iodine deficiency
E. Toxic multinodular goiter

9. Which of the following is the most common type of thyroid carcinoma?
A. Follicular carcinoma of thyroid
B. Poorly differentiated carcinoma of thyroid
C. Anaplastic carcinoma of thyroid
D. Medullary carcinoma of thyroid
E. Papillary carcinoma of thyroid

10. A 51-year-old man presents to the emergency room in congestive heart failure. His past medical history is significant for intermittent hypertensive attacks precipitated by emotional stress. Physical exam reveals an abdominal mass. Surgery is done. A right retroperitoneal mass is removed and H&E microscopic picture is shown below. The most likely diagnosis is:

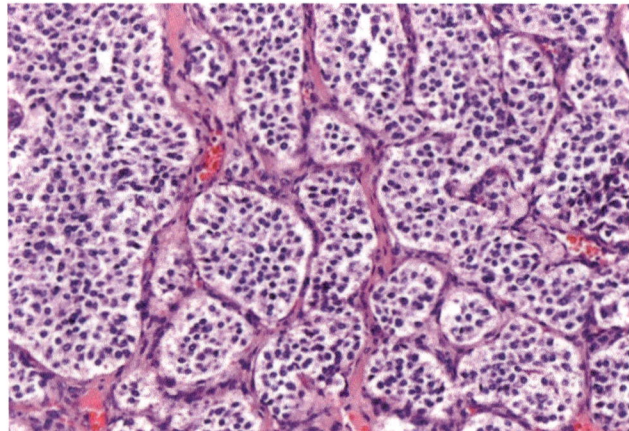

A. Renal cell carcinoma
B. Malignant fibrous histiocytoma
C. Neuroblastoma
D. Neurofibroma
E. Pheochromocytoma

11. Which of the following presents in the form of septicemic shock with sudden vascular collapse, DIC, and adrenal hemorrhage?
A. Waterhouse–Friderichsen syndrome
B. Adrenal crisis
C. Adrenal incidentaloma
D. Pheochromocytoma
E. Acute abdomen

12. A 35-year-old female comes to the office with the pain in the front of the neck. Physical examination shows tender, firm, enlarged thyroid gland. These symptoms are preceded by a viral illness. What is the diagnosis?
A. Riedel thyroiditis
B. Subacute thyroiditis
C. Hashimoto's thyroiditis
D. Graves disease

E. Thyroid lymphoma

13. A 47-year-old male patient comes to the physician office with symptoms of high blood pressure. Laboratory investigations reveal hypokalemia, elevated aldosterone, and decreased renin. What is the diagnosis?
A. Adrenal carcinoma
B. Bartter syndrome
C. Adrenogenital syndrome
D. Conn's syndrome
E. Iatrogenic Cushing syndrome

14. One month newborn male infant is brought to the pediatrician office by his mother with symptoms of poor feeding, very little crying, thickened facial features. What is the diagnosis?
A. Beckwith–Wiedemann syndrome
B. Congenital hypothyroidism (cretinism)
C. Panhypopituitarism
D. Hyperthyroidism
E. Perlman syndrome

15. A middle aged female comes to the physician office with features of palpitations, nervousness, diaphoresis, heat intolerance, weakness, tremors, diarrhea, weight loss despite a good appetite. Laboratory investigations show elevated free T4 and decreased TSH. What is the diagnosis?
A. Multinodular goiter
B. Hyperthyroidism
C. Hypothyroidism
D. Papillary thyroid carcinoma
E. Pheochromocytoma

16. A 4-year-old male presents with symptoms of virilization including pubic hair, growth spurt, adult body odor. Laboratory findings show elevated serum concentration of 17-hydroxyprogesterone. What is the diagnosis?
A. Adrenal hypoplasia
B. Androgen insensitivity syndrome
C. Denys–Drash syndrome
D. Congenital adrenal hyperplasia
E. Pseudohypoparathyroidism

17. Chronic renal failure, vitamin D deficiency, and malabsorption are characteristics of which of the following medical conditions?
A. Secondary hyperparathyroidism
B. Riedel thyroiditis
C. Papillary carcinoma
D. Hashimoto's thyroiditis
E. Graves' disease

18. A 42-year-old female has stridor and dysphagia due to a slowly enlarging neck mass. She is found to be hypocalcemic preoperatively. What is the diagnosis?
A. Radiation thyroiditis
B. Hashimoto's thyroiditis
C. Thyroid lymphoma

D. Thyroid agenesis

E. Riedel thyroiditis

19. Hypoglycemia with elevated insulin and low C-peptide levels suggests:

A. Exogenous insulin administration

B. Insulin secreting tumor

C. Glucagonoma

D. Somatostatinoma

E. Chronic pancreatitis

20. Decreased luteinizing hormone (LH), follicle stimulating hormone (FSH), and estradiol are found in which of the medical condition?

A. Celiac disease (Sprue)

B. Anorexia nervosa

C. Hypothyroidism

D. Irritable bowel syndrome (IBS)

E. Hyperthyroidism

21. Which of the following profile is associated with primary hyperparathyroidism?

A. Increased levels of ionized calcium and decreased levels of PTH

B. Decreased levels of ionized calcium and decreased levels of parathyroid stimulating hormone (PTH)

C. Increased levels of ionized calcium and increased levels of parathyroid stimulating hormone (PTH)

D. Decreased levels of ionized calcium and increased levels of PTH

E. Anyone of the above with primary hypocalcemia

22. A 60-year-old female has a serum calcium of 12 mg/dL. Neck exploration demonstrates three enlarged glands. What is the diagnosis?

A. Parathyroid adenoma

B. Parathyroid hyperplasia

C. Parathyroid carcinoma

D. Wermer's syndrome

E. Sipple's syndrome

Answers and Explanations

1. Answer: A. Autoimmune adrenalitis

Most common cause of Addison's disease is idiopathic, which is probably autoimmune. Clinically, patients present with weakness, weight loss, bronzing of the skin due to ACTH, dehydration, and hypotension. Other causes include tuberculosis (TB), fungal, viral, and amyloidosis. Autoimmune adrenalitis is usually associated with increased levels of 21-hydroxylase antibodies. It is a life threatening disorder that results from bilateral adrenal cortex destruction of adrenocortical hormones including cortisol, aldosterone. Over 90% of the gland is destroyed before symptomatic hypoadrenalism occurs. Histologically, the cortex is thin, and discontinuous with lipoid poor cells. There is patchy chronic inflammation centered on residual cortical tissue.

2. Answer: B. Neuroblastoma

Neuroblastoma is a neoplasm of the autonomic nervous system in the adrenal medulla. It produces catecholamines that can be detected in the urine as vanillylmandelic acid (VMA) and homovanillic acid (HVA). Gross appearance is solid or multinodular mass, deep red with small cysts and foci of necrosis and calcification. Microscopically, neuroblastoma is composed of small primitive neuroblasts separated by a pink fibrillar matrix. Groups of cells form Homer Wright rosettes around the fibrillar matrix. Prognosis is best in infants who present in the first 18 months of life. Many of these tumors seem to undergo a spontaneous remission or disappearance of the tumor without any treatment. Activation of the immune system is a key factor in the pathogenesis.

3. Answer: C. High dose dexamethasone suppression

The overnight high dose dexamethasone suppression test is an important test for the diagnosis of Cushing disease. It helps to distinguish patients with Cushing disease from most patients with the ectopic ACTH syndrome. High dose dexamethasone suppresses ACTH and cortisol secretion when Cushing's syndrome is caused by a pituitary adenoma (Cushing disease) but not when it is caused by ectopic secretion (small cell lung cancer).

4. Answer: B. Cushing's syndrome

Common cause of Cushing's syndrome is iatrogenic due to glucocorticoids and pituitary dependent Cushing's syndrome. Paraneoplastic hypercortisolism due to small lung cancer can also cause Cushing's syndrome. Common signs and symptoms of Cushing's syndrome are obesity/weight gain, buffalo hump or dorsocervical fat pad, proximal muscle wasting and weakness, moon face, plethora, facial hirsutism, and increased supraclavicular fat pads. Patients also present with lethargy, depression, hypertension, and abnormal glucose tolerance. Menstrual irregularities are reported in women. Dermatological changes include easy bruisability, purple striae on abdomen, skin atrophy, and hyperpigmentation in areas exposed to light. Initial diagnostic test for hypercortisolism is sensitive. Hypercortisolism is confirmed by finding elevated cortisol levels in a late night salivary sample or 24 h urine collection. ACTH secreted by small lung cancer is not inhibited by high dose exogenous corticosteroids, but pituitary ACTH secretion decreases via negative feedback.

5. Answer: D. Pituitary adenoma

Patient's symptoms indicate the possibility of a pituitary tumor. Pituitary adenomas arise in the anterior lobe of the pituitary. Microadenomas are tumors less than

10 mm in diameter. Macroadenomas are tumors larger than 10 mm. Prolactinoma is the most common type of pituitary adenoma. Lactotrophs of the pituitary gland secrete the hormone prolactin. Large pituitary tumors can cause mass effects leading to headaches. Visual field defects are due to the compression of the optic chiasm by suprasellar extension of tumor. Prolactinomas are the most frequent hyperfunctioning adenomas and account for 30% of all pituitary adenomas. Two-third of prolactin secreting tumors are macroadenomas. Prolactinomas patients present with amenorrhea, loss of libido, galactorrhea, menstrual irregularities, and infertility in women.

6. Answer: B. Medullary thyroid cancer, pheochromocytoma, and primary hyperparathyroidism

   Multiple endocrine neoplasia type 2 (MEN2) are of two types: MEN type 2A and MEN type 2B. MEN 2 have a genetic defect in RET proto-oncogene on chromosome 10. MEN type 2A is characterized by medullary thyroid cancer (MTC), parathyroid tumors, and pheochromocytoma. MEN type 2 B is more aggressive than MEN type 2A. MEN type 2 B has mucosal neuromas and a marfanoid habitus along with medullary thyroid cancer (MTC), and pheochromocytoma. They are inherited in an autosomal dominant manner.

7. Answer: B. Graves' disease

   Graves' autoimmune is an autoimmune hypothyroidism. Etiology is an antithyroid antibody called thyrotropin receptor antibodies (TRA), thyroid stimulating immunoglobulin (TRA) or thyroid stimulating autoantibodies. They bind to TSH receptors on follicular cells, leading to overstimulation of the thyroid with thyroid enlargement, overproduction of thyroid hormones, suppression of TSH production, and hyperthyroidism. It accounts for 70–80% of hyperthyroidism and more common in females. Most patients have both hyperthyroidism and goiter. Extrathyroidal manifestations include ophthalmopathy with proptosis caused by edema, lymphocytic infiltration, and accumulation of glycosaminoglycans in extraocular muscles. Histologically, it shows diffusely abnormal gland with crowded follicles without colloid. Cytoplasm of follicular cells is eosinophilic and cuboidal to columnar. Nuclei are round, dense, small, and basally oriented. Intralobular fibrosis is present, accentuating lobular appearance of the tissue. Autoimmune basis is supported by TRA antibodies, higher incidence of genetic predisposition to Graves' and other autoimmune diseases. There is also presence of HLA-Dr type II antigens on follicular cells.

8. Answer: C. Hashimoto's thyroiditis

   Chronic lymphocytic (Hashimoto's) thyroiditis is the most common cause of hypothyroidism in iodine sufficient regions such as developed countries. In contrast, worldwide hypothyroidism is due to an inadequate dietary intake of iodine. It is common in females with age range 45–65 years. Patients present with fatigue, weight gain, and constipation. Laboratory findings show low serum thyroxine (t4) levels and an elevated TSH. Elevated antiperoxidase antibody levels confirm the diagnosis. Pathology involves the formation of antithyroid antibodies that attack thyroid tissue leading to progressive fibrosis.

9. Answer: E. Papillary carcinoma of thyroid

   Papillary carcinoma is the most common type of thyroid carcinoma and accounts for 75–85% of all thyroid cancers. Patients present as an enlarging nodule in a clinically euthyroid state. Light microscopy shows branching papillary structures with psammoma bodies and "Orphan Annie eye" nuclei.

10. Answer: E. Pheochromocytoma

   Pheochromocytoma is an uncommon tumor. 90% are sporadic and 10% are familial. Familial occurrences are found in MEN 2A (most common), MEN 2 B, von Hippel-Lindau disease, and neurofibromatosis. There is broad age range with peak in the fifth decade of life. Hypertension is key clinical finding. Majority of patients have headaches, palpitations, sweating, fatigue, abdominal pain, diarrhea, constipation, and dyspnea. Grossly, there is multiplicity or bilaterality, which is seen in familial cases. They are usually ink-tan or red, with hemorrhage and cystic changes. Pheochromocytomas can appear histologically very variable. The tumor consists, in a typical case, of polygonal or spindle cells arranged in small nests (Zellballen), surrounded by substentacular cells. The nests are separated by a delicate fibrovascular stroma. The nuclei are round or oval and have prominent nucleoli. Malignancy is seen in approximately 10% of the cases of pheochromocytoma.

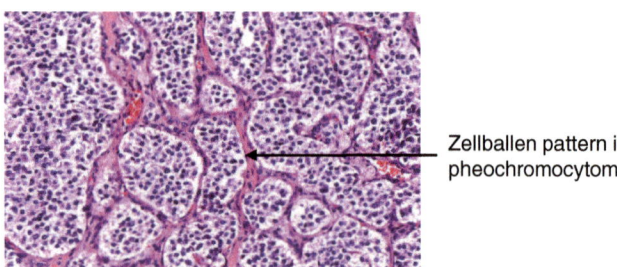
Zellballen pattern in pheochromocytoma

11. Answer: A. Waterhouse–Friderichsen syndrome

   Waterhouse–Friderichsen syndrome is a form of septicemic shock associated with sudden vascular collapse, disseminated intravascular coagulation (DIC) and adrenal hemorrhage. It is historically linked to meningococcemia. Other causes include streptococcus pneumoniae, haemophilus influenzae, and echovirus. It has a rapid onset and always fatal. Shock is not likely to be due to adrenal insufficiency. The adrenal hemorrhage is probably secondary to DIC. Grossly, adrenals are acutely congested and hemorrhagic, but normal in size. Histology shows a massive hemorrhage with necrosis along corticomedullary junctions.

12. Answer: B. Subacute thyroiditis

Subacute thyroiditis is also called Dequervain's thyroiditis. It is common in females between second and fifth decades of life. Patients present with neck pain which may be local to thyroid or radiate to jaw, ears, face following a viral illness. There may be malaise, fever, weight loss, myalgia, and fatigue. In early stage of the disease, there is hyperthyroid phase with elevated T4 and suppressed TSH. Histology shows early destruction of follicular cells with the leakage of colloid. Initially, follicles are colonized by neutrophilic infiltrate. Later lymphocytes, histiocytes and giant cells replace neutrophilic infiltrate. It resolves with follicle regeneration and minimal fibrosis. Patients may have a late hypothyroid function with self-limiting disease within 6 weeks. Laboratory findings show elevated ESR and CRP and decreased radioiodine uptake during the inflammatory phase. Most patients recover euthyroid.

13. Answer: D. Conn's syndrome

Conn's syndrome is adrenal cortical adenoma with hyperaldosteronism. The overproduction leads to retention of sodium resulting in hypertension. Laboratory findings show hypokalemia, low renin levels, and high aldosterone levels.

14. Answer: B. Congenital hypothyroidism (cretinism)

Congenital hypothyroidism (CH) occurs due to thyroid hormone deficiency in newborns. It may be due to anatomic defect in gland or iodine deficiency. Common signs and symptoms are enlarged anterior fontanelle, poor feeding and weight gain, decreased activity, jaundice, constipation, hypotonia, and hoarse cry. Laboratory findings show decreased levels of total or free T4 and elevated TSH. The term cretinism is associated with endemic goiter and severe iodine deficiency. There are impaired neurological function, learning disabilities, speech and hearing disorders, stunted development and gait disorders.

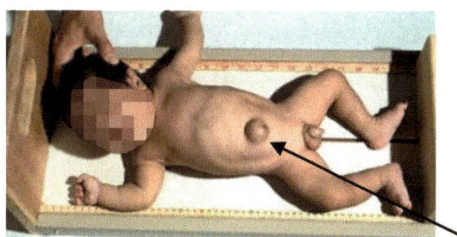

Umbilical hernia

15. Answer: B. Hyperthyroidism

The clinical and laboratory features point to hyperthyroidism. Most common cause of spontaneous hyperthyroidism is Grave's disease. Other causes of primary hyperthyroidism are toxic nodular or multinodular goiter, toxic adenoma. Causes of hyperthyroidism include pituitary adenoma and inappropriate feedback response to thyroid hormone or end-organ thyroid hormone resistance.

Thyroid function interpretation

TSH	Free T4	Free T3	Condition
Low	High	High	Hyperthyroidism
High	Low	Low	Primary hypothyroidism

16. Answer: D. Congenital adrenal hyperplasia

Congenital adrenal hyperplasia (CAH) is due to the deficiency of 21-hydroxylase. It is commonly inherited as an autosomal recessive disorder. Laboratory findings show an elevated serum concentration of 17-hydroxyprogesterone (17OHP), the normal substrate for 21-hydroxylase. There are clinical phenotypes: classic salt-losing, classic non-salt losing, and non-classic (late-onset). Males with salt-losing form present with failure to thrive, dehydration, hyponatremia, and hypokalemia usually at 7–14 days of life. Males with the classic non-salt-losing form present at 2–4 years of age with early virilization (increased linear growth, pubic hair, adult body odor). Females with the classic salt-losing and non-salt-losing form, present with genital atypia.

17. Answer: A. Secondary hyperparathyroidism

Secondary hyperparathyroidism is an adaptive increase in parathyroid hormone levels due to hypocalcemia and hyperphosphatemia associated with chronic renal failure. It can be associated with vitamin D deficiency or with malabsorption. It is differentiated from primary hyperparathyroidism in which there are increased levels of PTH and ionized calcium.

18. Answer: E. Riedel thyroiditis

Riedel thyroiditis is characterized by extensive fibrosis of the thyroid gland, causing compression and fibrosis of adjacent tissues. Riedel presentation includes a hard and firm mass associated with local symptoms and biochemical abnormalities such as hypoglycemia and hypothyroidism. The fibrotic gland is hard, often resembling a malignancy. Diagnosis of Riedel thyroiditis requires histopathological examination.

19. Answer: A. Exogenous insulin administration

The symptoms of hypoglycemia in patients, confirmed by Whipple triad require further evaluation and management. Whipple triad causes hypoglycemia (tremor, diaphoresis, confusion), a low plasma glucose level and relief of symptoms after the plasma glucose level is raised. Hypoglycemia due to excessive endogenous insulin production results in elevated levels of C-peptide. This may occur due to insulinomas (insulin producing tumors) or because of oral hypoglycemic agents. Exogenous insulin injection may cause hypoglycemia with increased insulin and low C-peptide.

20. Answer: B. Anorexia nervosa

Anorexia nervosa (AN) affects young women. Patients have a severe restriction of nutritional intake, despite extremely low weight. Some patients also binge eat or purge. Common manifestations are amenorrhea and infertility. Laboratory findings show decreased levels of follicle stimulating hormone, luteinizing hormone, and estradiol. Low estrogen may contribute to bone loss.

21. Answer: C. Increased levels of ionized calcium and increased levels of parathyroid stimulating hormone (PTH)

Primary hyperparathyroidism is a disorder that involves one or more of the parathyroid glands. Over secretion of parathyroid hormone causes hypercalcemia. Primary hyperparathyroidism is most commonly caused by an adenoma (80–95%), diffuse hyperplasia (10–15%), and rarely < 1% parathyroid cancer. The vast majority of patients present with asymptomatic hypercalcemia. Symptoms are related to the elevated calcium, and include kidney stones, weakness and fatigue, cognitive impairment. Treatment is surgery to remove the abnormal parathyroid tissue.

22. Answer: B. Parathyroid hyperplasia

Parathyroid hyperplasia is common in females between fifth to sixth decades of life. They may be asymptomatic or present with lethargy, weakness, depression, constipation, polydipsia. They are responsible for approximately 15% of the cases of hyperparathyroidism. Average serum calcium is high (more than the upper limit of calcium 10.5 mg/dL). Operative findings show 2 or more glands enlarged and may be quite asymmetrical. Cut surface shows homogeneous appearance. Microscopically, it usually involves chief cells. Water clear cell hyperplasia is rare and associated with a very high serum calcium.

Bibliography

1. Gossman W, Munir S, Waseem M. Addison disease. Treasure Island, FL: StatPearls; 2019.
2. Salman T. Spontaneous tumor regression. J Oncol Sci. 2016;2(1):1–4.
3. Lacroix A, et al. Dexamethasone suppression tests. Baltimore: Wolters Kluwer; 2017.
4. Wagner-Bartak NA, et al. Cushing syndrome: diagnostic workup and imaging features, with clinical and pathologic correlation. Am J Roentgenol. 2017;209(1):19–32.
5. Molitch ME. Diagnosis and treatment of pituitary adenomas a review. JAMA. 2017;317(5):516–24.
6. Melanie LR, Griffing GT. Multiple endocrine neoplasia type 2 (MEN2). Baltimore: Wolters Kluwer; 2018.
7. Mincer DL, Jialal I. Hashimoto thyroiditis. Treasure Island, FL: StatPearls; 2019.
8. Mount DB, et al. Hyponatremia and hyperkalemia in adrenal insufficiency. Baltimore: Wolters Kluwer; 2019.
9. Alrezk R, Suarez A, Tena I, Pacak K. Update of pheochromocytoma syndromes: genetics, biochemical evaluation, and imaging. Front Endocrinol. 2018;9:515.
10. Nishimura T, et al. Septic shock caused by Waterhouse–Friderichsen syndrome caused by *Neisseria meningitidis*. Surg Infect Case Rep. 2017;2(1):1.
11. Lee SL, Khardori R. Subacute thyroiditis. Baltimore: Wolters Kluwer; 2018.
12. De Leo S, et al. Hyperthyroidism. Lancet. 2016;388(10047):906–18.
13. Reddy V, et al. Atrial fibrillation and hyperthyroidism: a literature review. Indian Heart J. 2017;69(4):545–50.
14. Fuleihan GE. Primary hyperparathyroidism: diagnosis, differential diagnosis, and evaluation. Baltimore: Wolters Kluwer; 2019.
15. Falhammar H, et al. Riedel's thyroiditis: clinical presentation, treatment and outcomes. Endocrine. 2018;60(1):185–92.
16. John Service F, et al. Hypoglycemia in adults without diabetes mellitus: diagnostic approach. Baltimore: Wolters Kluwer; 2019.

Skip Disorders

Multiple Choice Questions

1. An 8-year-old girl presents with a 1 cm red nodule on her upper thigh. She noticed this nodule 8 weeks ago. Biopsy is done and microscopic picture shows spindle shaped pleomorphic melanocytes in the epidermal nests. What is the diagnosis?
   A. Spitz nevus
   B. Melanocytic nevus
   C. Congenital nevus
   D. Dysplastic nevus
   E. Melanoma

2. A 6-year-old male child is brought to the pediatrician office with symptoms of severe pruritus on the sides and webs of the fingers. Pruritus is worse at night. What is the diagnosis?
   A. Allergic contact dermatitis
   B. Atopic dermatitis
   C. Irritant contact dermatitis
   D. Scabies
   E. Pediatric atopic dermatitis

3. Characteristic racquet-shaped intracytoplasmic granules known as Birbeck granules are seen in which of the following cells?
   A. Epithelioid
   B. Melanocytes
   C. Langerhans cells
   D. Monocytes
   E. Markel cells

4. A 10-year-old male presents with irregular completely depigmented patches. Biopsy is done and the micro scopic picture of affected areas are devoid of melanocytes. What is the diagnosis?
   A. Melasma
   B. Vitiligo
   C. Freckles (ephelides)
   D. Benign lentigo
   E. Congenital nevus

5. Which of the following skin condition is associated with internal malignancy?
   A. Seborrheic keratoses
   B. Acanthosis nigricans
   C. Psoriasis
   D. Dysplastic nevi
   E. Nevocellular nevus

6. Characteristic skin lesions pruritic, purple/pink, polygonal papules, and plaques are found in which of the following skin condition?
   A. Lichen nitidus
   B. Pityriasis rosea
   C. Lichen planus
   D. Plaque psoriasis
   E. Tinea corporis

7. What is Mycosis fungoides?
   A. Cutaneous B-cell lymphoma
   B. Cutaneous T-cell lymphoma
   C. Proliferation of Langerhans cells
   D. Benign squamoproliferative neoplasm
   E. Benign tumor of melanocytes

8. A middle aged woman presents with well-demarcated erythematous plaques with a silvery scale on knees, elbows, and scalp. Nail beds show pitting and discoloration. What is the diagnosis?
   A. Acanthosis nigricans
   B. Seborrheic keratoses
   C. Psoriasis
   D. Histiocytosis X
   E. Mycosis fungoides

9. Which of the following is precursor lesion of squamous cell carcinoma?
   A. Acanthosis nigricans
   B. Seborrheic keratoses
   C. Histiocytosis X
   D. Mycosis fungoides
   E. Actinic keratosis

V. K. Kohli et al., *Comprehensive Multiple-Choice Questions in Pathology*, https://doi.org/10.1007/978-3-031-08767-7_19

10. An elderly man presents with skin blisters on his trunk and groin. Skin biopsy is done and microscopic picture shows papillary dermal edema, epidermal split, perivascular lymphohistiocytic infiltrate accompanied by conspicuous eosinophils. What is the diagnosis?
    A. Pemphigus vulgaris
    B. Bullous pemphigoid
    C. Porphyria cutanea tarda
    D. Drug-induced bullous disorders
    E. Contact dermatitis

11. A middle aged man comes to the office with red skin lesions as shown in the photograph. What is the diagnosis?

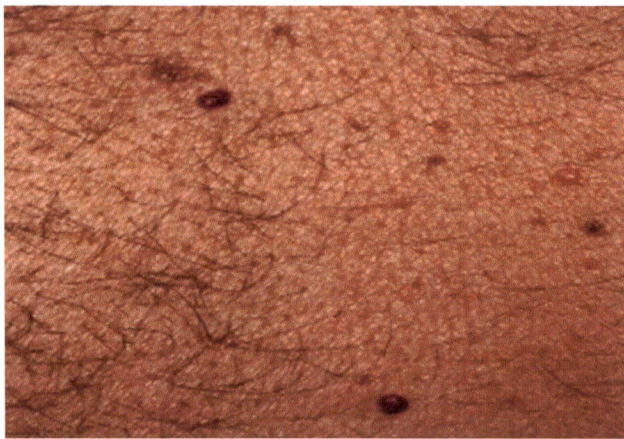

    A. Angiokeratoma (especially on genitals [scrotal, vulvar])
    B. Lobular capillary angioma
    C. Nodular melanoma
    D. Metastatic carcinoma
    E. Cherry angioma

12. A 58-year-old male presents with an asymmetric, irregular border, variegated color, large diameter, enlarging nodule on the face for the last 6 months. What is the diagnosis?
    A. Squamous cell carcinoma
    B. Malignant melanoma
    C. Basal cell carcinoma
    D. Seborrheic keratosis
    E. Acanthosis nigricans

13. Bullous impetigo is a superficial infection caused by which organism?
    A. Proteus vulgaris
    B. Staphylococcus aureus
    C. Pseudomonas aeruginosa
    D. Staphylococcus viridans
    E. Campylobacter jejuni

14. A 55-year-old man presents with pearly papules on the right side of the nose. Biopsy is done and microscopic findings show invasive nests of basaloid cells with a palisading growth pattern. What is the diagnosis?

    A. Squamous cell carcinoma
    B. Basal cell carcinoma
    C. Actinic keratosis
    D. Bowen disease
    E. Malignant melanoma

15. Excessive tissue response to dermal injury characterized by local fibroblast proliferation and overproduction of collagen is known as?
    A. Keloid
    B. Nodular scleroderma
    C. Dermatofibrosarcoma protuberans
    D. Giant cell fibroblastoma
    E. Squamous cell carcinoma

16. A patient with gluten intolerance complains of an itchy vesicular eruption on the back. A skin biopsy shows microabscess within the tips of the dermal papillae. Direct immunofluorescence demonstrates IgA deposition at the tips of dermal papillae. Which of the following is the most likely diagnosis?
    A. Epidermolysis bullosa
    B. Pemphigus vulgaris
    C. Bullous pemphigoid
    D. Porphyria cutanea tarda
    E. Dermatitis herpetiformis

17. A 55-year-old man comes to the physician office with a tan and brown, round lesion with a well-demarcated border and stuck-on appearance. Microscopic examination shows small cells resembling basal cells, with pigmentation, hyperkeratosis, and keratin-containing cysts. What is the diagnosis?
    A. Verruca vulgaris
    B. Seborrheic keratosis
    C. Melanocytic nevi
    D. Squamous cell carcinoma
    E. Melanoma

18. Which of the following morphologic changes is most consistent with allergic rather than irritant contact dermatitis?
    A. Lymphocytic exocytosis
    B. Papillary dermal edema
    C. Eosinophilic infiltration
    D. Perivascular lymphocytes
    E. Spongiosis

19. Which of the following bullous diseases is pathogenetically related to autoantibodies against antigens of epidermal intercellular junctions?
    A. Pemphigus vulgaris
    B. Bullous pemphigoid
    C. Dermatitis herpetiformis
    D. Erythema multiforme
    E. Pemphigus foliaceus

20. A 28-year-old male presents with a rash on his lower extremities. Physical examination shows multiple macular lesions with a red-blue discoloration. Biopsy shows

proliferation of thin walled angulated vessels and hemosiderin deposits throughout the dermis. What is the diagnosis?

A. Spindle cells hemangioendothelioma
B. Angiosarcoma
C. Bacillary angiomatosis
D. Kaposi sarcoma
E. Microvenular hemangioma

21. A 52-year-old male presents with a mass in the scalp for the last 6 months. Mass is dome shaped nodule with a smooth surface. Biopsy is done and the microscopic picture shows aggregates of basaloid cells that looks like a jigsaw puzzle. What is the diagnosis?

A. Squamous cell carcinoma
B. Cylindroma
C. Basal cell carcinoma
D. Trichoepithelioma
E. Nodular melanoma

22. A 42-year-old sexually active man undergoes biopsy which shows changes of subacute spongiotic dermatitis. The clinical diagnosis is pityriasis rosea. Which of the following features would favor a diagnosis of syphilis over that of pityriasis rosea?

A. Parakeratosis
B. Plasma cell infiltration
C. Hyperkeratosis
D. Parivascular lymphocytosis
E. Spongiosis

Answers and Explanations

1. Answer: A. Spitz nevus

Spitz nevus is common in children. It is a symmetric well-circumscribed melanocytic lesion arising in the epidermis and extending into the dermis. Patients usually present with small, pink, or reddish nodules usually on the head and neck region. Light microscopy shows large epithelioid or spindle shaped pleomorphic melanocytes with eosinophilic cytoplasm.

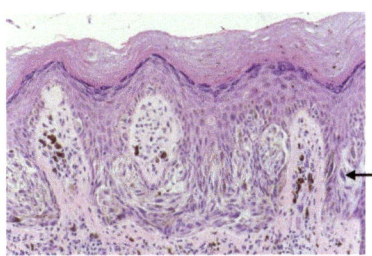
Spindle shaped pleomorphic melanocytes

2. Answer: D. Scabies

Scabies is an infection of the skin caused by *Sarcoptes scabiei*. It can infect individuals of any age. Classical symptoms of scabies include pruritic, erythematous lesions. These lesions are often found on the hands and in between the fingers. Patients usually present with severe pruritus which is worst in the night.

3. Answer: C. Langerhans cells

The Birbeck granule or Langerhans granule is usually seen in the cytoplasm of Langerhans cells. Langerhans cells are usually found in the epidermis. Electron microscopic shows Birbeck granules (tennis racket-shaped).

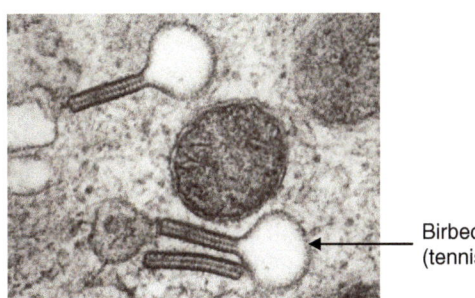
Birbeck granules (tennis racket-shaped)

4. Answer: B. Vitiligo

Vitiligo is autoimmune destruction of melanocytes. It leads to patchy areas of complete depigmentation. It may affect any race with a familial predisposition. Lesions can appear at any age and anywhere on the body but common sites are the face and areas around the orifices. It may also involve genitals and hands. Patients usually present with depigmented patches and macules. It lacks signs of inflammation.

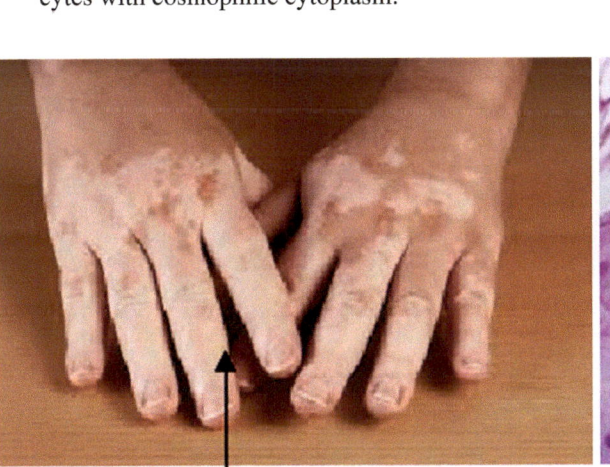
Vitiligo on hands

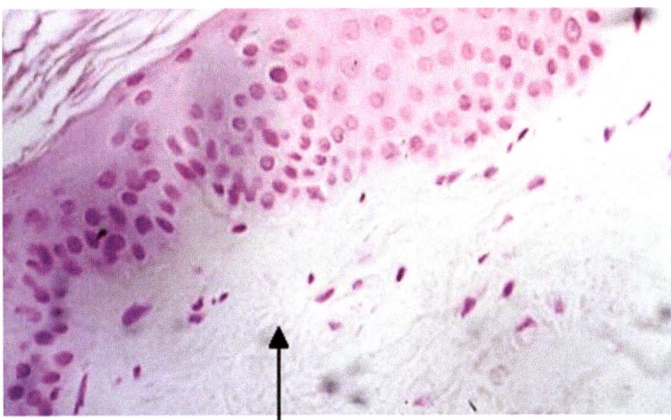
Absence of melanin and melanocytes

5. Answer: B. Acanthosis nigricans

Acanthosis nigricans is thickened hyperpigmented skin in axilla and groin. It is caused by hyperplasia of the stratum spinosum. Patients usually present with a velvety, light-brown patch often in the axilla on the back of the neck. Acanthosis nigricans is usually associated with insulin resistance (e.g., Diabetes Mellitus) and underlying malignancy. Majority of the acanthosis nigricans-associated tumors includes abdominal adenocarcinomas (gastric adenocarcinomas).

6. Answer: C. Lichen planus

Lichen planus is a self-limited, nonmalignant mucocutaneous disease of unknown cause that most commonly affects middle-aged adults. It results in classic Wickham's striae, which are white, lacelike pattern on the top of papules or plaques. It is associated with chronic hepatitis C. Common sites involved are wrists, elbows, and oral mucosa. Light microscopy shows hyperkeratosis, lymphocytic infiltrates at the demopepidemal junction. There may be civatte bodies (apoptotic keratinocytes) in the lower epidermis and saw-tooth shaped rete ridges.

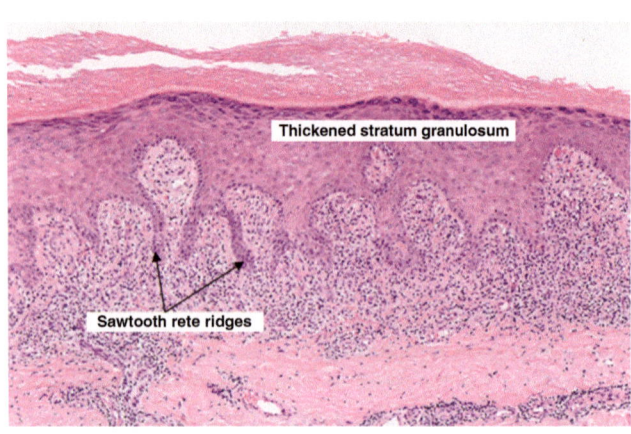
Thickened stratum granulosum
Sawtooth rete ridges

7. Answer: B. Cutaneous T-cell lymphoma

In cutaneous T-cell lymphoma (CTCL, mycosis fungoides), neoplastic mature T-cells proliferate in the dermis and epidermis. Mononuclear T-cells infiltrate into the epidermis characteristics of this lesion. The dermal infiltrates is usually sparse and superficial. It is common in male adults more than 40 years old. Patients present rash of scaly red patches, plaques, or nodules. Leukemic form of the disease called Sezary syndrome.

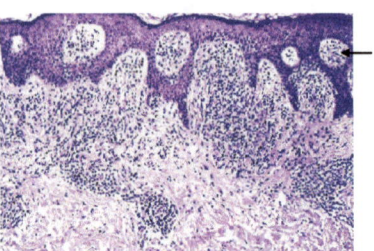
Mononuclear T-cells infiltrate into the epidermis

8. Answer: C. Psoriasis

Psoriasis is a common inflammatory skin disorder caused by unregulated proliferation of keratinocytes. It is identified by well demarcated, erythematous papules, and plaques with silvery scales. These areas are usually found on extensor surfaces, such as knees and elbows. Silver scale, when removed, results in pinpoint bleeding (Auspitz sign). Light microscopy shows parakeratosis. Psoriasis is characterized by stratum corneum that has retained nuclei. Psoriatic arthritis is found in approximately 10% of the patients.

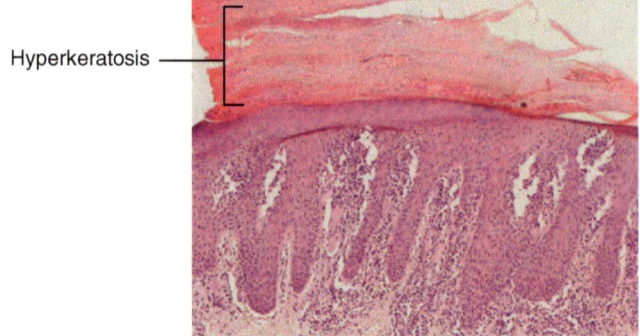
Hyperkeratosis

9. Answer: E. Actinic keratosis

Actinic keratosis is premalignant lesions to squamous cell carcinoma. It is due to the sun-induced dysplasia of the keratinocytes. Lesions are usually <1 cm in size and skin colored with a sandpaper consistency. Grossly, they are seen rough red papules on the face, arms, and hands. Cutaneous horns can develop due to too much deposition of keratin.

10. Answer: B. Bullous pemphigoid

In Bullous pemphigoid autoantibodies are targeting against hemidesmosomes at the basement membrane. It is predominantly seen in elderly patients. Common clinical features are tense bullae below the epidermis. They can be found throughout the body but usually spare the oral mucosa. Immunofluorescence shows linear IgG at basement membrane. Microscopic picture shows epidermal split with a viable roof and eosinophils. This pattern is characteristic of bullous pemphigoid.

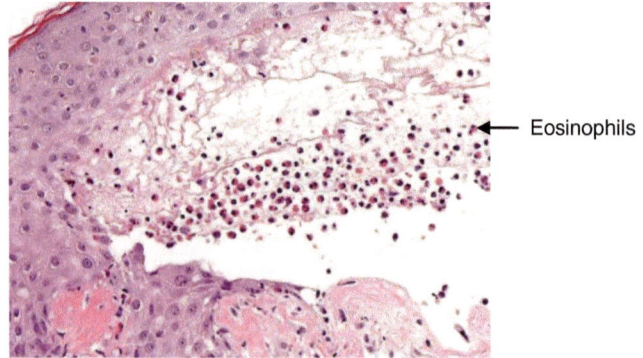
Eosinophils

11. Answer: E. Cherry angioma

Cherry angiomas are common benign vascular lesions. Patients usually present with small red papules and macules. Cherry angiomas do not require any treatment.

12. Answer: B. Malignant melanoma

Malignant melanoma is usually seen between 42 and 72 years of age. Common risk factors are sunlight exposure, sunburn, light-skin individuals, and dysplastic nevus. Grossly, melanomas are asymmetrical in shape, irregular border, variability of color, diameter > 0.5–1 cm and evolution in appearance and size with passes of time. The common sites are upper back in males and back and legs in females. On light microscopy, tumor cells are found in nests with large nuclei and prominent nucleoli. The most prognostic indicator in malignant melanoma is depth of invasion (Breslow thickness). Immunostains commonly used to diagnose malignant melanoma are S-100 and HMB-45. Treatment is usually wide surgical excision.

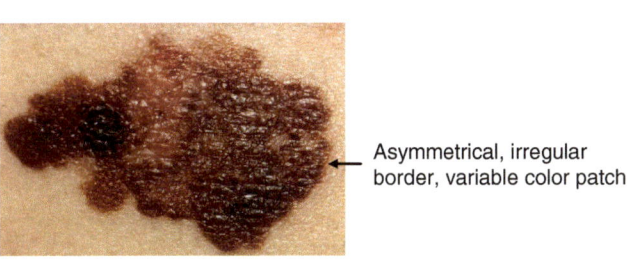

Asymmetrical, irregular border, variable color patch

13. Answer: B. *Staphylococcus aureus*

Impetigo is common in children. It is a cutaneous infection caused by *Staphylococcus aureus*.

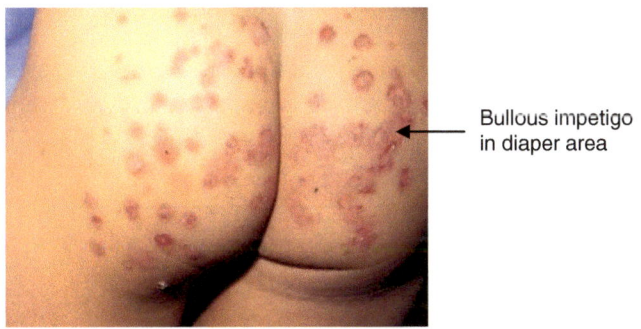

Bullous impetigo in diaper area

14. Answer: B. Basal cell carcinoma

Basal cell carcinoma is a common skin tumor in middle-aged or elderly individuals. Common risk factors are chronic sun exposure, fair complexion, immunosuppression, and xeroderma pigmentosum. It tends to involve sun-exposed areas and usually involve on the upper part of the face. Grossly, it presents as a pearly papules, often with overlying telangiectatic vessels. Microscopic examination shows invasive nests of darkly staining basaloid cells with a palisading arrangement of

nuclei. It grows slowly, locally aggressive rarely metastasize. Patients are usually cured by surgical resection of the tumor.

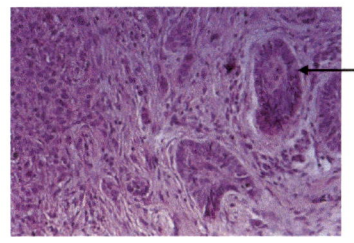

Invasive nests of darkly staining basaloid cells with a palisading arrangement of nuclei

15. Answer: A. Keloid

Keloids are overactive fibroblastic reaction to injury. They are mostly common in darkly pigmented skin. Keloids usually reoccur despite corticosteroid treatment or surgical intervention. Some common sites of keloids are the upper chest, upper back, head, and neck, especially on the ear. On light microscopy, keloids show fibrous tissue containing thickened, eosinophilic collagen bundles.

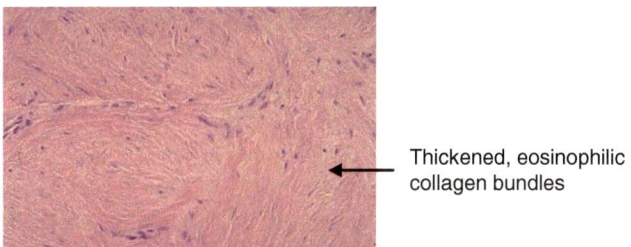

Thickened, eosinophilic collagen bundles

16. Answer: E. Dermatitis herpetiformis

The most characteristic clinical manifestations are clusters of extremely pruritic vesicles and bullae on the back, often in association with gluten-sensitivity enteropathy (celiac disease). Hypersensitivity to gliadin, a protein of gluten, is thought to play a crucial pathogenic role, and clinical manifestations resolve on a gluten-free diet. Microabscesses within the tips of dermal papillae and IgA/IgG deposition by direct immunofluorescence are diagnostic features. Patients of dermatitis herpetiformis (DH) present with intense pruritic skin eruptions leading to the formation of papules and vesicles. Common clinical manifestations are excoriations and erosions due to pruritus. Dermatitis herpetiformis, being a lifelong condition requires continuing treatment with spontaneous remission in a minority of patients.

17. Answer: B. Seborrheic keratosis

Seborrheic keratosis is a common benign lesion that occurs on the trunk of adults. It is common after the age of 50 years. It may also be present on other sites like head, neck, and extremities. Common clinical manifestations are "stuck-on," warty well-circumscribed lesions. Patients usually present with round or oval lesions with a dull, verrucous surface. Chronic irritation may lead to pruritus and bleeding. Light microscopy shows the proliferation of keratinocytes, with small keratin-filled cysts. However, the sudden appearance of numerous foci of seborrheic keratosis (the paraneoplastic sign of Leser–Trelat) is often a sign of underlying visceral malignancy.

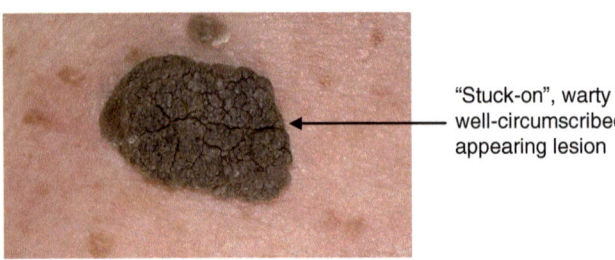

"Stuck-on", warty well-circumscribed appearing lesion

18. Answer: C. Eosinophilic infiltration

Contact dermatitis manifests with a similar picture of eczematous/spongiotic dermatitis. Allergic form results from prior sensitization to specific allergens and is accompanied by eosinophilic infiltration. The nonallergic form is a nonimmune mediated response to irritants such as soaps and detergents. Contact dermatitis is a common localized inflammatory response of the skin to the wide range of chemical and physical agents. It is a common form of an occupational dermatitis. Mechanism of contact dermatitis is due to damage of keratinocytes, activation of innate immunity, and release of inflammatory cytokines.

19. Answer: A. Pemphigus vulgaris

Pemphigus vulgaris is an autoimmune blistering disorder affecting the mucosa and skin. Common sites are scalp, face, groin, and trunk. Earlier lesions appear as superficial vesicles and bullae that are suprabasal. They get ruptured when touched. The mechanism of bulla development in pemphigus vulgaris is acantholysis. Acantholysis causes dissolution and lysis of the intercellular adhesion sites within a squamous epithelial surface. It leads to intraepidermal bullae formation. Autoantibodies against epidermal desmosomal proteins such as demoglein-3 mediate the immune mechanism leading to destruction of the intercellular junction. Depending on the level of intraepidermal cleavage, pemphigus can be superficial (foliaceus and erythematosus) or deep (vulgaris and vegetans).

20. Answer: D. Kaposi sarcoma

Kaposi sarcoma is a vascular tumor that has well-defined growth pattern. It is common in HIV positive patients. Human herpesvirus 8 has also been implicated in the development of Kaposi sarcoma.

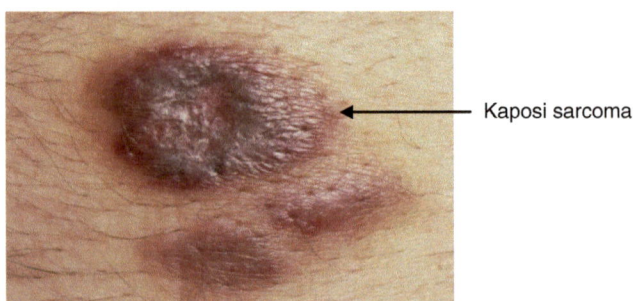

Kaposi sarcoma

21. Answer: B. Cylindroma

Eccrine cylindroma (turban tumor) is a sweat gland adenoma. It is commonly located in the scalp. Cylindroma is characterized by aggregates of basaloid cells. These aggregates of basaloid cells are usually surrounded by eosinophilic basement membrane. Basaloid cells are arranged in a circular pattern which looks like blue balls in the dermis.

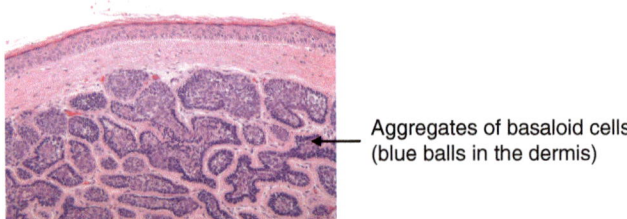

Aggregates of basaloid cells (blue balls in the dermis)

22. Answer: B. Plasma cell infiltration

Secondary syphilis of the skin can be macular or papular. Macular lesions are nonspecific. Papular lesions of later stages show swelling and hyperplasia of endothelial cells in dermal vessels. There is a plasma cell-rich perivascular infiltrate. Some common manifestations of secondary syphilis are mucous patches and condyloma lata. These lesions are infectious. Risk of transmission through cutaneous lesions of secondary syphilis is low because of the presence of few treponemes.

Bibliography

1. Chranioti AA, et al. Retrospective study of choroidal melanomas. Indian J Cancer. 2016;53(1):190–2.
2. Beth G, et al. Approach to the patient with pustular skin lesions. Baltimore: Wolters Kluwer; 2019.
3. Kenneth LM. Clinical manifestations, pathologic features, and diagnosis of Langerhans cell histiocytosis. Baltimore: Wolters Kluwer; 2019.
4. Grimes PE. Vitiligo: pathogenesis, clinical features, and diagnosis. Baltimore: Wolters Kluwer; 2019.
5. Sander I. Acanthosis nigricans. Amsterdam: Elsevier; 2019.
6. Goldstein BG, Goldstein AO, Mostow E. Lichen planus. Baltimore: Wolters Kluwer; 2019.

7. Denis D, Beneton N, Laribi K, Maillard H. Management of mycosis fungoides-type cutaneous T-cell lymphoma (MF-CTCL): focus on chlormethine gel. Cancer Manag Res. 2019;11:2241.

8. Feldman SR. Epidemiology, clinical manifestations, and diagnosis of psoriasis. Baltimore: Wolters Kluwer; 2019.

9. Padilla RS. Epidemiology, natural history, and diagnosis of actinic keratosis. Baltimore: Wolters Kluwer; 2019.

10. Baigrie D, Nookala V. Bullous pemphigoid. Treasure Island, FL: StatPearls; 2018.

11. Craft N, Fox LP, Goldsmith LA, Tharp MD. Cherry hemangioma—skin. Philadelphia: Lippincott Williams & Wilkins; 2019.

12. Shah AC, et al. Eruptive xanthoma: a rare cutaneous marker of secondary hyperlipidemia. J Integr Health Sci. 2014;2(1):40–1.

13. Pereira LB. Impetigo—review. An Bras Dermatol. 2014;89(2):293–9.

14. Krooks J, et al. Langerhans cell histiocytosis in children: diagnosis, differential diagnosis, treatment, sequelae, and standardized follow-up. J Am Acad Dermatol. 2018;78(6):1047–56.

15. Goldstein BG, et al. Keloids and hypertrophic scars. Baltimore: Wolters Kluwer; 2019.

16. Goldstein BG, et al. Overview of benign lesions of the skin. Baltimore: Wolters Kluwer; 2019.

17. Weston WL, Howe W. Atopic dermatitis (eczema): pathogenesis, clinical manifestations, and diagnosis. Baltimore: Wolters Kluwer; 2019.

18. Lewin J. What is ecchymosis? Baltimore: Wolters Kluwer; 2018.

19. Romero RJ, et al. Hand, foot, and mouth disease and herpangina. Baltimore: Wolters Kluwer; 2019.

20. Hunt R. Acquired melanocytic nevi (moles). Baltimore: Wolters Kluwer; 2019.

Bones, Joints, and Soft Tissue Disorders

20

Multiple Choice Questions

1. A 17-year-old male presents with a 1 cm tumor in the femur bone. He also has severe pain, worse at night and relieved by over the counter anti-inflammatory agents. Which of the following is the most likely diagnosis?
   - A. Osteoblastoma
   - B. Osteosarcoma
   - C. Osteoid osteoma
   - D. Chondroblastoma
   - E. Chondrosarcoma

2. Tophus is the pathognomonic lesion of which of the following conditions?
   - A. Multiple myeloma
   - B. Cystinosis
   - C. Gout
   - D. Eale's disease
   - E. Rheumatoid arthritis

3. H&E microscopic picture of bone tumor of distal femur of 35-year-old female is shown below. What is the diagnosis?

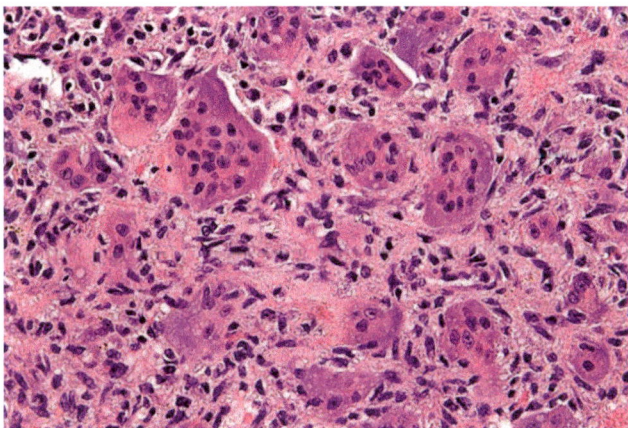

   - A. Osteoblastoma
   - B. Giant cell tumor of bone.

C. Osteogenic sarcoma
D. Adamantinoma
E. Chondroid chordoma

4. A 22-year-old male presents with back pain. The pain is not relieved by over the counter anti-inflammatory agents. There is no history of trauma or any weakness in extremities. Laboratory studies are unremarkable. An X-ray of spine shows lytic expansile lesion with cortical thinning at L4 vertebra measuring 1.5 cm. Patient undergoes surgical resection of the lesion. Microscopic pictures with H&E stain are shown below. What is the diagnosis?

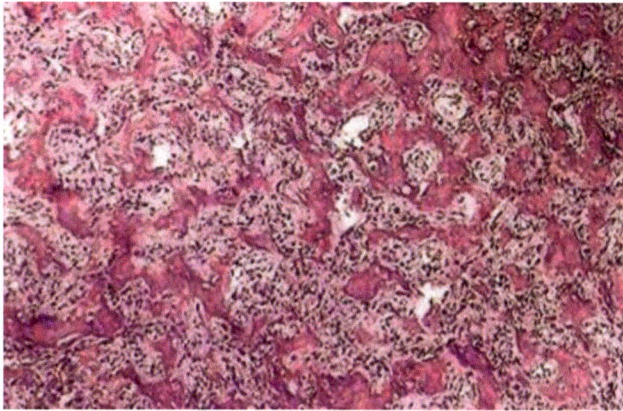

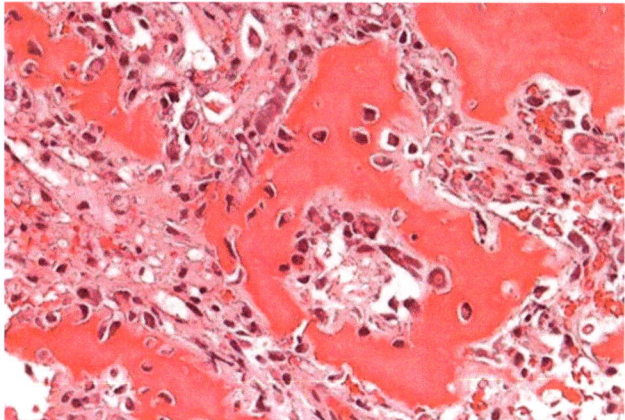

A. Chondrosarcoma
B. Benign fibrous histiocytoma
C. Hemangioma
D. Osteoblastoma
E. Giant cell tumor of bone

5. What is the characteristic radiographic finding of Ewing sarcoma?
   A. Onion peel appearance
   B. Lytic lesions
   C. Sunburst appearance
   D. Moth eaten appearance
   E. Soap bubble appearance

6. A 30-year-old woman comes to the office with symptoms of right hip pain. She is a patient of sickle cell disease. Which of the following is the cause of patient's pain?
   A. Rheumatoid arthritis
   B. Osteoarthritis
   C. Osteoporosis
   D. Avascular necrosis
   E. Septic arthritis

7. A 18-year-old male teenager comes to the physician office with clinical features of localized pain and swelling around the knee. X-ray findings show Codman's triangle (periosteal elevation), sunburst pattern, and bone destruction. What is the diagnosis?
   A. Ewing sarcoma
   B. Giant cell tumor of bone
   C. Osteosarcoma
   D. Osteoblastoma
   E. Rhabdomyosarcoma

8. What are the laboratory findings in Paget disease of bone?

	Calcium	Phosphorus	Alkaline phosphatase
A.	Increased	Normal	Normal
B.	Normal	Normal	Increased
C.	Normal	Decreased	Increased
D.	Decreased	Decreased	Increased
E.	Normal	Normal	Normal

9. A 45-year-old male comes to the physician office with clinical presentation of enlarging mass with pain and swelling of the right shoulder girdle. Biopsy of the mass is done. Microscopic findings show atypical chondro-

cytes and chondroblasts, often with multiple nuclei in a lacuna. What is the diagnosis?
   A. Osteoclastoma
   B. Chondrosarcoma
   C. Chondroblastoma
   D. Chondromyxoid fibroma
   E. Fibrosarcoma

10. Microscopic picture of a 16-year-old male teenager is shown below. What is the diagnosis?

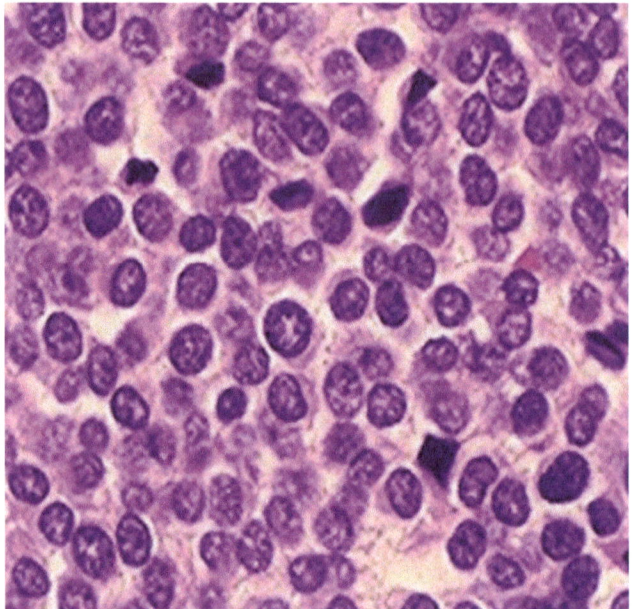

   A. Chondrosarcoma
   B. Osteosarcoma
   C. Ewing sarcoma
   D. Rhabdomyosarcoma
   E. Osteoblastoma

11. Swan neck deformity in a 65-year-old arthritis patient is shown below. What is the diagnosis?

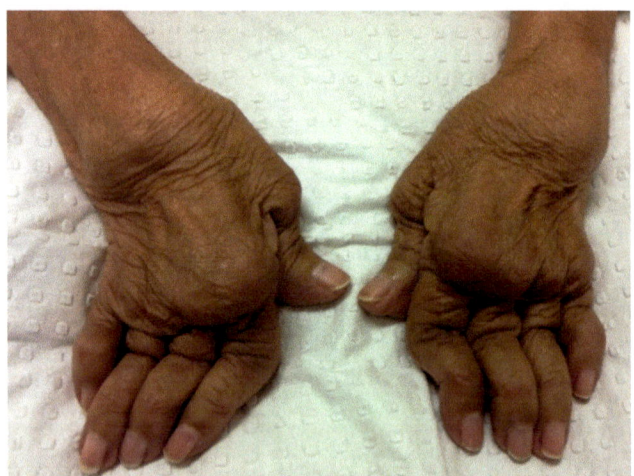

A. Rheumatoid arthritis
B. Osteoarthritis
C. Ankylosing spondylitis
D. Viral polyarthritis
E. Psoriatic arthritis

12. Microscopic pictures of a bone tumor in a male teenager with swelling around the knee are shown below. What is the diagnosis?

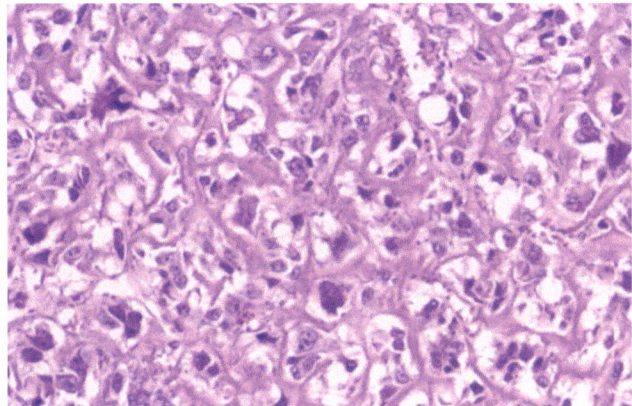

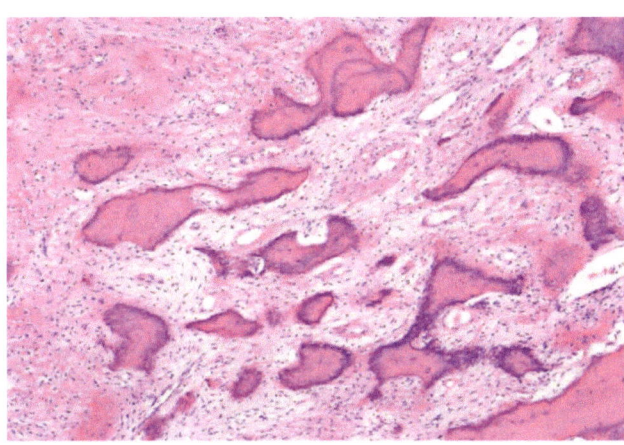

A. Chondrosarcoma
B. Histiocytosis
C. Osteosarcoma
D. Nonrhabdomyosarcoma soft tissue sarcomas
E. Osteoclastoma

13. A 42-year-old woman presented with history of asymptomatic progressive nodular lesion over abdomen since 8 years. An incisional biopsy was performed. H&E microscopic picture showing spindle shaped tumor cells arranged in storiform pattern in the dermis is shown below. What is the diagnosis?

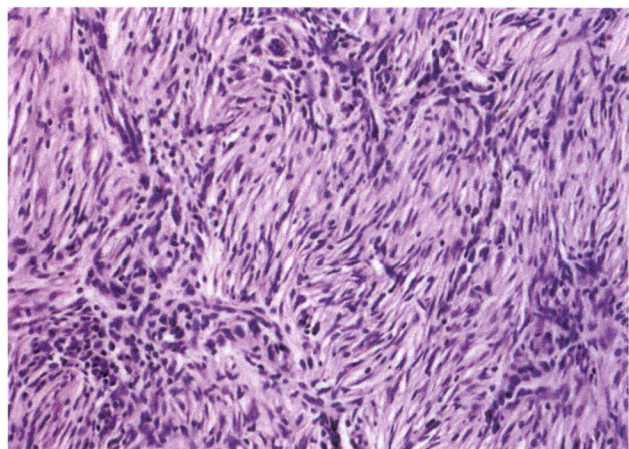

A. Dermal fibrous histiocytoma
B. Myxoid liposarcoma
C. Dermatofibrosarcoma protuberans
D. Plexiform fibrohistiocytic tumor
E. Fibrosarcoma

14. Trabecular bone loss is seen in which of the following condition?
A. Osteomalacia
B. Osteoporosis
C. Hyperparathyroidism
D. Mastocytosis
E. Paget Disease

15. A soft tumor is excised from a 40-year-old woman. Microscopic examination shows nests of polygonal cells with abundant cytoplasm separated by fibrovascular tissue. What is the diagnosis?
A. Alveolar rhabdomyosarcoma
B. Metastatic carcinoma
C. Metastatic melanoma
D. Alveolar soft part sarcoma
E. Paraganglioma

16. Which of the following organism that commonly causes pyogenic osteomyelitis?
A. Escherichia coli
B. Streptococci
C. Staphylococcus aureus
D. Gonococci
E. Haemophilus influenzae

17. A 42-year-old woman presents with a small axillary mass. She had the mass for the last several years without any change. On physical examination, 4 cm mass is seen which is soft, nontender and freely mobile. Excisional biopsy is done and microscopic picture is shown below. What is the diagnosis?

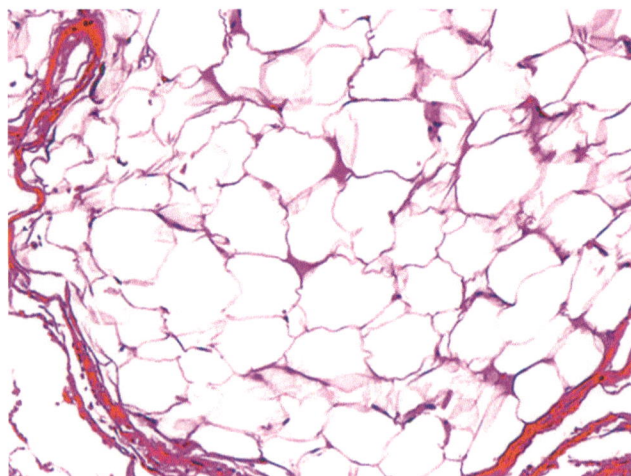

A. Liposarcoma
B. Leiomyosarcoma
C. Rhabdomyosarcoma
D. Fibrous histiocytoma
E. Solitary fibrous tumor

19. A 29-year-old presents with a painless, sternal mass. H&E photomicrograph is shown below. Which of the following is the most likely diagnosis?

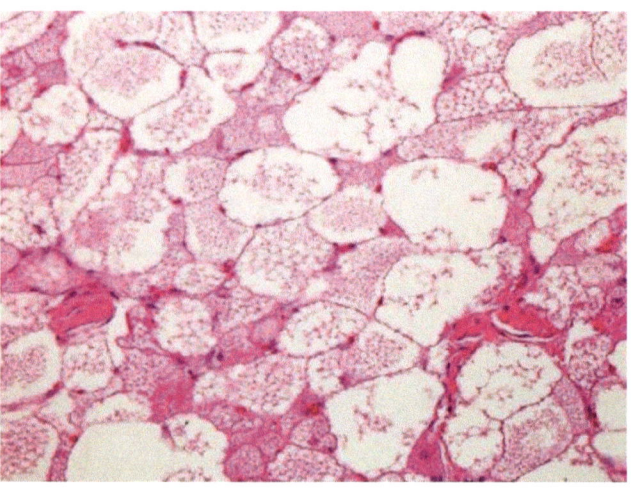

A. Hibernoma
B. Lipoma
C. Sebaceous cyst
D. Atypical lipomatous tumor
E. Liposarcoma

18. A 66-year-old male presents with a painless, enlarging mass on the left thigh. Physical examination shows a soft, nontender mass on the anterior left thigh. MRI shows a fatty, soft tissue mass with lobulated margins. Surgical resection is done and microscopic pictures are shown below. What is the diagnosis?

A. Rhabdomyoma
B. Lipoma
C. Angiolipoma
D. Fibroma
E. Hibernoma

20. Radiograph of the skull with punched out radiolucent lesions are seen. What is the diagnosis?

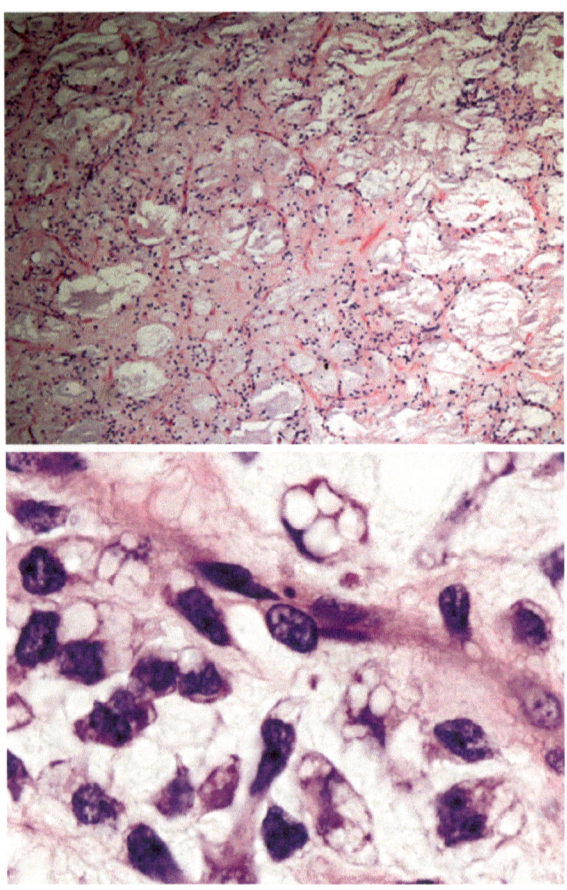

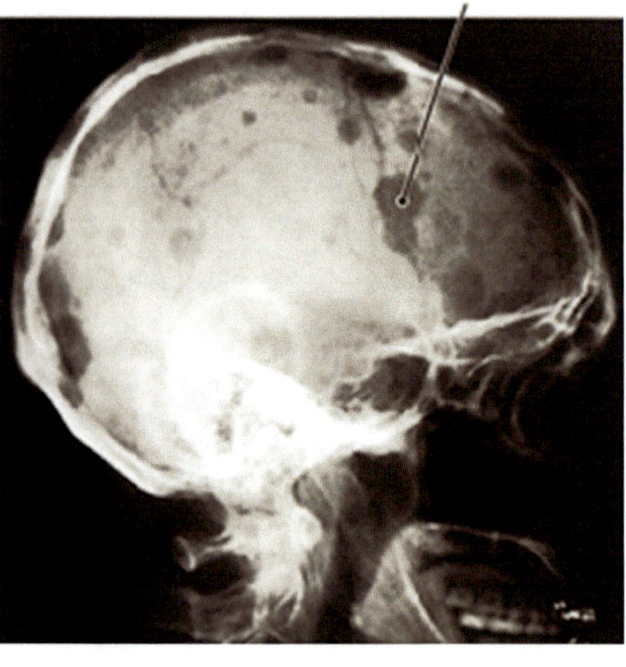

A. Primary (malignant) lymphoma of bone

B. Multiple myeloma

C. Metastatic bone disease

D. Monoclonal gammopathies of undetermined significance

E. Waldenstrom macroglobulinemia

21. Photographs with symmetric bowing of the femurs and tibias are shown below. What is the diagnosis?

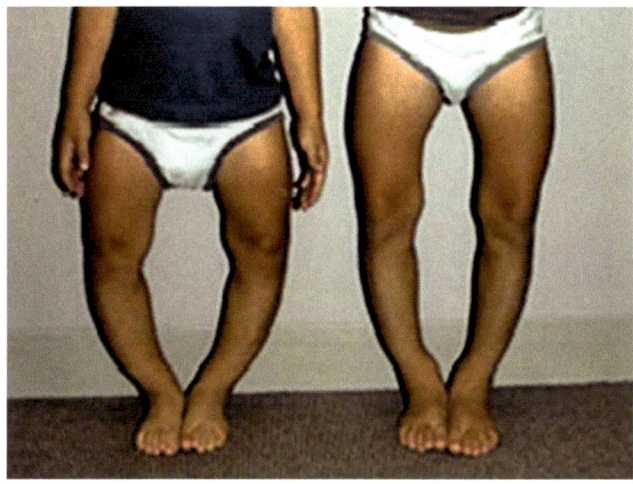

A. Hypophosphatasia

B. Metaphyseal dysostosis

C. Rickets

D. Blount syndrome

E. Fanconi syndrome

22. Which of the following diseases is because of type-I collagen defect?

A. Rickets

B. Osteopetrosis

C. Osteogenesis imperfecta

D. Osteomalacia

E. Wilson disease

23. A 32-year-old male presents with a slow growing maxillary mass. Excisional biopsy is done by an oral surgeon. H&E photomicrograph is shown below. What is the diagnosis?

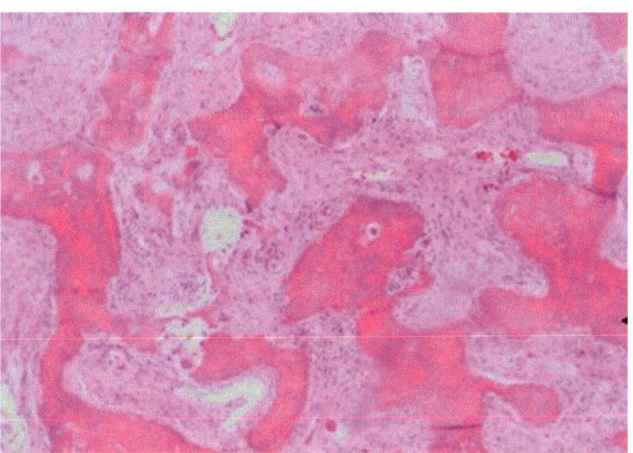

A. Calcifying aponeurotic fibroma

B. Osteofibrous osteosarcoma

C. Fibrous dysplasia

D. Fibroblastic osteosarcoma

E. Dermatofibrosarcoma protuberans

24. A 24-year-old male presents to his physician office with a large mass in his left thigh. Wide surgical excision is done. Microscopic pictures are shown below. What is the diagnosis?

A. Leiomyosarcoma

B. Desmoid tumor

C. Myxoid liposarcoma

D. Dermatofibroma

E. Nodular fasciitis

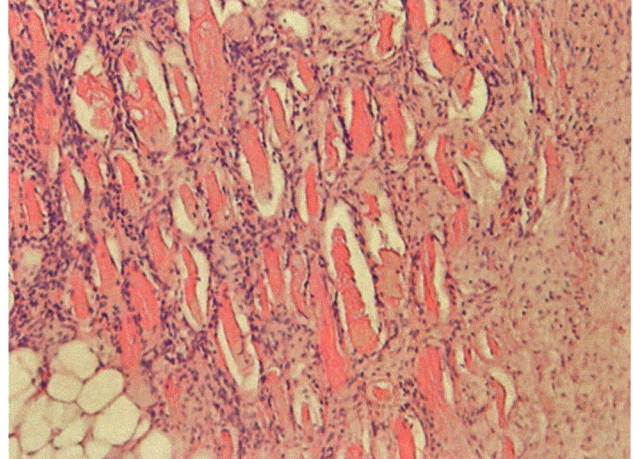

25. A 29-year-old male presents with pain and swelling of his left knee for 10 months. Physical examination, plain radiographs, and laboratory studies are unremarkable. CT reveals an enhancing soft tissue mass of heterogeneous density. What is the diagnosis?

A. Synovial sarcoma

B. Ewing sarcoma

C. Myxoid chondrosarcoma

D. Clear cell sarcoma

E. Rhabdomyosarcoma.

26. A 39-year-old man presents with a small nodule of 4 cm on the right forearm. The nodule has grown rapidly over the last 3 weeks. Excision of the nodule is done and H&E photomicrograph is shown below. Which of the following is the most likely diagnosis?

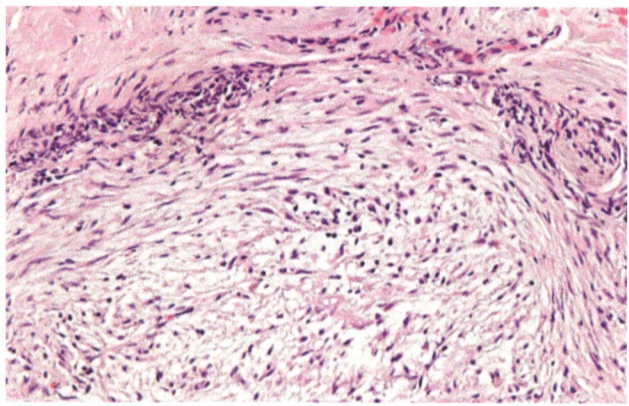

A. Solitary fibrous tumor
B. Neurofibroma
C. Nodular fasciitis
D. Keloid scar
E. Fibrosarcoma

27. A 26-year-old male presents with right knee pain. The pain has worsened since an injury to the right knee 2 months back while playing football. X-ray shows well circumscribed lesion on the epiphyseal plate of the right knee. The biopsy is shown below. What is the diagnosis?

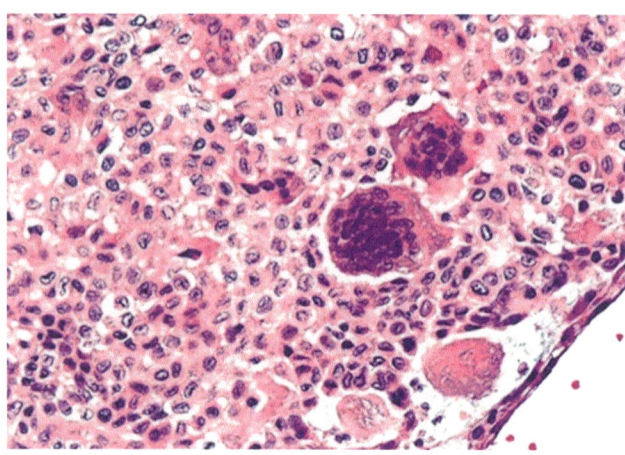

A. Osteochondroma
B. Chondromyxoid fibroma
C. Chondrosarcoma
D. Osteoblastoma
E. Chondroblastoma.

28. A 40-year-old patient comes to the physician office with symptoms of pain in the spine, fever, night sweats, and weight loss. On physical examination, there is spinal tenderness upon palpation of the thoracolumbar junction. A biopsy of lumbar vertebra (L1)

is done. H&E microscopic findings are shown below. What is the diagnosis?

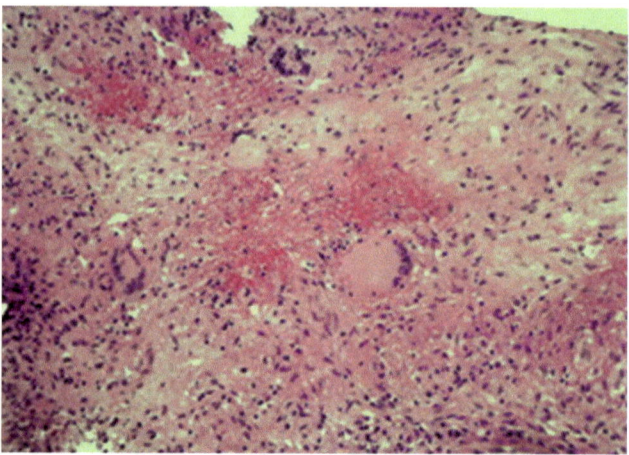

A. Pyogenic osteomyelitis
B. Spinal cord abscess
C. Spinal tumor
D. Tuberculous osteomyelitis
E. Multiple myeloma

29. Heberden's nodes and Bouchard's nodes are found in which of the following bone disease?
A. Rheumatoid arthritis
B. Osteoarthritis
C. Ankylosing spondylitis
D. Psoriatic arthritis
E. Gout

30. Deposition of calcium pyrophosphate crystals are found in which of the following bone diseases?
A. Pseudogout
B. Gout
C. Lyme disease
D. Ankylosing spondylitis
E. Psoriatic arthritis

Answers and Explanations

1. Answer: C. Osteoid osteoma

Osteoid osteoma is a benign bone producing tumor of limited growth potential. Classic history is severe pain, worse at night and relieved by anti-inflammatory agents. It is common in adolescent boys. It is similar to osteoblastoma but measures less than 1.5 cm. Light microscopy shows random anastomosing woven/bone rimmed by innocuous activated osteoblasts and occasional osteoclasts with rich fibrovascular stroma.

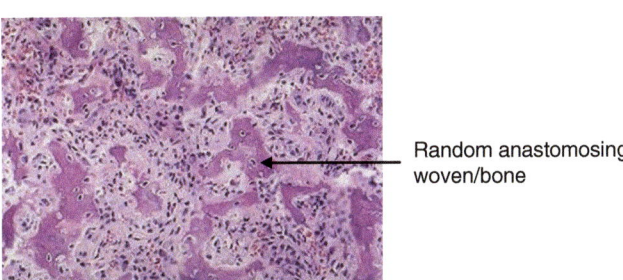

Random anastomosing woven/bone

2. Answer: C. Gout

Gout is a monosodium urate crystal deposition. It is reflected by hyperuricemia, with serum urate concentrations exceeding 6.8 mg/dL. Clinical manifestations include recurrent flares of arthritis (gout flare), chronic gouty arthritis, and tophaceous deposits due to the accumulation of urate crystals. Gout is more common in males than females. Hyperuricemia is due to excessive urate production and impairment of renal uric acid secretion. A gout flare occurs in lower extremities and is monoarticular with inflammation. Factors provoking gout flares include trauma, fatty foods, alcohol consumption, and ingestions of drugs (thiazide and loop diuretics). Typical gout flare includes clinical features of severe pain, redness, swelling, and disability. About 80% of the initial flares occur at the base of the great toe (first metatarsophalangeal joint). Involvement in ankle or wrist is more common in recurrent gout flare. There is uncommon involvement of axial joints. Tophaceous gout is collections of solid urate with inflammatory and destructive changes in the surrounding connective tissue.

3. Answer: B. Giant cell tumor of bone

Giant cell tumor of bone is more common in females between 30 and 50 years. It occurs commonly in distal femur, proximal tibia, and distal radius. It is a locally aggressive destructive tumor. Light microscopy shows biphasic lesion with stromal cells and osteoclast like giant cells. Tumor cells are mononuclear with minimal, ill-defined cytoplasm.

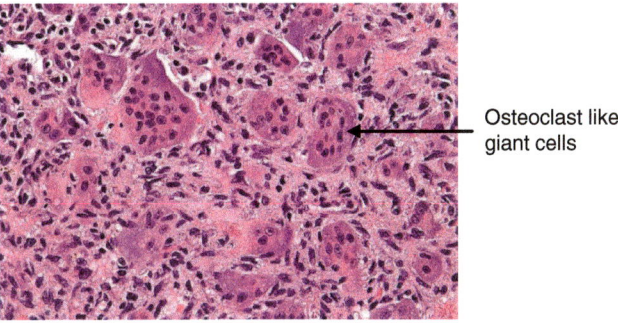

Osteoclast like giant cells

4. Answer: D. Osteoblastoma

Osteoblastoma is a benign bone producing lesion and > 1–2 cm. It has a predilection for the spine in young male patients. Clinically and radiologically, it is similar to osteoid osteoma. Osteoblastoma is differentiated from osteoid osteoma based on the size of the lesion and microscopic appearance. Light microscopy examination shows nidus of anastomosing bone trabeculae rimmed by osteoblasts without evidence of spindle cells or permeation.

5. Answer: A. Onion peel appearance

In Ewing sarcoma, radiographic appearance is moth eaten or permeative. There is onion skin periosteal reaction with new bone formation. It is common in males in first and second decades. Ewing sarcoma is the second most common malignant tumor in children after osteosarcoma.

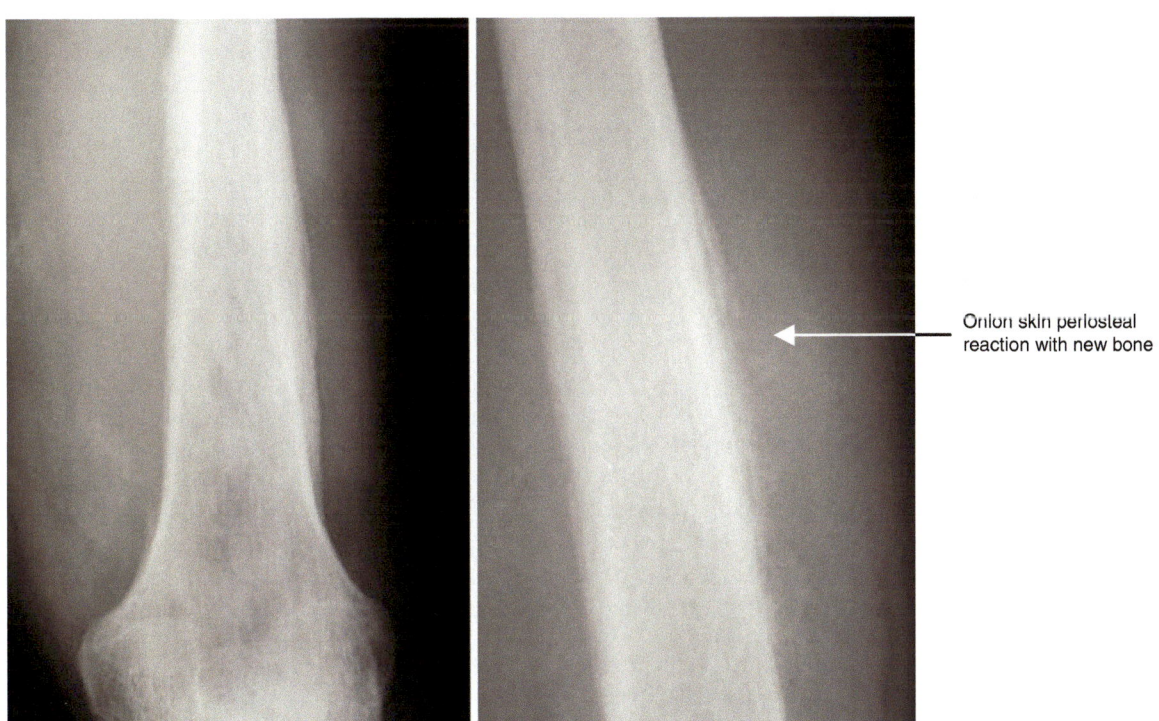

Onion skin periosteal reaction with new bone

6. Answer: D. Avascular necrosis

   Osteonecrosis, vaso-occlusive, and septic arthritis are some of the orthopedic complications of sickle cell disease (SCD). Osteonecrosis (avascular necrosis) occurs in about 10% of patients with SCD. Common sites are humeral head and femoral head. The area above the knee is also affected frequently. Medullary infarcts occur in the diaphysis of a long bone leading to necrosis in the epiphysis and causing a subchondral bone to collapse. Osteonecrosis causes severe pain with decreased mobility. Femoral head osteonecrosis is a risk factor for osteonecrosis of the humeral head. There is a decreased range of motion and pain with a passive range of motion. Hemoglobin to hematocrit ratio and a surrogate for mean corpuscular hemoglobin concentration is highly associated with osteonecrosis. All patients with SCD with hip pain should be evaluated for avascular necrosis.

7. Answer: C. Osteosarcoma

   Osteosarcoma is common in males between second and third decades. Skeletal distribution includes distal femur, proximal tibia and proximal humerus. X-ray findings show destructive, blastic, lytic lesions with a soft tissue mass. There is periosteal elevation with the formation of Codman triangle. Radial or sunburst pattern is seen due to the ossification of associated soft tissue.

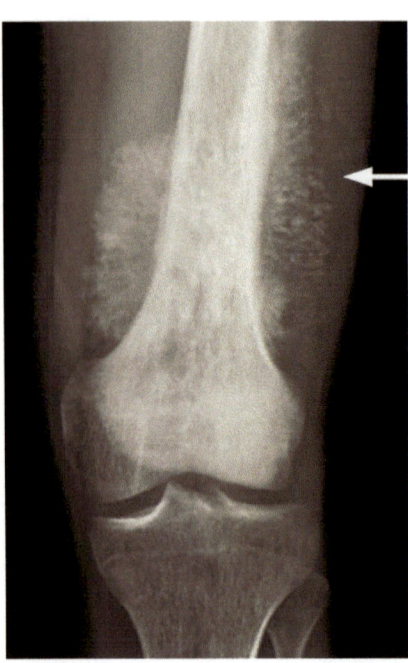

Sun-burst appearance

8. Answer: B: Calcium-normal, phosphorus-normal, alkaline phosphatase-increased

   Paget disease of bone (PDB) is commonly found in aging bone. It is common in men after the age of 55 years. PDB patients are at increased risk of bone neoplasms, especially osteosarcoma. Abnormalities of the osteoclasts are found in PDB. This contributes to accelerated bone turnover and bone remodeling. Pathogenesis involves genetic and environmental causes. In Paget disease of bone (PDB), serum calcium and phosphorus are normal in most patients. The serum alkaline phosphatase is frequently elevated. Elevated serum alkaline phosphatase causes the formation of a new bone. Skull, vertebral column, and long bones are commonly involved in PDB. Common manifestations are bone pain, bone deformities, and arthritis. X-ray shows bony deformities with thickening of cortical and trabecular bone.

9. Answer: B. Chondrosarcoma

   Chondrosarcoma is a primary, intramedullary, malignant tumor in which the neoplastic cells produce a pure cartilaginous matrix. It is common in males between the fourth and sixth decades. Radiologically, tumor is geographic, lobulated, with cortical thinning and endosteal scalloping. Light microscopy shows disorganized, hypercellular tumor cells with more than occasional binuclear chondrocytes. Tumor cells infiltrate between the trabeculae of normal bone. Chondrosarcomas are graded on a scale of I–III.

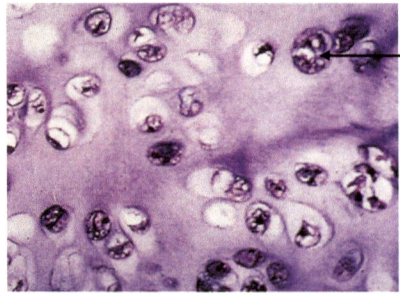

— Binuclear chondrocytes

10. Answer: C. Ewing sarcoma

    Ewing sarcoma is a malignant bone tumor of children. It arises in the diaphysis of the long bones. Femur bone is the commonest site. It occurs in the 10–15 years range. Light microscopy shows sheets of undifferentiated small round cells and presence of Homer Wright pseudorosettes. Tumor cells are separated by fibrous septae. Tumor cells invade surrounding tissues. There is diffuse immunostaining for CD99.

11. Answer: A. Rheumatoid arthritis

    In rheumatoid arthritis, there is fixed flexion of the distal interphalangeal joint and hyperextension of the proximal interphalangeal joint leading to swan neck deformity. Classic features include joint enlargement and ulnar deviation at the metacarpophalangeal joints. There is destruction of cartilage and bone. The joint space is replaced by a synovial pannus causing a destructive process. Pannus results from synovial derived fibroblast like cells. Cells in pannus produce proteinases that cause the destruction of the extracellular matrix of the cartilage. Over time, blood vessels and other cell types transform pannus into a fibrous tissue (inactive pannus). Cartilage and bone destruction can lead to joint instability causing fibrous ankylosis.

12. Answer: C. Osteosarcoma

Osteosarcoma involves the metaphysis of long bones and common in children and young adults.

Histologically, osteosarcoma is composed of poorly formed trabecular bone due to disorganized osteoid production. It is a highly cellular tumor with spindle shaped tumor cells. Tumor cells show atypia and nuclear polymorphism.

13. Answer: C. Dermatofibrosarcoma protuberans

Dermatofibrosarcoma protuberans (DFSP) is a nodular cutaneous tumor. DFSP presents during early or middle adult life as a nodular cutaneous mass. There is a slow and persistent growth over a long period, often several years. Common locations are trunk or groin. Light microscopy shows spindle cells arranged in a distinct storiform pattern. Tumor diffusely infiltrates the dermis and subcutis. CD34 immunochemical stain is used as a diagnostic marker of DFSP.

14. Answer: B. Osteoporosis

There occurs a trabecular loss with aging in both sexes. Osteoporosis is more pronounced in women. Estrogen decline after menopause promotes a trabecular loss. There is low bone mass and skeletal fragility with an increased risk of fractures because of decreased bone strength. Low BMD Z-scores require further evaluation for secondary causes of osteoporosis. The most common clinical manifestation is a vertebral fracture. Hip fractures are also common. A BMD T-score of 2.5 SD or below is suggestive of osteoporosis. Risk factors include smoking, excessive alcohol, poor nutrition and physical inactivity.

15. Answer: D. Alveolar soft part sarcoma

Alveolar soft part sarcoma (ASPS), a rare tumor, occurs in young females. Majority of cases are found in lower extremities and head/neck. Grossly, it is poorly defined, soft and yellow. There can be hemorrhagic and necrotic areas as well. Light microscopy shows nests of polygonal cells with abundant cytoplasm separated by fibrovascular tissue. 5-Year survival rate is about 60%.

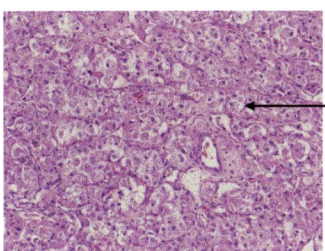

Nests of polygonal cells with abundant cytoplasm separated by fibrovascular tissue

16. Answer: C. *Staphylococcus aureus*

Infection of the bone is osteomyelitis. Mechanisms can be hematogenous or nonhematogenous. Cause of nonhomogeneous osteomyelitis is infection to bone from adjacent soft tissues. Microorganisms cause hematogenous osteomyelitis. Bone infections are commonly caused by certain pyogenic bacteria. Pyogenic osteomyelitis is caused by Staphylococcus aureus in about 80–90% of the cases. Biopsy of the involved bone is done to establish the diagnosis. Positive blood cultures and X-ray findings are helpful in making a diagnosis of osteomyelitis caused by *Staphylococcus aureus*. In that case, bone biopsy is not required.

17. Answer: B. Lipoma

Lipoma is a common benign tumor. The tumor arises from the subcutaneous fat in middle aged adults. Lipomas are found in any part of the body. Soft subcutaneous lipomas range in size from 1 to 10 cm. Common sites are trunk and upper extremities. Ultrasound is useful to distinguish a lipoma from an epidermoid cyst. Histologically, lipoma is composed of mature, well differentiated adipocytes with a fibrous capsule. Treatment is surgical removal of the fat cells and fibrous capsule.

18. Answer: A. Liposarcoma

In adults, liposarcoma is one of the most common soft tissue sarcoma. Liposarcomas are usually large and occur most frequently in lower extremities, retroperitoneal mesenteric region, and shoulder area. Grossly, they are well circumscribed but not encapsulated. The common tumor cells are lipoblasts. Lipoblasts include an indented or sharply scalloped hyperchromatic nuclei. Well differentiated liposarcoma is the most common tumor with a peak incidence between 60 and 70 years. Men and women are equally affected. Dedifferentiation in liposarcoma is considered as precursor lesion of high grade liposarcoma. 5-Year survival rate is between 25 and 90% at different locations.

19. Answer: E. Hibernoma

Hibernoma is a benign, brown fat tumor. It is a slow growing tumor and common in males. Hibernoma has predilections for the limbs and trunk. On light microscopy, tumor consists of cells with eosinophilic cytoplasm and several small vacuoles.

20. Answer: B. Multiple myeloma

Neoplastic proliferation of plasma cells producing a monoclonal immunoglobulin causes multiple myeloma. There is a proliferation of plasma cells in the bone marrow resulting in extensive skeletal osteolytic lesions. Multiple myeloma patients present with increased total serum protein concentration, anemia, hypercalcemia, and acute renal failure.

21. Answer: C. Rickets

Vitamin D is essential for phosphorus and calcium homeostasis. Risk factors include inadequate sun exposure and inadequate intake. The clinical manifestations include frontal bossing, craniotabes. There is also an enlargement of the costochondral junction leading to deformity (rachitic rosary), and bowing of legs. There is an excess of unmineralized osteoid matrix and epiphyseal cartilage due to vitamin D deficiency.

22. Answer: C. Osteogenesis imperfecta

Osteogenesis imperfecta (OI) is caused by impaired synthesis of type 1 collagen. In most patients, it is inherited as an autosomal dominant disorder. Type 1 collagen defect causes brittle bones that are prone to fractures with minimal or no trauma. Besides fractures clinical manifestations include skull deformities, increased laxity of the joints and skin, easy bruisability, hearing loss, blue sclera, and small malformed teeth.

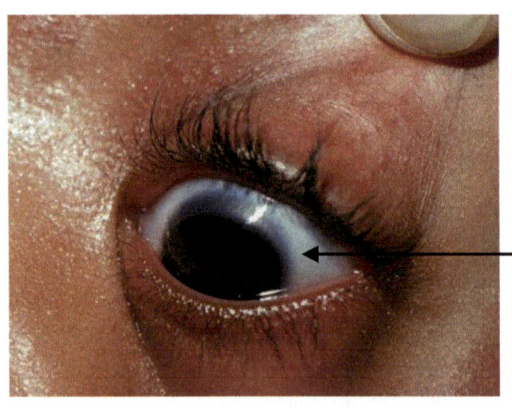

Blue sclera

23. Answer: C. Fibrous dysplasia

Fibrous dysplasia is common in males between 20 and 40 age range. Light microscopy shows curvilinear irregular trabeculae of metaplastic bony islands without osteoblastic rimming and surrounding interstitial fibrous stroma. It is a medullary lesion involving the craniofacial bones, femur, or ribs.

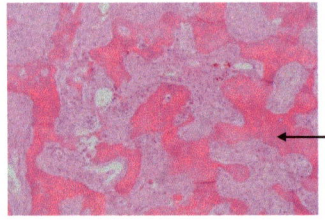

Curvilinear irregular trabeculae of metaplastic bony islands without osteoblastic rimming

24. Answer: B. Desmoid tumor

Desmoid tumor may be extra abdominal, abdominal, or intra-abdominal. Patients present as large, infiltrative masses which may be painful. Histologically, the tumor is composed of plump fibroblasts arranged in fascicles and infiltrating the adjacent tissue.

25. Answer: A. Synovial sarcoma

Synovial sarcoma occurs commonly between the ages of 20 and 50. The lower extremity is the most common site. Synovial sarcoma may be biphasic or monophasic. Biphasic synovial sarcoma is composed of spindle and epithelial cells. Monophasic tumors are composed of spindle cell components. The prognosis is poor. 5 year, survival rate is between 30 and 60%.

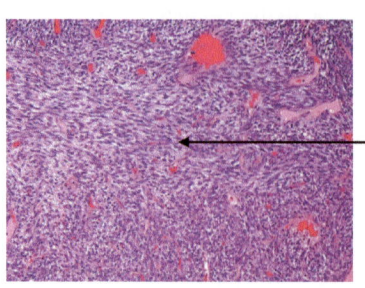

Biphasic synovial sarcoma is composed of spindle and epithelial cells

26. Answer: C. Nodular fasciitis

Nodular fasciitis is a reactive process and its rapid growth helps distinguish this highly cellular lesion from sarcomatous tumors. On light microscopy, different zones are identifiable: a peripheral capillary rich zone, an intermediate myxoid area, and a central hypocellular core. Cellular components are heterogeneous which include fibroblasts, myofibroblasts, inflammatory cells, and vascular endothelial cells.

27. Answer: E. Chondroblastoma

Chondroblastoma is a benign cartilage tumor. It is more common in males between second and third decades. Skeleton distribution is epiphysis of femur, tibia, and humerus bones. Light microscopy shows biphasic pattern. Tumor cells are oval chondroblasts with abundant cytoplasm. Matrix is cobblestone with pink to blue cartilage. The presence of chicken wire shaped calcifications is a diagnostic feature. Chicken wire calcifications signify chondroid differentiation.

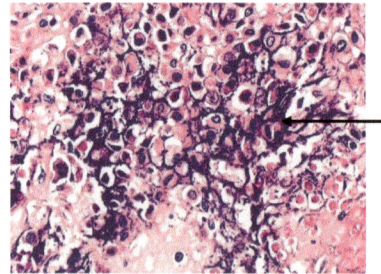

Chicken wire calcifications

28. Answer: D. Tuberculous osteomyelitis

The most common form of skeletal tuberculosis is tuberculous spondylitis (Pott's disease). Lower thoracic and upper lumbar region are commonly affected. Patients present with local pain, and abnormal erect posture.

29. Answer: B. Osteoarthritis

Osteoarthritis (OA) is the most common form of arthritis. There is progressive erosion of articular cartilage. Osteoarthritis has a predilection for the knees, hips, interphalangeal joints. Heberden's and Bouchard's nodes with the underlying interphalangeal Osteoarthritis make up nodal osteoarthritis. Women are frequently affected around the menopause. Heberden's nodes are bony growths on distal interphalangeal joints (DIP) close to fingernail. Bony bumps on the middle joint of the finger (PIP joint) are called Bouchard's nodes.

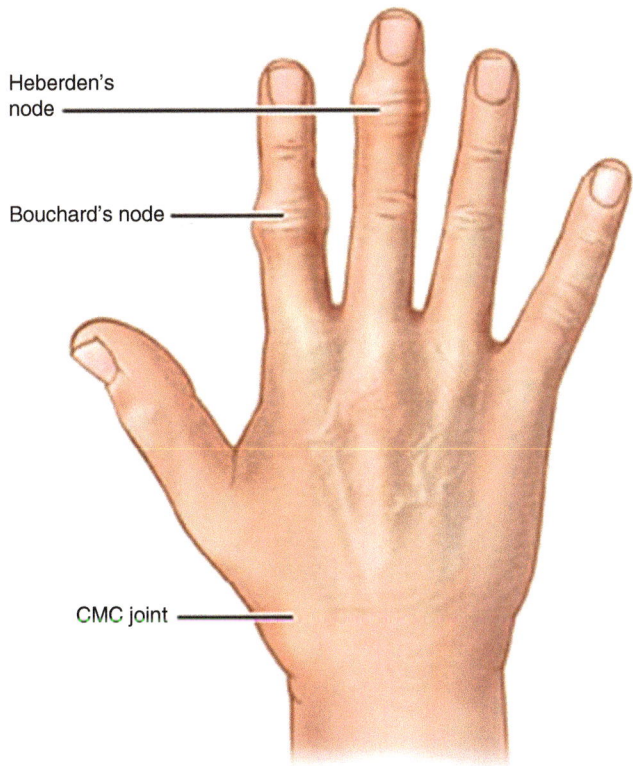

30. Answer: A. Pseudogout

Pseudogout is an attack of inflammatory arthritis caused by calcium pyrophosphate crystal (CPP) deposition in synovial fluid. CPP crystal arthritis is more common in men. Patients present with pain, joint swelling, and erythema. The presence of rhomboid-shaped calcium pyrophosphate crystals in synovial fluid analysis is diagnostic for pseudogout. CPP deposition consequences include acute inflammatory arthritis, inflammatory, and degenerative chronic arthropathies. Crystal pyrophosphate deposition (CPPD) diseases are pseudogout and chondrocalcinosis. Acute CPP crystal arthritis causes acute or subacute arthritis. In acute CPP crystal arthritis, the knee joint is involved in approximately 50% of cases. First episodes of acute CPP crystal arthritis persist longer. These episodes are self-limited and last days to weeks.

Bibliography

1. Welch WC, et al. Spinal cord tumors. Baltimore: Wolters Kluwer; 2019.
2. Michael AB, et al. Pathophysiology of gout. Oxford: Oxford University Press; 2019.
3. Verma S, et al. Multiarticular tophaceous gout with severe joint destruction: a pictorial overview with a twist. Indian J Dermatol. 2014;59(6):609–11.
4. O'Donnell P. Giant cell tumor. Baltimore: Wolters Kluwer; 2019.
5. Kravets I. Pagets disease of bone: diagnosis and treatment. Am J Med. 2018;131(11):1298–303.
6. Thomas FD, et al. Clinical presentation, staging, and prognostic factors of the Ewing sarcoma family of tumors. Baltimore: Wolters Kluwer; 2019.
7. George A, et al. Acute and chronic bone complications of sickle cell disease. Baltimore: Wolters Kluwer; 2019.
8. Ridley WE, Xiang H, Han J, Ridley LJ. Swan neck deformity. J Med Imaging Radiat Oncol. 2018;62:159–60.
9. Charles RF, et al. Clinical manifestations and diagnosis of Paget disease of bone. Baltimore: Wolters Kluwer; 2019.
10. Gelderblom AJ, et al. Chondrosarcoma. Baltimore: Wolters Kluwer; 2019.
11. Rekhi B, Mridha A, Kattoor J. Small round cell lesions of the bone: diagnostic approach, differential diagnoses and impact on treatment. Indian J Pathol Microbiol. 2019;62(2):199–205.
12. Wang LL, Gebhardt MC, Rainusso N. Osteosarcoma: epidemiology, pathogenesis, clinical presentation, diagnosis, and histology. Baltimore: Wolters Kluwer; 2019.
13. Durfee RA, Mohammed M, Luu HH. Review of osteosarcoma and current management. Rheumatol Ther. 2016;3(2):221–43.
14. Malkud S, Dyavannanavar V. Dermatofibrosarcoma protuberans. Indian Dermatol Online J. 2017;8(6):495–7.
15. Pruksapong C, Satayasoontorn K. Alveolar soft part sarcoma of flexor tendon. J Surg Case Rep. 2017;2017(12):rjx240.
16. Birt MC, et al. Osteomyelitis: recent advances in pathophysiology and therapeutic strategies. J Orthop. 2017;14(1):45–52.
17. Sexton DJ, et al. Skeletal tuberculosis. Baltimore: Wolters Kluwer; 2019.
18. Jayker SS, Prakash CJ, Arkeswara MY, Ansari MN, Hashim SM, Achappa P. Osteitis fibrosa cystica of tibia as initial manifestation of primary hyperparathyroidism. J Case Rep. 2017;7(1):1–14.
19. Miller M, et al. Clinical manifestations of dermatomyositis and polymyositis in adults. Baltimore: Wolters Kluwer; 2019.
20. Rajkumar SV, et al. Multiple myeloma: clinical features, laboratory manifestations, and diagnosis. Literature review current through. Baltimore: Wolters Kluwer; 2019.
21. Thomas C, et al. Overview of rickets in children. Literature review current through. Baltimore: Wolters Kluwer; 2019.
22. Bacino CA, Hahn S, TePas E. Achondroplasia. Baltimore: Wolters Kluwer; 2019.
23. Bacino CA, Hahn S, TePas E. Skeletal dysplasias: specific disorders. Baltimore: Wolters Kluwer; 2019.
24. Humeniuk Arasiewicz M, Stryjewska Makuch G, Janik MA, Kolebacz B. Giant fronto-ethmoidal osteoma—selection of an optimal surgical procedure. Braz J Otorhinolaryngol. 2018;84(2):232–9.
25. Dawson NA, et al. Overview of the treatment of castration-resistant prostate cancer (CRPC). Baltimore: Wolters Kluwer; 2019.
26. Lebowitz D, et al. TB determined: tuberculous osteomyelitis. Am J Med. 2014;127(3):198–201.
27. Rosenthal AK, Dalbeth N, Romain PL. Clinical manifestations and diagnosis of calcium pyrophosphate crystal deposition (CPPD) disease. Baltimore: Wolters Kluwer; 2019.
28. Beary JF, et al. Osteogenesis imperfecta: clinical features and diagnosis. Baltimore: Wolters Kluwer; 2019.

Multiple Choice Questions

1. Which muscular dystrophy is the cause of mutations in the dystrophin gene?
   A. Becker muscular dystrophy
   B. Guillain–Barre syndrome
   C. Duchenne muscular dystrophy
   D. Inflammatory myopathies
   E. Dermatomyositis

2. A 35-year-old woman present with muscular weakness affecting the facial muscles, ptosis, and diplopia. Laboratory findings show autoantibodies against the acetylcholine (ACh) receptors. What is the diagnosis?
   A. Eaton–Lambert syndrome
   B. Myasthenia gravis
   C. Botulism
   D. Basilar artery thrombosis
   E. Cavernous sinus syndrome

3. A 42-year-old man presents with muscular weakness with an ascending paralysis. He had a viral illness for the last 10 days. Physical examination shows loss of deep tendon reflexes. A lumbar puncture is done and CSF contains increased levels of protein with minimal cellular reaction. What is the diagnosis?
   A. Transverse myelitis
   B. Chronic inflammatory demyelinating polyneuropathy
   C. Guillain–Barre syndrome
   D. Vascular injury
   E. Conversion disorder

4. A 22-year-old male presents with muscle weakness, which is most pronounced in the proximal muscles. Deltoid muscle biopsy is done and staining of the biopsy shows dystrophin is present, but in an abnormal form. What is the diagnosis?
   A. Amyotrophic lateral sclerosis
   B. Becker muscular dystrophy
   C. Myasthenia gravis

   D. Polymyositis
   E. Duchenne muscular dystrophy

5. A 49-year-old woman presents with symptoms of bilateral proximal muscle weakness, skin rash of the upper eyelids, periorbital edema, and inflamed muscles. Muscle biopsy shows perimysial and vascular lymphocytic inflammation, perifascicular fiber atrophy. What is the diagnosis?
   A. Polymyositis
   B. Dermatomyositis
   C. Inclusion body myositis
   D. Myasthenia gravis
   E. Eaton–Lambert syndrome

6. A 39-year-old woman comes to the physician office with clinical feature of flat, light brown spots on the skin, freckling in the armpits or groin area, tiny bumps on the iris of the eye and soft, pea-sized bumps on or under the skin. What is the diagnosis?
   A. Neurofibromatosis type 2 (NF-2)
   B. Neurofibromatosis type 1 (NF-1)
   C. Schwannomatosis
   D. McCune–Albright syndrome
   E. Sturge–Weber syndrome

7. A 57-year-old male presents with difficulty in carrying out daily activities, including walking. There is weakness in the feet, hands, legs, and ankles. Patient is wheelchair bound. Biopsy of one of the muscles of the thigh shows only atrophy of the myofibers. What is the diagnosis?
   A. Paraneoplastic neuropathy
   B. Multifocal acquired demyelinating neuropathy
   C. Monoclonal gammopathies
   D. Spinal cord arteriovenous malformation
   E. Amyotrophic lateral sclerosis

8. A 54-year-old female presents with bilateral proximal muscle weakness. Biopsy of one of the muscles is done and microscopic findings show endomysial lymphocytic inflammation, skeletal muscle fiber degeneration and regeneration. What is the diagnosis?

A. Polymyositis
B. Myasthenia gravis
C. Diabetic polyradiculopathy
D. Eosinophilic myositis
E. Myositis ossificans

9. A 65-year-old man with the diagnosis of small cell lung carcinoma comes to the physician office with proximal muscular weakness. What is the diagnosis?
   A. Dermatomyositis
   B. Amyotrophic lateral sclerosis
   C. Inclusion body myositis
   D. Multiple sclerosis
   E. Lambert–Eaton syndrome

10. Which of the following is a form of compressive neuropathy in which plantar nerve is trapped between metatarsal heads?
    A. Stress fracture
    B. Tendon sheath ganglion
    C. Morton neuroma
    D. Strain of the plantar capsule
    E. Nerve-sheath tumor

11. Which of the following medical conditions result from entrapment of the medial nerve beneath the flexor retinaculum at the wrist?
    A. Acute compartment syndrome
    B. Diabetic neuropathy
    C. Multiple sclerosis
    D. Carpal tunnel syndrome (CTS)
    E. Syringomyelia

12. Which of the following medical condition is seen in patients with immunological diseases?
    A. Cervical myelopathy
    B. Chronic inflammatory demyelinating polyneuropathy (CIDP)
    C. Diabetic neuropathy
    D. Charcot–Marie-Tooth disease
    E. Lambert–Eaton myasthenic syndrome

13. Which of the following drug is responsible for causing myopathy with creatine kinase level more than ten times normal?
    A. Carbamazepine
    B. Gabapentin
    C. Oxcarbazepine
    D. Lovastatin
    E. Pregabalin

14. Which of the following medical condition is consistent with sensory neuropathy?
    A. Chronic pancreatitis
    B. Diabetes mellitus
    C. Cystic fibrosis
    D. Prader–Willi syndrome
    E. Multiple sclerosis

15. Which of the following disease is a form of spinal muscular atrophy resulting from loss of motor neurons in infancy?
    A. Transverse myelitis
    B. Werdnig–Hoffmann disease
    C. Muscular dystrophy
    D. Polymyositis
    E. Inflammatory myopathy

16. Which of the following is a congenital myopathy that is present in childhood and may be nonprogressive or slowly progressive?
    A. Metabolic myopathies
    B. Spinal muscular atrophy
    C. Nemaline rod myopathy
    D. Amyotrophic lateral sclerosis.
    E. Polymyositis

17. Deficiency of lysosomal acid alpha-glucosidase causes which of the following disease?
    A. Myotonic dystrophy
    B. Pompe disease
    C. McArdle disease
    D. Spinal muscular atrophy
    E. Mitochondrial myopathy

18. Which of the following autosomal recessive condition results from the deficiency in muscle phosphorylase and does not produce progressive weakness?
    A. McArdle disease
    B. Spinal muscular atrophy
    C. Mitochondrial myopathy
    D. Becker muscular dystrophy
    E. Amyotrophic lateral sclerosis

19. In which disease, type II muscle fiber atrophy can occur with glucocorticoid excess?
    A. Myasthenia gravis
    B. Cushing's syndrome
    C. Amyotrophic lateral sclerosis
    D. Mitochondrial myopathy
    E. Diabetes mellitus

20. Which of the virus after infection becomes dormant in dorsal root ganglia?
    A. Varicella Zoster virus
    B. Epstein–Barr virus
    C. Rhinovirus
    D. Adenovirus
    E. Cytomegalovirus

Answers and Explanations

1. Answer: C. Duchenne muscular dystrophy
   Duchenne muscular dystrophy (DMD) is a complete loss of dystrophin gene on chromosome Xp21. Duchenne

muscular dystrophy is essential for membrane integrity in skeletal muscle. It is inherited as an X-linked recessive trait. Patients present with weakness with difficulty in ambulation. Affected patients become wheelchair bound. Common complications are orthopedic and cardiac. Death occurs due to respiratory muscle weakness or cardiomyopathy usually in the twenties. Patients may also exhibit the Gower sign in which patients stand from a sitting position by first getting on their hands and feet. Elevated creatinine phosphokinase is specific for muscular dystrophy (250 times above normal). Histologically, there is muscle fiber degeneration and proliferation of adipose tissue.

2. Answer: B. Myasthenia gravis

Myasthenia gravis is an autoimmune disease in which antibodies attack the nicotinic ACh receptors. In myasthenia gravis, acetylcholine receptor (AChR) antibodies are found in about 80–85% of patients. Patients present with weakness which worsen during the periods of activity and improve during the period of rest. If left untreated, myasthenia gravis can lead to respiratory failure. Diagnosis is confirmed by Tensilon test. Administration of edrophonium a short acting ACh inhibitor rapidly improves symptoms in myasthenia gravis.

3. Answer: C. Guillain–Barre syndrome

Guillain–Barre syndrome is inflammatory autoimmune destruction of Schwann cells. It causes the demyelination of peripheral motor ventral roots and cranial nerve often associated with infections. Patients present with symmetric and ascending, rapidly progressive muscle weakness that begins in the distal lower extremities with or without paresthesias. It can lead to flaccid, neuromuscular paralysis. Lower extremity deep tendon reflexes are diminished. A history of antecedent respiratory or gastrointestinal infection, 2–4 weeks prior is common. CSF shows an elevated protein and normal amount of white blood cells (albuminocytologic dissociation). There is an increased risk of respiratory muscle paralysis over time. It may result in cardiac dysrhythmias, hypertension, and hypotension. Bilateral facial paralysis occurs in about 50% of the patients. There is a deep aching pain in weakened muscles.

4. Answer: B. Becker muscular dystrophy

In Becker muscular dystrophy (BMD) mutations involve truncation of dystrophin. This lead to a functional though less-active protein. This is a milder disease variant. Patients symptoms are milder and can be delayed by decades. It is a hereditary disorder that follows male distribution pattern. BMD is usually milder than Duchenne muscular dystrophy (DMD). Diagnosis can be confirmed by identifying the defects in the dystrophin gene and muscle biopsy specimens staining with dystrophin.

5. Answer: B. Dermatomyositis

Dermatomyositis (DM) is an inflammatory muscle disorder. It is characterized primarily by proximal muscle weakness. This prominent rash that occurs in dermatomyositis. It commonly affects women between 40 and 60 years old. It is a rare autoimmune condition that leads to microangiopathy and muscle fiber ischemia through antibody-mediated damage. Lungs, heart, and esophagus are some organs that may be affected.

6. Answer: B. Neurofibromatosis type 1 (NF-1)

Neurofibromatosis type 1 (NF-1) is cutaneous manifestations that include cafe-au-lait macules (hyperpigmented macules). It is inherited as an autosomal dominant disorder. It is due to inactivation mutations in the NF-1 tumor suppressor gene, leading to a neurogenic tissue overgrowth. They are typically six or more, occur in 100% of affected individuals before 2 years old. Lisch nodules (pigmented iris hamartomas), and freckling in the axillary or inguinal region (Crowe sign). NF-1 skin tumors are produced from neural crest cells. Plexiform, neurofibromas may undergo malignant transformation to neurofibrosarcoma. NF-1 is usually associated with optic pathway glioma and pheochromocytoma.

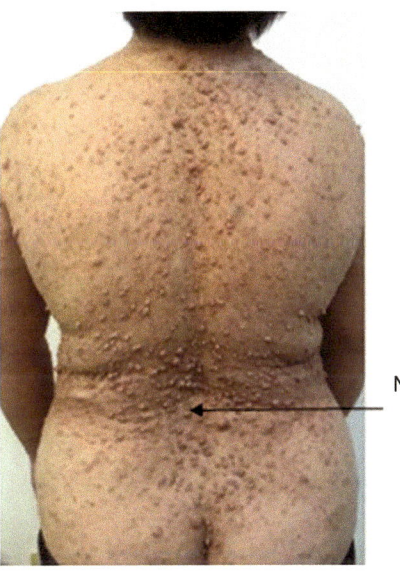

Numerous pedunculated cutaneous nodules on the back

7. Answer: E. Amyotrophic lateral sclerosis

Amyotrophic lateral sclerosis is associated with LMN and UMN signs. There is sparing of sensation. Onset is usually at 40–60 years age. It is the most common motor neuron disease. Patients present with muscle weakness, disability and eventually death occurs. Diagnosis is based on clinical criteria.

8. Answer: A. Polymyositis

Polymyositis is an inflammatory muscle disorder causing proximal muscle weakness. The clinical distinction between polymyositis (PM) and dermatomyositis

(DM) is the prominent rash that occurs in DM. Patients present with symmetrical, proximal muscle weakness. Laboratory findings show elevated levels of skeletal muscle enzyme.

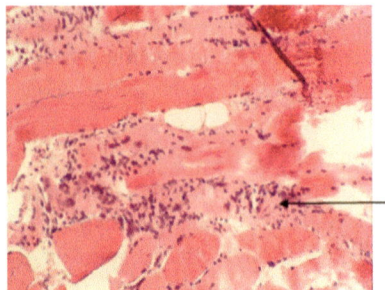

Endomysial inflammatory infiltrate and muscle fiber necrosis.

9. Answer: E. Lambert–Eaton syndrome

Lambert–Eaton myasthenic syndrome is an autoimmune disease, in which antibodies attack presynaptic voltage gated Ca^{2+} channels of the neuromuscular junction. Proximal muscle weakness, and depressed tendon reflexes are present in Lambert–Eaton myasthenic syndrome (LEMS).

10. Answer: C. Morton neuroma

Morton neuroma is also called intermetatarsal neuroma of the foot. Patients usually present with tingling, burning, numbness, and pain. It feels like there is something inside the ball of the foot. Pain usually radiates forward from the metatarsal heads to the third and fourth toes. Walking on hard surface and wearing high heeled shoes aggravates the pain. On physical examination, there is tenderness in the plantar aspect of the third and fourth metatarsals. There is clicking sensation when palpating the involved interspace. Diagnosis is confirmed by imaging studies.

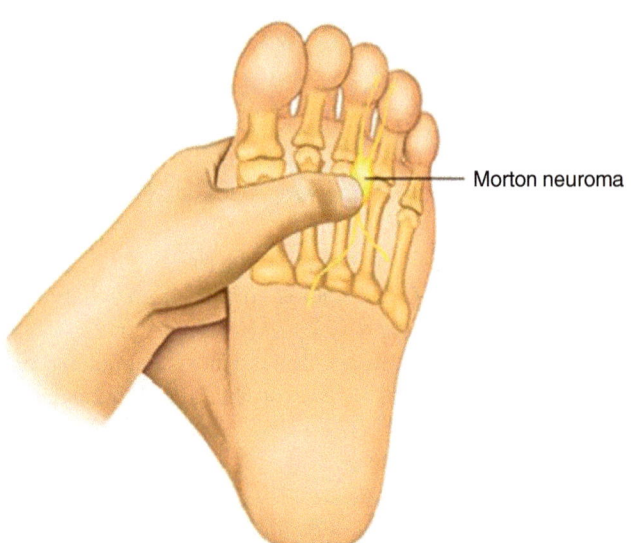

Morton neuroma

11. Answer: D. Carpal tunnel syndrome (CTS)

CTS occur due to compression of the median nerve passing through pronator teres under flexor retinaculum in the carpal tunnel. Patient presents with tingling, numbness, pain, paresthesia, and weakness in the median nerve distribution. CTS is a common cause of compressive focal mononeuropathy. Symptoms of CTS are worse at night and often awaken patients from sleep.

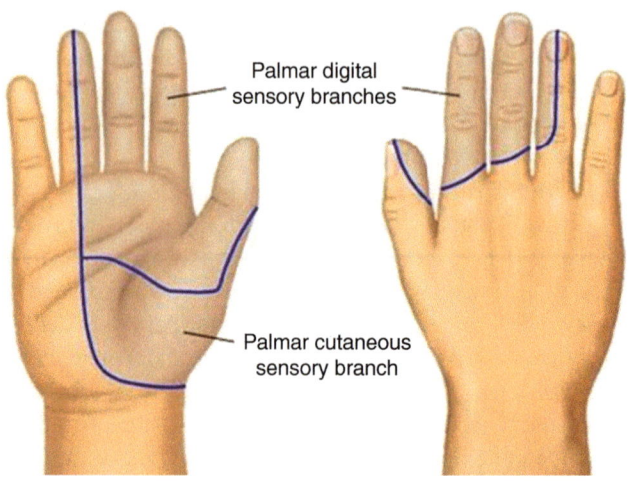

Palmar digital sensory branches

Palmar cutaneous sensory branch

12. Answer: B. Chronic inflammatory demyelinating polyneuropathy (CIDP)

CIDP is a rare neurological, acquired, immune-mediated neuropathy. It commonly affects peripheral nerves and nerve roots. There is a relapsing-remitting or progressive course. CIDP usually responds to glucocorticoids. Pathological features of demyelination are found in CIDP. Patients present with symmetric, motor-predominant neuropathy. It affects both proximal and distal muscles leading to weakness. Diagnosis is confirmed by electrodiagnostic findings and nerve biopsy.

13. Answer: D. Lovastatin

Statins are commonly used drugs for the treatment of hypercholesterolemia. Patients usually present with mild myalgias with or without mild weakness. Severe side effects of statins are myotoxicity which include myopathy, myalgia, myositis or rhabdomyolysis. The creatine kinase (CK) levels are elevated (greater than 10 times the normal upper limit). The most severe adverse effect of statins is rhabdomyolysis that can cause renal failure, disseminated intravascular coagulation, and death. Different mechanisms including direct myotoxicity, immunologically induced inflammatory myopathy or a combination of multiple mechanisms have been described. The only effective treatment of myopathy induced by statin is to discontinue the statin.

14. Answer: B. Diabetes mellitus

In diabetes mellitus, the commonest type of neuropathy seen is a distal symmetric sensorimotor polyneuropathy. It is also called diabetic neuropathy. There is progressive loss of distal sensation which correlate with the loss of sensory axons. Motor weakness and motor axonal loss occur in severe cases. In diabetes mellitus, there is classic stocking-glove sensory loss.

15. Answer: B. Werdnig–Hoffmann disease

Werdnig–Hoffmann disease is an autosomal recessive disease that manifests at birth as a floppy baby, tongue fasciculations, lower motor neuron (LMN) disease. It is also called infantile spinal muscular atrophy (SMA). There is degeneration of anterior horns. Upper motor neuron (UMN)/corticospinal tract are not degenerated. There is a defect in the gene that normally turns of perinatal programmed cell death. Patient presents with progressive muscle weakness and atrophy. There are four phenotypes (0 through 4) of spinal muscular atrophy (SMA) depending upon the onset of age and clinical course. Symptoms progress rapidly, and death usually occurs before 2 years of age due to respiratory failure.

16. Answer: C. Nemaline rod myopathy

Nemaline rod myopathy is a rare congenital myopathy. Nemaline rod myopathy demonstrates tangles of small rod-shaped granules. These tangles are commonly found in the type I fibers. Although it is present from birth, their expression is delayed until later in childhood. There are characteristic rod bodies in muscle which appear threadlike in longitudinal sections. The presentation in newborns is relatively mild, but can be severe. This generalized weakness and hypotonia involving the face, bulbar and respiratory muscles are seen in severe form of the disease. The milder form presents with a relatively less facial weakness and diaphragm impairment.

17. Answer: B. Pompe disease

In Pompe disease (type II glycogenosis), there is an enzyme deficiency of α-1,4-glucosidase (acid maltase). It is a type II glycogen storage disease. There are different forms of Pompe disease: infantile form, juvenile and adult form. Liver, heart, and skeletal muscle are common organs where glycogen is accumulated. Infantile form (early onset) presents with cardiomyopathy, severe generalized hypotonia. Death usually occurs within the first year or two of life without treatment. Juvenile and adult form (late onset) present with skeletal myopathy in a limb-girdle distribution. It has a protracted course leading to respiratory failure. It is inherited in an autosomal recessive disorder.

18. Answer: A. McArdle disease

In McArdle syndrome (type V glycogenosis), there is an enzyme deficiency muscle phosphorylase leading to the accumulation of glycogen in skeletal muscle. It is usually present in adolescence or early adulthood. Patients present with muscle cramps, muscle weakness following exercise, muscle swelling, fatigue and exercise intolerance. Laboratory findings show elevated creatine kinase and myoglobinuria. It is inherited as an autosomal recessive disorder. Mutations in the muscle isoform of phosphorylase (muscle glycogen phosphorylase, PVGM), are located on chromosome 11q13.

19. Answer: B. Cushing's syndrome

The common type of myopathy induced by the drug is due to glucocorticoids. Around 60% of Cushing's syndrome patients have muscle weakness. Glycolytic, fast-twitch muscle fibers (type IIb fibers) are usually affected. Diagnostic approach of patients involves evaluation for endogenous or exogenous glucocorticoid use. In acute phase of the drug-induced myopathy creatine kinase and aldolase are elevated.

20. Answer: A. Varicella Zoster virus

Infection due to Varicella Zoster virus has two clinically distinct types (chickenpox and shingles). Chickenpox infection present with vesicular lesions on an erythematous base in different stages of development. Lesions are commonly present on face and trunk. Herpes zoster (shingles) occurs due to the reactivation of latent virus which usually gain access to sensory ganglia. There is painful, unilateral vesicular eruption in a dermatomal distribution in Herpes zoster.

Bibliography

1. Venugopal V, Pavlakis S. Duchenne muscular dystrophy. Treasure Island: StatPearls; 2019.
2. Chu ECP, Bellin D. Remission of myasthenia gravis following cervical adjustment. AME Case Rep. 2019;3:9.
3. Nguyen TP, Taylor RS. Guillain Barre syndrome. Treasure Island: StatPearls Publishing; 2018.
4. Mandac BR, Kishner S. Becker muscular dystrophy. Gaithersburg: GARD; 2019.
5. Okogbaa J, Batiste L. Dermatomyositis: an acute flare and current treatments. Clin Med Insights Case Rep. 2019;12:5370.
6. Ho T-H, Lee J-T, Liu T-C, Lin J-C, Yang F-C. Neurofibromatosis type 1. QJM Int J Med. 2019;112(4):307.
7. Riancho J, et al. Amyotrophic lateral sclerosis: a complex syndrome that needs an integrated research approach. Neural Regen Res. 2019;14:193.
8. Seetharaman M, Herbert SD. Polymyositis. Treasure Island: StatPearls; 2018.
9. Stickler DE, Lorenzo N. Lambert–Eaton Myasthenic syndrome (LEMS). Treasure Island: StatPearls; 2019.

10. Fields KB. Evaluation and diagnosis of common causes of forefoot pain in adults. Baltimore: Wolters Kluwer; 2019.
11. Kothari MJ. Carpal tunnel syndrome: Clinical manifestations and diagnosis. Baltimore: Wolters Kluwer; 2019.
12. Lewis RA. Chronic inflammatory demyelinating polyneuropathy: etiology, clinical features, and diagnosis. Neurophysiol Clin. 2019;34(2):71–9.
13. Miller ML. Drug-induced myopathies. Baltimore: Wolters Kluwer; 2019.
14. Feldman EL. Epidemiology and classification of diabetic neuropathy. Baltimore: Wolters Kluwer; 2019.
15. Bodamer OA. Spinal muscular atrophy. Waltham: UptoDate; 2019.
16. Merritt JL II. Lysosomal acid alpha-glucosidase deficiency (Pompe disease, glycogen storage disease II, acid maltase deficiency). Waltham: UptoDate; 2019.
17. Merritt JL II. Myophosphorylase deficiency (glycogen storage disease V, McArdle disease). Treasure Island: StatPearls; 2019.
18. Gupta A, Gupta Y. Glucocorticoid-induced myopathy: pathophysiology, diagnosis, and treatment. Indian J Endocrinol Metab. 2019;17(5):913.
19. Albrecht MA, Levin MJ. Epidemiology, clinical manifestations, and diagnosis of herpes zoster. Baltimore: Wolters Kluwer; 2019.

Central Nervous System

Multiple Choice Questions

1. A 33-year-old man presents with headache, nausea, vomiting, ataxia, and vertigo. Fundus examination shows papilledema. MRI shows posterior fossa tumor. The mass is removed and microscopic picture shows tumor cells arranged in a rosette pattern. What is the diagnosis?
   A. Astrocytoma
   B. Ependymoma
   C. Meningioma
   D. Schwannoma
   E. Medulloblastoma

2. A 45-year-old woman presents with unilateral headache. CT scan shows a mass which is surgically removed. Microscopic examination shows cellular whorls and psammoma bodies. What is the diagnosis?
   A. Hemangioblastoma
   B. Ependymoma
   C. Meningioma
   D. Glioblastoma
   E. Medulloblastoma

3. A 9-year-old boy presents with symptoms of headaches, nausea, vomiting, double vision, and unsteady walk. CT scan head shows mass in a cerebellar vermis and dilation of the cerebral ventricles. Biopsy of the mass is done and microscopic finding shows dark staining tumor cells with round nuclei. What is the diagnosis?
   A. Ependymoma
   B. Meningioma
   C. Medulloblastoma
   D. Craniopharyngioma
   E. Oligodendroglioma

4. A 34-year-old man presents with headaches and focal seizures. MRI of the brain shows a ring-enhancing mass in the right cerebral hemisphere. H&E picture is shown below. What is the diagnosis?

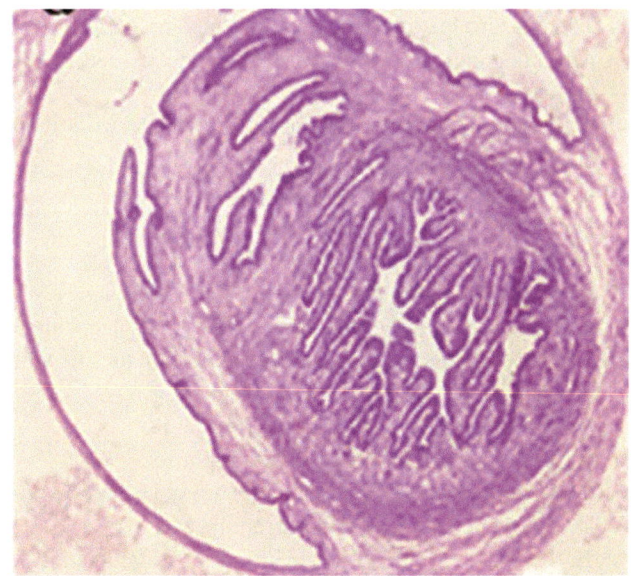

   A. Echinococcosis
   B. Encysted taenia solium larva
   C. Coenurosis
   D. Tuberculoma
   E. Toxoplasmosis

5. Which genetic abnormalities is commonly seen in meningiomas?
   A. Chromosome 10p13-p14 deletion
   B. TBX1 gene mutation
   C. p53 mutations
   D. Estrogen receptor mutations
   E. Deletions on chromosome 22

6. Which of the following virus is present in hippocampal pyramidal neurons as eosinophilic cytoplasmic inclusions?
   A. Rabies virus
   B. Enteroviruses
   C. Coxsackieviruses

© The Author(s), under exclusive license to Springer Nature Switzerland AG 2022
V. K. Kohli et al., *Comprehensive Multiple-Choice Questions in Pathology*, https://doi.org/10.1007/978-3-031-08767-7_22

D. Herpes simplex virus

E. Echoviruses

7. Which is the best answer regarding hemorrhage in the subependymal germinal plate next to the lateral ventricles in premature babies?

A. 34 weeks gestation

B. 28 weeks gestation

C. 38 weeks gestation

D. 40 weeks gestation

E. 44 weeks gestation

8. A middle-aged woman presents with involuntary, jerky movements of the face, and extremities. Her husband also complains that the patient is also having behavioral abnormalities including aggressiveness and depression. There is also history of dementia. Which of the following neuroimaging findings is most likely to be seen in this patient?

A. Atrophy of caudate nucleus

B. Atrophy of putamen

C. Atrophy of caudate and putamen

D. Neurofibrillary tangles

E. Atrophy of cingulate gyrus

9. A patient develops flu-like signs and symptoms, fever, and headache and he is diagnosed as viral encephalitis. What are the histological features characteristics of viral encephalitis?

A. Intranuclear and cytoplasmic inclusions

B. Inflammation of brains by neutrophils

C. Lymphocytes and macrophages around blood vessels

D. Microglial nodules and neuronophagia

E. Myelin loss, gliosis and neutrophilic inflammation

10. Subependymal giant cell astrocytomas (SEGA) are associated with which of the following underlying conditions?

A. West syndrome

B. Neurofibromatosis 1 (NF1)

C. Von Hippel–Lindau disease

D. Tuberous sclerosis

E. Lennox–Gastaut syndrome

11. A 62-year-old woman presents with sudden onset of headache, cognitive symptoms, dementia, and problems with the vision. Computed tomography (CT) is done and a biopsy is also performed. Biopsy of brain shows eosinophilic structure. What is the diagnosis?

A. Frontal lobe syndromes

B. Frontal and temporal lobe dementia

C. Intracranial hemorrhage

D. Multiple cavernoma syndrome

E. Cerebral amyloid angiopathy (CAA)

12. Rapid correction of chronic hyponatremia may lead to which of the following conditions?

A. Neuromyelitis optica spectrum disorder

B. Multiple sclerosis

C. Transverse myelitis

D. Osmotic demyelination syndrome

E. Metabolic disorder

13. A 59-year-old man has experienced headaches for the first time in his life for the last 1 month. He has noticed speech difficulties, weakness on the left side. MRI of the brain shows a 5 cm irregular mass in the cerebral hemisphere. Stereotactic biopsies of the masses is done. Microscopically biopsy shows pleomorphic cells positive for glial fibrillary acidic protein (GFAP). What is the diagnosis?

A. Medulloblastoma

B. Ependymoma

C. Schwannoma

D. Glioblastoma

E. Meningioma

14. A 49-year-old male with acute myeloid leukemia (AML) presents with fever, headache, fatigue, weakness, and nausea. What is the diagnosis?

A. Acanthamoeba encephalitis

B. Aspergillosis

C. Histoplasmosis

D. Nocardiosis

E. Toxoplasmosis

15. Inclusions in oligodendrocytes are a feature of:

A. Herpes simplex virus

B. Progressive multifocal leukoencephalopathy

C. Creutzfeldt–Jakob disease

D. Chronic inflammatory demyelinating polyneuropathy (CIDP)

E. Pick disease

16. Obstruction to the flow of CSF at the aqueduct of sylvius will lead to enlargement of:

A. All of the ventricles

B. Only lateral ventricle

C. Only fourth ventricle

D. Both lateral and third ventricles

E. Only third ventricle

17. A 54-year-old man has an intradural cauda equina tumor. What is the most likely diagnosis?

A. Ependymoma

B. Paraganglioma

C. Glioblastoma

D. Astrocytoma

E. Oligodendroglioma

18. A 71-year-old female presents with increased memory loss and confusion. There is also difficulty with language, problems with reading, writing, and working with numbers according to her daughter. Microscopic picture of this disease shows neurofibrillary tangles and sensile plaques. What is the diagnosis?

A. Alzheimer disease

B. Vascular dementia

C. Lewy body dementia

D. Frontotemporal dementia

E. Mixed dementia

19. Mononeuropathy, especially affecting the oculomotor nerve (cranial nerve III) occurs in which of the following medical conditions?
    A. Hypertension
    B. Diabetes mellitus
    C. Cancer
    D. Coronary heart disease
    E. Metastatic tumor

20. A 69-year-old male smoker with a prosthetic mitral valve undergoes a tooth extraction. Patient later develops a low-grade fever (39 °C) and neurologic deficits. He subsequently dies. Microscopic picture shows necrosis and abscess of the brain. What is the diagnosis?
    A. Acute meningitis
    B. Multiple brain abscesses
    C. Meningoencephalitis
    D. Metastatic lung cancer
    E. Pale infarct

21. A 42-year-old male presents with headache, seizure. Imaging studies show a mass in the frontal lobe. Histologically, the gray matter is being infiltrated by tumor cells. Tumor cells with vesicular nuclei and perinuclear halos. What is the diagnosis?
    A. Classic oligodendroglioma
    B. Medulloblastoma
    C. Glioblastoma
    D. Astrocytoma
    E. Ependymoma

22. Which of the following tumor arises from Rathke's pouch?
    A. Oligodendroglioma
    B. Craniopharyngioma
    C. Meningioma
    D. Schwannoma
    E. Medulloblastoma

23. A 40-year old man presents with symptoms of tinnitus and hearing loss. CT scan shows a mass at the cerebellopontine angle. What is the appropriate diagnosis?
    A. Morton neuroma
    B. Mucosal neuromatosis
    C. Palisaded encapsulated neuroma
    D. Neurofibroma
    E. Schwannoma

24. A 45-year-old female presents with slurred speech, fatigue, dizziness, tingling or pain in parts of the body. Physical examination shows intention tremors and nystagmus. These symptoms are relapsing-remitting for the last 1 year. What is the diagnosis?
    A. Sarcoidosis
    B. Transverse myelitis
    C. Vasculitis
    D. Multiple sclerosis
    E. Progressive multifocal leukoencephalitis

25. Hyperacusis (increased sensitivity to sound) is an indication of damage to which of the following cranial nerve?
    A. Facial nerve (CN VII)
    B. Oculomotor nerve (CN III)
    C. Vagus nerve (CN X)
    D. Vestibulocochlear nerve (CN VIII)
    E. Glossopharyngeal nerve (CN IX)

26. A 45-year-old HIV positive patient presents with headache, fever, muscle aches, and pains. MRI shows a ring-enhancing lesion. What is the diagnosis?
    A. Toxoplasmosis
    B. Brain abscess
    C. Histoplasmosis
    D. Lymphoma
    E. Gliomas

27. Photograph of an infant who died soon after birth is shown below. What is the diagnosis?

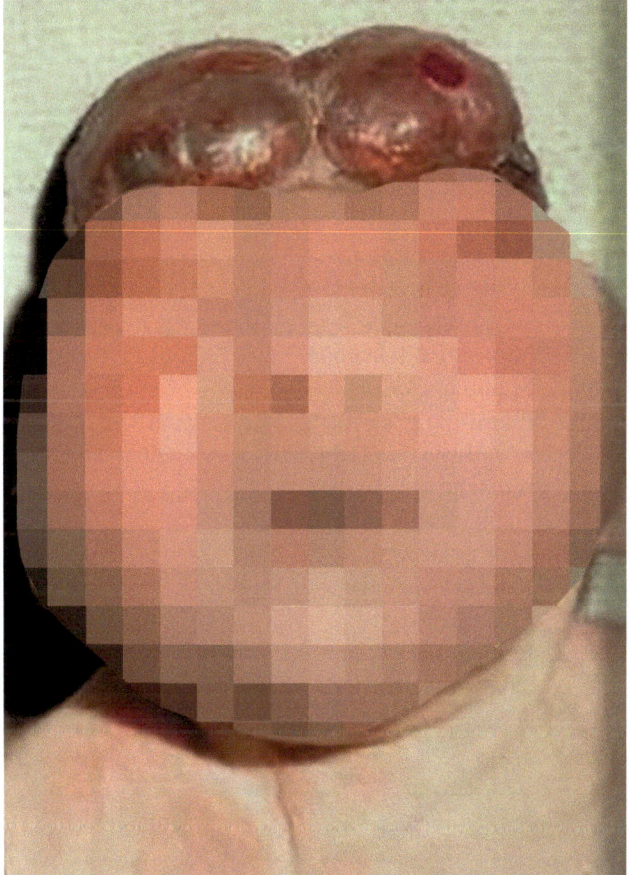

    A. Anencephaly
    B. Down syndrome
    C. Fetal alcohol syndrome
    D. Pediatric craniosynostosis
    E. Rett syndrome

28. A 55-year-old male patient with a history of chronic medical condition is brought to the emergency depart-

ment by his wife. CT scan of the head shows hemorrhages in the basal ganglia. What is the diagnosis?

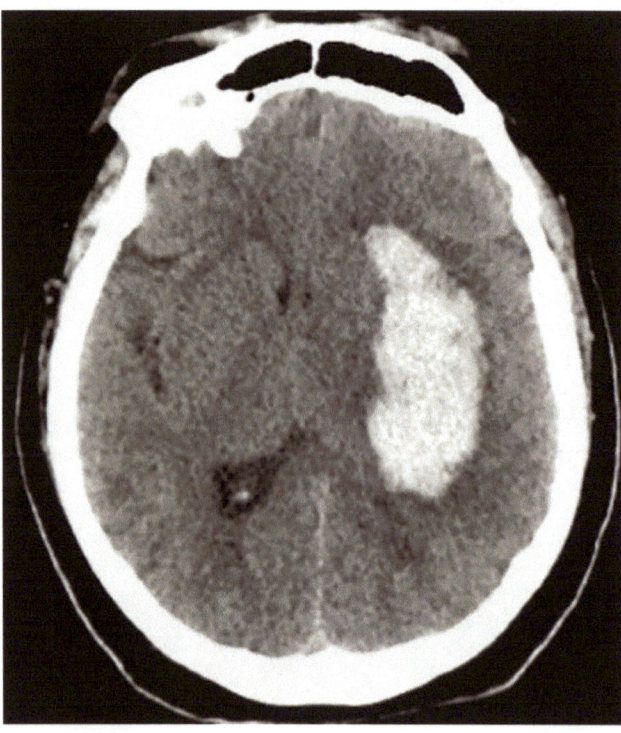

A. Pheochromocytoma
B. Systemic hypertension
C. Acute vasculitis
D. Myocardial Infarction
E. Multiple sclerosis

29. A 32-year-old male patient presents with visual impairment, diplopia, headache. MRI shows sellar mass. What is the diagnosis?
A. Glioblastoma multiforme
B. Low-grade astrocytoma
C. Pituitary adenoma
D. Meningioma
E. Primary CNS lymphoma

30. A 47-year-old HIV positive patients present with frequent headaches. MRI shows a brain mass. What is the diagnosis?
A. Actinomycosis
B. Aspergillosis
C. Nocardia abscess
D. Histoplasmosis
E. Kaposi sarcoma

31. A hemangioblastoma is a benign, highly vascular tumor of the brain. Hemangioblastoma is seen in which of the following diseases?
A. Multiple endocrine neoplasia, type 2
B. Neurofibromatosis
C. Pheochromocytoma
D. Tuberous sclerosis complex
E. Von Hippel–Lindau disease

32. Which of the following is the most frequent cause of subarachnoid hemorrhage?
A. Trigeminal neuralgia
B. Cavernous sinus syndrome
C. Migraine headache
D. Saccular aneurysm
E. Pituitary tumor

33. Which of the following hemorrhage is because of rupture of bridging veins?
A. Subdural hemorrhage
B. Epidural hemorrhage
C. Subarachnoid hemorrhage
D. Intracerebral hemorrhage
E. Pontine hemorrhage

34. An 11-year-old boy presents with headaches, blurring of vision, and speech difficulty of gradual onset. CT scan of the head shows a small 5 cm cystic mass in the right cerebral hemisphere. Mass is removed and histologically, it is composed of tumor cells with hyperchromatic nuclei. Cells stain for glial fibrillary acidic protein (GFAP). What is the diagnosis?
A. Tuberculoma
B. Meningioma
C. Ependymoma
D. Medulloblastoma
E. Astrocytoma

Answers and Explanations

1. Answer: B. Ependymoma
    There are four subtypes of ependymomas according to World Health Organization (WHO):

Tumor classification	Tumor grade
Subependymoma	I
Myxopapillary ependymoma	I
Classic ependymoma	II
Anaplastic ependymoma	III

Intracranial ependymomas present as periventricular tumors. The most common location is posterior fossa (often in contact with fourth ventricle). Histologically, ependymoma consists of the tumor cells which are arranged in a perivascular pseudorosettes and true ependymal rosette.

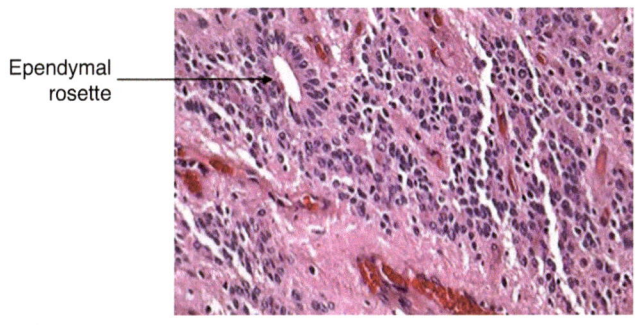

Ependymal rosette

2. : C. Meningioma

Meningiomas are relatively common neoplasms derived from meningothelial cells of the arachnoid. The World Health organization (WHO) classified meningiomas in three groups:

Meningioma subtypes	WHO grade
Meningiomas with low risk of recurrence or aggressive growth:	
(Fibrous, transitional, psammomatous, angiomatous, microcystic, secretory, lymphoplasmacytic-rich, metaplastic)	I
Meningiomas with greater likelihood of recurrence and/or aggressive behavior	
Atypical, clear cell, and chordoid meningiomas.	II
Anaplastic, papillary, and rhabdoid meningiomas (malignant)	III

Histologically, tumors is composed of spindle cells arranged in a concentric whorled pattern. There are also laminated calcifications called psammoma bodies.

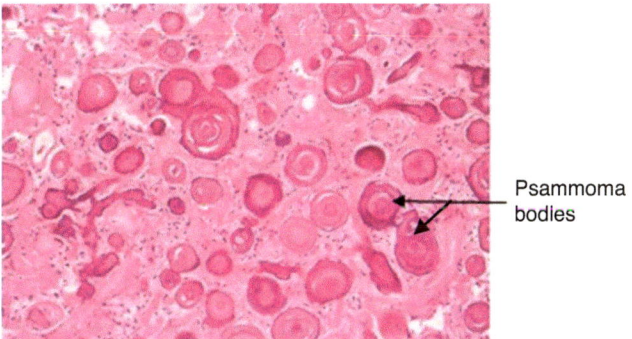

Psammoma bodies

with round or oval nuclei and little cytoplasm. Platelet-derived growth factor receptor alpha (PDGFR-a) has been found to be upregulated and overexpressed in the metastatic tumors.

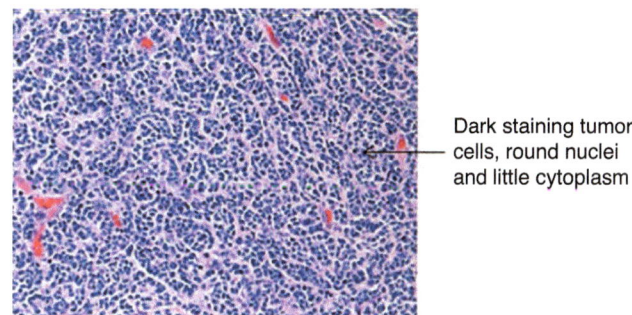

Dark staining tumor cells, round nuclei and little cytoplasm

3. Answer: C. Medulloblastoma

Medulloblastoma is the most common malignant tumor of childhood. This tumor is found exclusively in the cerebellum. Patients present with headache, nausea, and vomiting. Papilledema is a common symptom due to increased intracranial pressure. Gait disturbances, nystagmus, dysmetria are usually a reflection of cerebellar dysfunction. Histologically, medulloblastoma is highly cellular tumor. Tumor cells show abundant dark staining

4. Answer: B. Encysted taenia solium larva

The most common form of cysticercosis is intraparenchymal neurocysticercosis caused by tapeworm (taenia solium). Common symptoms are headache, seizures. Less common manifestations are altered vision, focal neurologic signs, and meningitis. Many cases are identified incidentally via imaging studies. Eating undercooked pork infected with taenia solium may lead to neurocysticercosis.

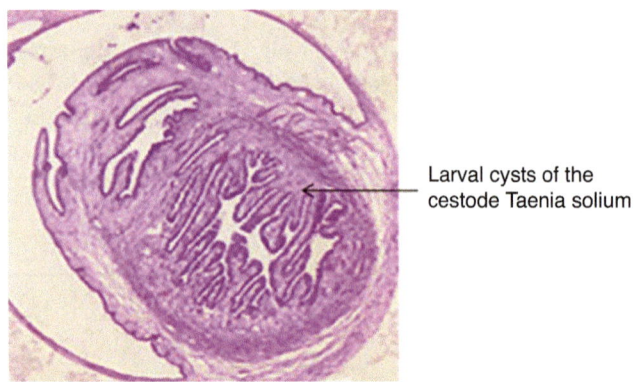

Larval cysts of the cestode Taenia solium

5. Answer: E. Deletions on chromosome 22

Chromosome 22 deletions can be seen in meningiomas. Although some meningiomas express estrogen receptors. They do no show mutations in ER genes.

6. Answer: A. Rabies virus

Rabies is contracted from the bite of an infected animal. Virus replicates locally in skeletal muscle spindles and ascends to CNS via peripheral nerves. Symptom free interval may last from weeks to months. Presence of intracytoplasmic eosinophilic negri bodies are characteristic findings, seen in large neurons (Purkinje cells).

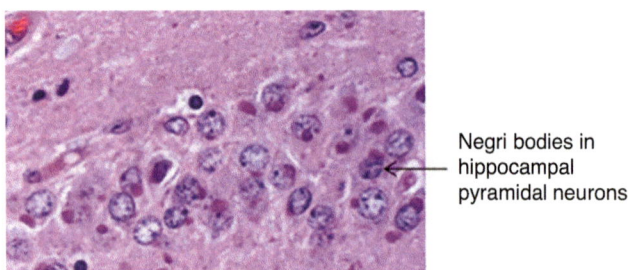

Negri bodies in hippocampal pyramidal neurons

7. Answer: B. 28 Weeks gestation

In premature babies, hemorrhage within the germinal matrix is a common complication. Peak incidence of germinal matrix hemorrhage is between 23 and 28 weeks. Germinal matrix hemorrhage commonly occurs in the subependymal germinal matrix with or without rupture into the lateral ventricle.

8. Answer: C. Atrophy of caudate and putamen

Huntington disease has an autosomal dominant inheritance. It is a progressive neurodegenerative disease. Clinically, HD is characterized by neurological, psychiatric, and cognitive symptoms. Neurological symptoms include chorea, dystonia, slowing of the eye movement, and gait abnormality. Psychiatric symptoms are apathy, irritability, depression, delusions, and paranoia. Cognitive symptoms are poor judgment, inflexibility of thought, decreased concentration, memory loss, and subcortical dementia. There is an increased number of CAG repeats in the Huntington (HTT) gene. There is decrease in GABA and acetylcholine in caudate nuclei. Neuroimaging studies show atrophy of the corpus striatum involving the caudate and putamen.

9. Answer: D. Microglial nodules and neuronophagia

The microscopic findings in viral encephalitis are microglial nodules, neuronophagia, and chronic inflammation around blood vessels. Neuronophagia is clusters of microglial cells encircling degenerating neurons. Activated microglial cells also form clusters around small foci of necrotic brain tissue called microglial nodules.

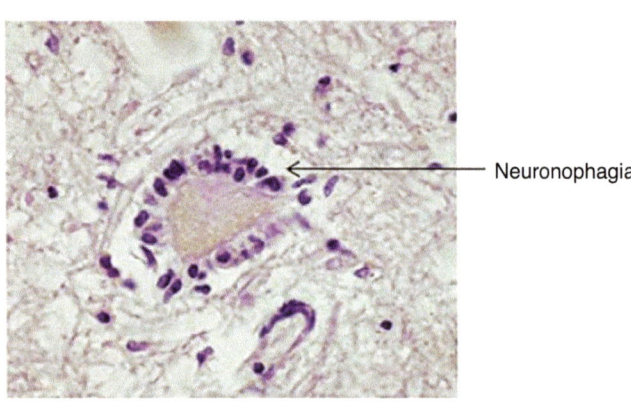

Neuronophagia

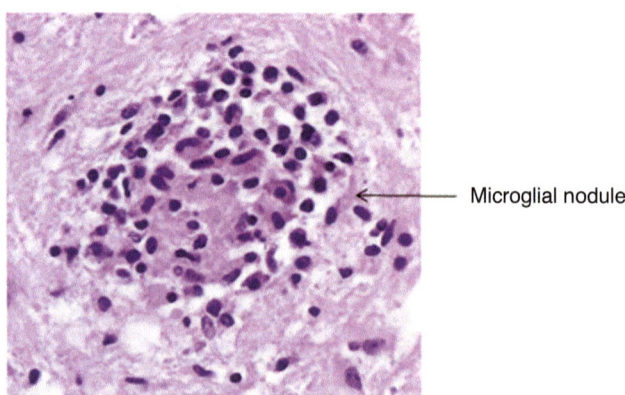

Microglial nodule

10. Answer: D. Tuberous sclerosis

Subependymal giant cell astrocytomas (SEGA) are low astrocytic brain tumor (astrocytoma). It commonly

arises within the ventricles of the brain. Subependymal giant cell astrocytoma is pathognomonic for tuberous sclerosis. The tumor suppressor genes TBC1 on the

9q34 chromosome and TSC2 on the 16p13 chromosome encode tuberin and hamartin in the SEGA associated with tuberous sclerosis.

11. Answer: E. Cerebral amyloid angiopathy (CAA)

Presence of amyloid plaque is a pathological finding which is most consistent with cerebral amyloid angiopathy (CAA) in conjunction with Alzheimer's disease. Congo red is the stain for amyloid. Under polarized light, it gives apple green birefringence. CAA is associated with a greatly increased risk of brain hemorrhage.

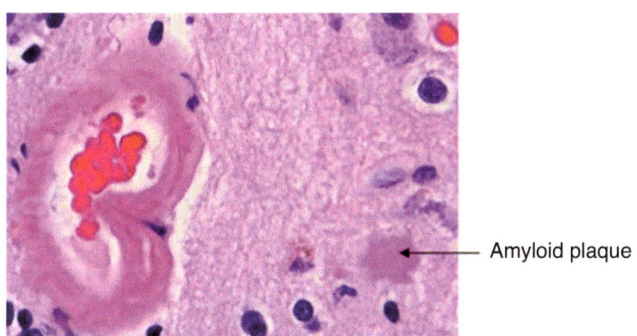

Amyloid plaque

12. Answer: D. Osmotic demyelination syndrome

Osmotic demyelination syndrome (central pontine myelinolysis) is demyelination of neurons due to overly rapid correction of chronic (more than 2 days) hyponatremia. During prolonged hyponatremia, neurons compensate by reducing intracellular osmolytes to present cellular swelling. Upon rapid correction, the neurons are hypotonic relative to the suddenly normal serum osmolality. Fluid moves out of neurons into the extracellular compartment, leading to demyelination. The uncontrolled cell shrinkage leads to the degeneration of astrocytes and oligodendrocytes. Demyelination commonly affects the pons. Symptoms of osmotic demyelination syndrome, manifest 2–6 days. Patients usually present with spastic quadriplegia, pseudobulbar palsy. There may also present with dysphagia, dysarthria, tongue paresis. Osmotic demyelination syndrome usually occurs in patients with the sodium concentration is less than 105 mEq/L.

13. Answer: D. Glioblastoma

Glioblastoma (previously called glioblastoma multiforme) is the highest grade and most aggressive form of astrocytoma. The tumor is composed of densely-packed pleomorphic astrocytes, with areas of necrosis and vascular proliferation. Necrosis is usually present in a serpentine pattern. Tumor cells collect at the edges of the areas of necrosis in a pseudopalisading pattern.

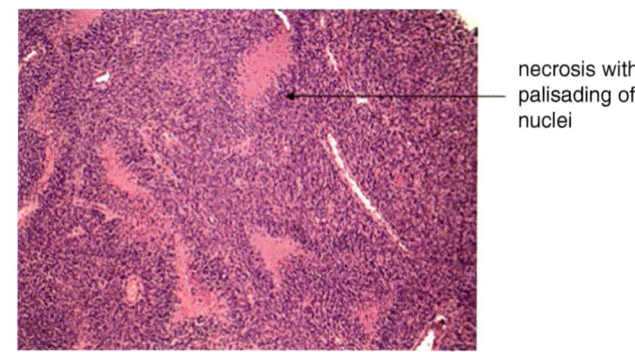

necrosis with palisading of nuclei

14. Answer: A. Acanthamoeba encephalitis

Immunocompromised patients are prone to develop acanthamoeba encephalitis. Histologically, brain parenchyma is infiltrated by scattered neutrophils and lymphocytes. There is also a population of abnormal cells that look like somewhat lake macrophages. These cells have a prominent centrally located nucleus. These are acanthamoeba trophozoites, which cause opportunistic encephalitis in immunocompromised patients.

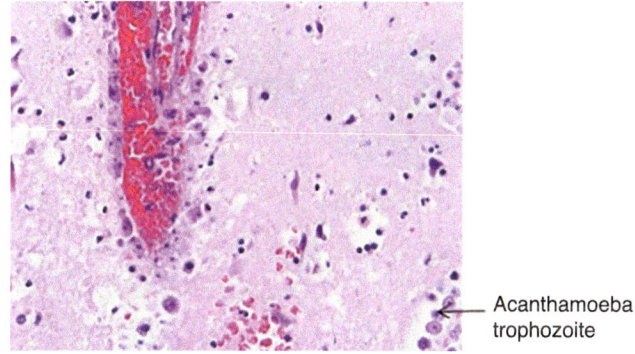

Acanthamoeba trophozoite

15. Answer: B. Progressive multifocal leukoencephalopathy

Progressive multifocal leukoencephalopathy is an opportunistic infection caused by a papovavirus called JC virus. This virus is a nonenveloped double stranded DNA polyomavirus. Patients present with speech disturbance (aphasia), cortical blindness, conjugate gaze abnormalities, and weakness (hemiparesis). Histologically, there are abnormal cells that can be identified as both oligodendrocytes and astrocytes. There are large atypical astrocytes. There are also oligodendroglial cells with enlarged, glassy nuclei. These two findings lead to the diagnosis of progressive multifocal leukoencephalopathy (PML). JC virus multiplies in oligodendrocytes of immunodeficient patients such as AIDS. Confirmation of infection with the JC virus is done with immunohistochemistry, in situ hybridization for the JC virus and imaging studies (MRI).

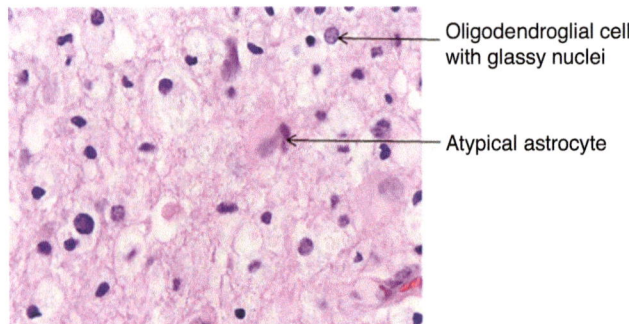

Oligodendroglial cell with glassy nuclei

Atypical astrocyte

16. Answer: D. Both lateral and third ventricles

The cerebral aqueduct of Sylvius is a canal that passes through the midbrain and connects the third with the fourth ventricle. It allows cerebrospinal fluid to pass between them. Tumors such as pinealoma in the midbrain may occlude the aqueduct. The result is blockage of CSF flow resulting in enlargement of the ventricles sometimes called triventricular hydrocephalus.

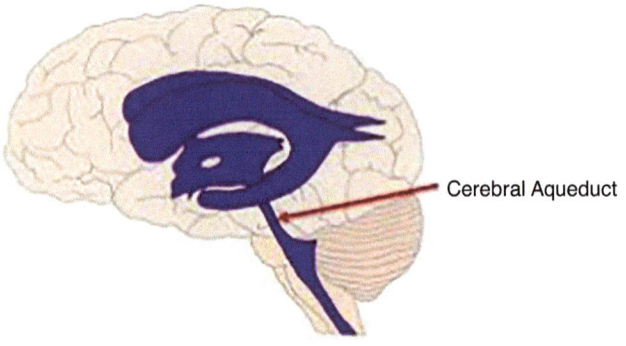

Cerebral Aqueduct

17. Answer: B. Paraganglioma

Spinal paragangliomas are almost always found in the cauda equina/filum terminale region of the spinal cord. It arises most frequently in adults between fourth and sixth decade of life. Histologically the paraganglioma includes nested zellballen pattern of polygonal cells. Polygonal cells have round nuclei with fine chromatin and granular eosinophilic cytoplasm.

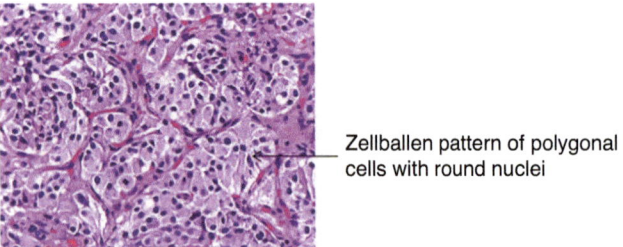

Zellballen pattern of polygonal cells with round nuclei

18. Answer: A. Alzheimer disease

Alzheimer disease is a disorder of older age. It accounts for about two-thirds of cases of adult dementia. The early memory loss in Alzheimer disease is antero-grade long-term episodic amnesia. Other early clinical findings are disorientation, dysgraphia, and language impairment. Late clinical features include impairment of vocabulary and concepts (semantic memory). Alzheimer disease is characterized by significant decreased acetyl-choline concentrations in hippocampus and neocortex triggered by the degeneration of cholinergic neurons. For learning and memory, acetylcholine is essential. Histologically, the common findings found in the brain are neurofibrillary tangles and senile plaques. In MRI, brain atrophy is best seen in temporoparietal lobes and hippocampus.

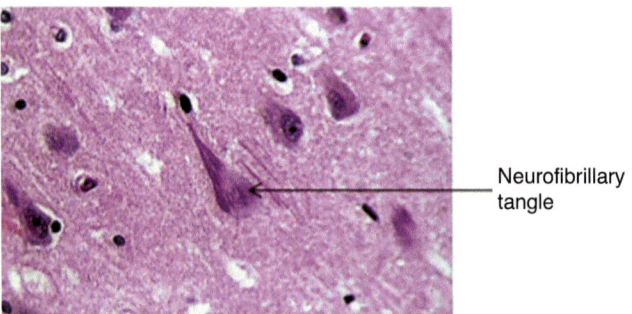

Neurofibrillary tangle

19. Answer: B. Diabetes mellitus

Most common neuropathy is diabetic polyneuropa-thy. Common cranial nerve involvement due to diabetic neuropathies includes oculomotor nerve (cranial nerve III). Patients with oculomotor nerve (cranial nerve III) usually present with an acute onset diplopia. The affected eye shows down and out position due to the unopposed action of the superior oblique and lateral rectus. In dia-betic neuropathy, there is peripheral neuropathy (loss of pain and vibratory sensation in the leg which is charac-teristic of stocking distribution). Diabetes also causes autonomic neuropathy (sexual impotence, delayed gas-tric emptying).

20. Answer: B. Multiple brain abscesses

Brain abscess is defined as local infection within the brain parenchyma. Common causes are infections, trauma, and surgery. Common routes of invasion of brain by bacteria are direct and hematogenous spread. Common pathogens isolated from brain abscess are usu-ally staphylococcus and streptococcus. Histologically, there is inflammatory exudates, necrosis, and abscess of the brain. MRI is the study of choice in brain abscess.

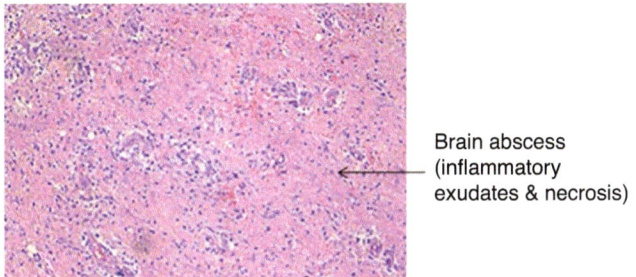

Brain abscess (inflammatory exudates & necrosis)

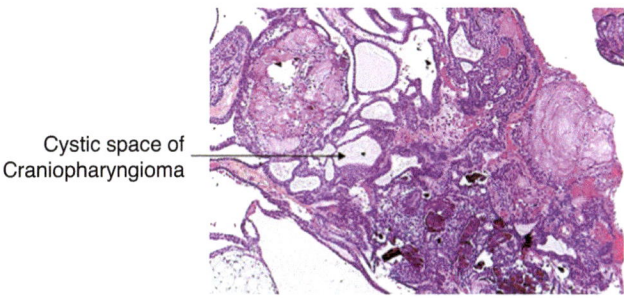

Cystic space of Craniopharyngioma

21. Answer: A. Classic oligodendroglioma

Oligodendroglioma tumor is commonly seen in the white matter of the frontal lobes. Patient present with headache and seizure. Common sites are frontal lobe and temporal lobe. Histologically, it is composed of diffusely infiltrating monomorphic cells with uniform vesicular nuclei and perinuclear halos. Other features of this tumor include thin capillaries, forming a branching network (chicken-wire) and myxoid change. These findings are suggestive of classic oligodendroglioma, WHO Grade II. The common genetic alteration in oligodendroglioma is 1p19q co-deletion. This deletion occurs in approximately 50–80% of oligodendrogliomas and associated with a better response to chemotherapy and longer survival.

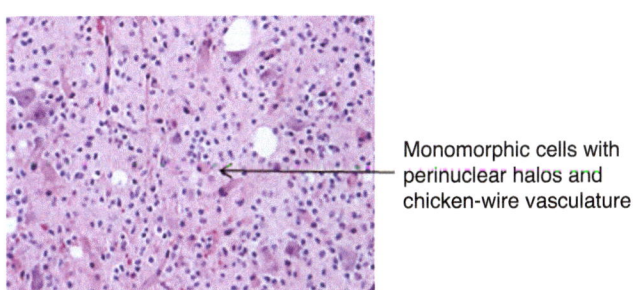

Monomorphic cells with perinuclear halos and chicken-wire vasculature

22. Answer: B. Craniopharyngioma

Craniopharyngiomas, also referred to Rathke's pouch tumors arise in the suprasellar region. WHO classifies them into two types, adamantinomatous (Pediatric type) and papillary (Adult type). On microscopic examination, it contains both solid and cystic components. The cysts are filled with brownish-yellow fluid due to the presence of cholesterol crystals.

23. Answer: E. Schwannoma

Schwannomas occur at the cerebellopontine angle, attached to the eighth nerve. They are well circumscribed masses and easily separated from the nerve to which they are attached. On microscopic examination, two histologic patterns coexist. The Antoni A regions consist of spindle cells with pink cytoplasm. Nuclear palisading is a typical feature and results in the formation of Verocay bodies. Antoni A alternate with looser Antoni B tissue. Antoni B is composed of cells which show clear, vacuolated cytoplasm due to lipid accumulation.

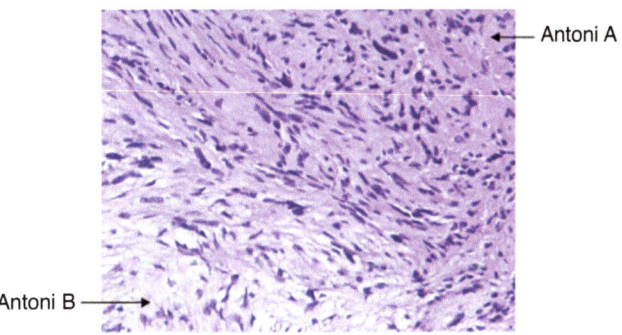

Antoni A

Antoni B

24. Answer: D. Multiple sclerosis

Multiple sclerosis (MS) is a chronic relapsing–remitting inflammatory immune disorder. There are recurring episodes of demyelination of axons in the brain and spinal cord which characterize multiple sclerosis. It is more common in females and commonly affects between the age of 20 and 50 years. Patients usually present with charcot triad consisting of scanning speech, intention tremor, and internuclear ophthalmoplegia/nystagmus. It is associated with HLA-DR2. In acute lesions of multiple sclerosis, there are well circumscribed plaques, with loss of myelin. Histologically, there is phagocytosis of myelin by macrophages and chronic inflammation. There is preservation of axons in initial stages. Axons show remyelination and there is no signs of inflammation in chronic lesions. Imaging studies demonstrate multiple bright signal abnormalities in white matter.

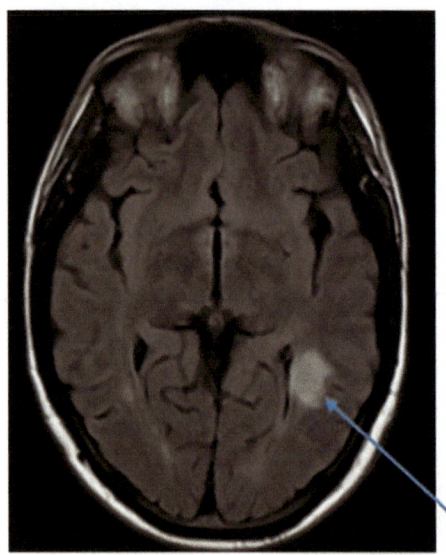

Well circumscribed plaque (MRI)

25. Answer: A. Facial nerve (CN VII)

Common cause of facial nerve (CN VII) palsy is due to nerve compression usually by a mass in the posterior fossa. Patients present with a headache that is worse in the morning due to increased intracranial pressure. Common causes of facial nerve palsy include iatrogenic trauma, stroke, idiopathic Bell's palsy, neoplasm or granulomatous meningitis. Supranuclear lesion occurs as a result of damage to the upper motor neuron (UMN) of the facial nerve. Common cause of supranuclear lesion is a lacunar stroke in the posterior limb of the internal capsule. UMN lesion leads to paralysis of the contralateral lower face only, sparing the upper face and forehead. Infranuclear lesion leads to paralysis of the ipsilateral upper and lower face. Patients usually present with mouth droop, flattening of nasolabial fold, inability to close eye, and smoothing of the brow on the damaged side. Idiopathic facial nerve palsy is referred to as Bell's palsy.

26. Answer: A. Toxoplasmosis

In toxoplasmosis, MRI shows ring-enhancing lesions. Similar lesions can be seen in lymphomas, gliomas, and in multiple sclerosis. Histologically, there are abundant

inflammatory cells, including neutrophils, lymphocytes, and macrophages. There are focal areas of necrosis in the background. *Toxoplasma gondii* is an obligate intracellular protozoan.

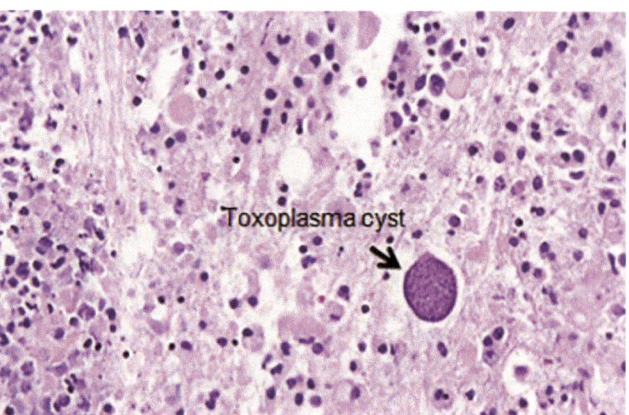

Toxoplasma cyst

27. Answer: A. Anencephaly

Anencephaly is due to neural tube defects leading to the absence of a large part of the skull along with the cerebral hemispheres of the brain. Infants usually die within a few hours or days after birth. Screening of alpha-fetoprotein (AFP) in the mother's blood, and ultrasound should be done to diagnose this neural tube defects before birth. Supplementation with folic acid in women of childbearing age reduces neural tube defects.

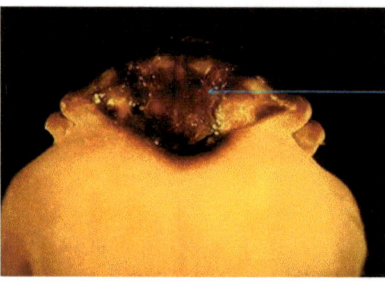

Anencephaly (most of the cranium is absent: exposing residual neural tissue)

28. Answer: B. Systemic hypertension

Hypertension is the most common cause of intracerebral hemorrhage (ICH). Hypertensive hemorrhages occur in the territory of penetrator arteries. Basal ganglia (putamen or caudate), thalamus, pons, and cerebellum are the common sites of hypertensive ICH. Common causes are trauma, infarct, amyloid angiography diabetes, hypertension (Charcot–Bouchard aneurysm). Charcot–Bouchard aneurysms usually occur in small blood vessels and commonly found in the lenticulostriate vessels of the basal ganglia.

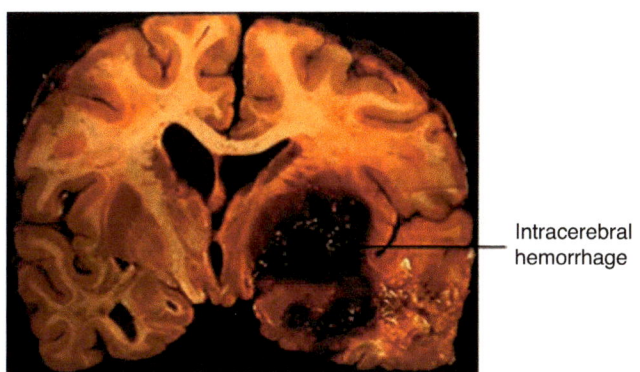

Intracerebral hemorrhage

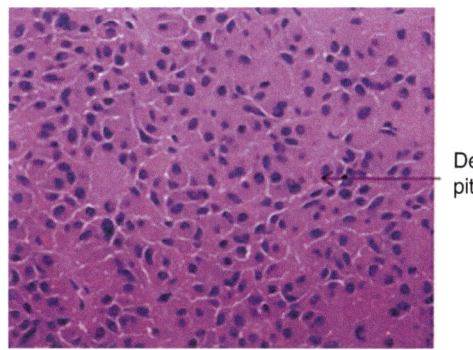

Densely granulated pituitary adenoma

29. Answer: C. Pituitary adenoma

Pituitary adenoma represents 15–20% of intracranial neoplasms of adenohypophysis. Most common neurologic symptoms include headache, diplopia. Histologically adenomas show uniform morphology and cell type with uncommon cytologic atypia.

30. Answer: C. Nocardia abscess

Nocardia is thin filamentous organisms that are GMS positive and gram positive. Nocardia is gram-positive bacilli with branching filaments. The most difficult differential diagnosis is with actinomyces, another Gram-positive bacilli with branching filaments that can also cause CNS infections. To distinguish between nocardia and actinomyces histologic section, an acid-fast stain should be performed. Nocardia is at least partially acid fast while actinomyces are not acid-fast.

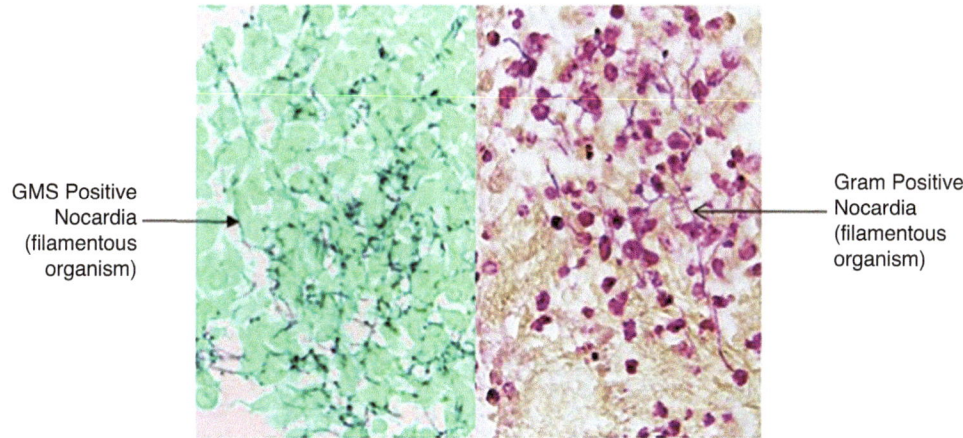

GMS Positive Nocardia (filamentous organism)

Gram Positive Nocardia (filamentous organism)

31. Answer: E. Von Hippel–Lindau disease

Varieties of tumors may be found in autosomal dominant Von Hippel–Lindau disease. They are retinal angioma (retinal hemangioblastoma), hemangioblastomas of the brain and spinal cord, clear cell renal cell carcinomas, and pheochromocytomas.

32. Answer: D. Saccular aneurysm

Subarachnoid hemorrhage (SAH) commonly results from the rupture of saccular aneurysms. Patients usually present with an abrupt onset of the worst headache of

life, confusion, and loss of consciousness. Common risk factors are cigarette smoking and hypertension. Other risk factors include hereditary syndromes (Ehlers–Danlos syndrome). Family members of patients with intracranial aneurysm are at increased risk of having an aneurysm. There is bloody xanthochromic spinal tap (yellow discoloration from the degradation of red blood cells). Imaging studies reveal blood in the subarachnoid space. Overall, a third of patients survive with good recovery. A third of them will recover with a stroke or a disability and a third will die. Patients with SAH can suffer short- and/or long-term deficiencies due to bleed or treatment.

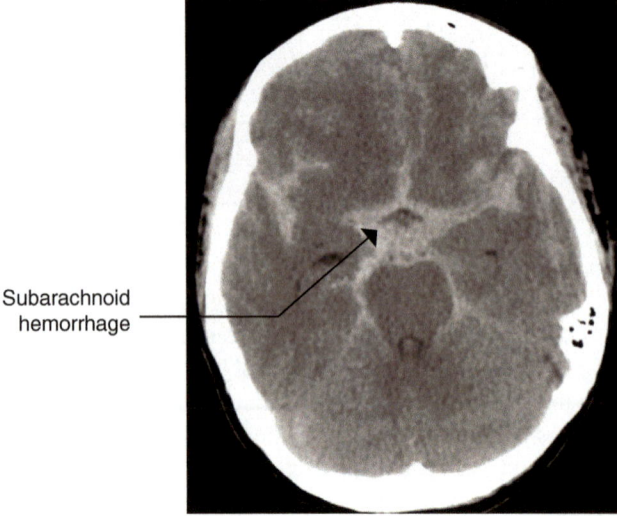

Subarachnoid hemorrhage

33. Answer: A. Subdural hemorrhage

Subdural hematoma (SDH) occurs because of the disruption of the bridging cortical veins. Older adults and those with a history of chronic alcohol abuse are at high risk of SDH due to cerebral atrophy. On imaging studies, SDH is demonstrated as crescent-shaped hypodensities that cross suture lines.

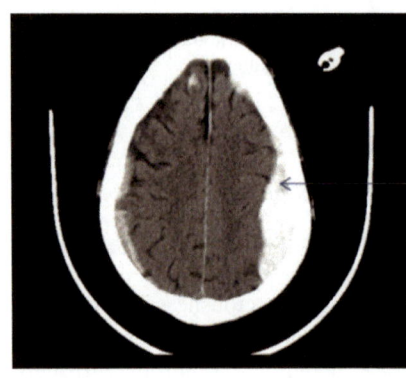

Subdural hematoma (right hemisphere)

34. Answer: E. Astrocytoma

Astrocytoma account for 70% of neuroglial tumors and are located in the frontal lobe of adults and the cerebellum of children. Histologically, the astrocytic tumors consist of tumor cells with elongated hyperchromatic nuclei. Histologically, there is a strong positivity for glial fibrillary acidic protein (GFAP) in the cytoplasm. Astrocytic tumors are usually diffusely infiltrating lesions. Astrocytoma is of different types: grade II, grade III, and grade IV tumors. Molecular abnormalities (ATRX mutations) are seen in approximately 75% of astrocytomas grade II and III.

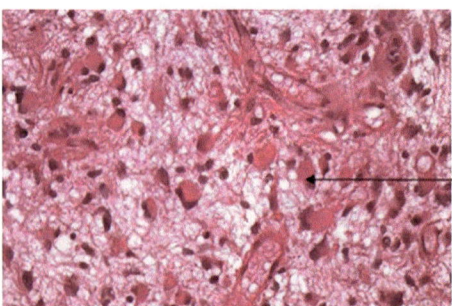

Tumour cell with eosinophilic cytoplasm

Bibliography

1. Upadhyaya SA, et al. Intracranial ependymoma and other ependymal tumors. Baltimore: Wolters Kluwer; 2019.
2. Park JK, et al. Epidemiology, pathology, clinical features, and diagnosis of meningioma. Baltimore: Wolters Kluwer; 2019.
3. Pomeroy SL, et al. Clinical presentation, diagnosis, and risk stratification of medulloblastoma. Baltimore: Wolters Kluwer; 2019.
4. Pellegatta M, Taveggia C. The complex work of proteases and secretases in Wallerian degeneration: beyond neuregulin-1. Front Cell Neurosci. 2019;13:93.
5. Vodopivec I, Rizzo JF. Ophthalmic manifestations of giant cell arteritis. Rheumatology (Oxford). 2018;57(suppl_2):263–72.
6. Suja MS, et al. Role of apoptosis in rabies viral encephalitis: a comparative study in mice, canine, and human brain with a review of literature. Pathol Res Int. 2011;2011:374286.
7. Dawes WJ, Zhang X, Fancy SPJ, Rowitch D, Marino S. Moderate-grade germinal matrix haemorrhage activates cell division in the neonatal mouse subventricular zone. Dev Neurosci. 2016;38:430–44.
8. Suchowersky O, Hurtig HI, Eichler AF. Huntington disease: clinical features and diagnosis. Baltimore: Wolters Kluwer; 2019.
9. Chen Z, Zhong D, Li G. The role of microglia in viral encephalitis: a review. J Neuroinflamm. 2019;16:76.
10. Schmohl JU, Vallera DA. CD133, selectively targeting the root of cancer. Toxins (Basel). 2016;8(6):165.
11. Ravi SM, Lutsep HL. Cerebral amyloid angiopathy. Baltimore: Wolters Kluwer; 2019.
12. Cox GM, Perfect JR. Epidemiology, clinical manifestations, and diagnosis of *Cryptococcus neoformans* meningoencephalitis in HIV-infected patients. Baltimore: Wolters Kluwer; 2019.
13. Cenciarini M, Valentino M, Belia S, et al. Dexamethasone in glioblastoma multiforme therapy: mechanisms and controversies. Front Mol Neurosci. 2019;12:65.
14. Outeiro TF, Koss DJ, Erskine D, et al. Dementia with Lewy bodies: an update and outlook. Mol Neurodegener. 2019;14(1):5.
15. Al Balushi A, Singh NN. Progressive multifocal leukoencephalopathy in HIV. Baltimore: Wolters Kluwer; 2016.
16. Corbett JJ, Haines DE. The ventricles, choroid plexus, and cerebrospinal fluid. In: Fundamental neuroscience for basic and clinical applications. Philadelphia: Elsevier; 2018.
17. Dublish S, Singh P. Bacterial meningitis: bugs' story. Indian Pediatr. 2018;55:903–4.
18. Garg R, Biller J. Recent advances in spontaneous intracerebral hemorrhage. F1000Res. 2019;8:16357.
19. Zhou W, Shao X, Jiang X. A clinical report of two cases of cryptogenic brain abscess and a relevant literature review. Front Neurosci. 2019;12:1054.
20. Farooqui A, Khalekar Y, Farooqui J, Kasat V. Schwannoma of floor of mouth: a case report. J Indian Acad Oral Med Radiol. 2017;29(2):135–7.

Multiple Choice Questions

1. What is the most common cause of corneal dendritic ulcers?
   A. Chlamydia trachomatis
   B. Staphylococcus aureus
   C. Haemophilus influenzae
   D. Herpes simplex virus
   E. Pseudomonas aeruginosa

2. A 65-year-old male patient presents with a sensation of flashes or specks of dust in the vision (floaters), blurry vision in one eye, loss of peripheral vision in the left eye. Fundus examination shows dark uveal mass. What is the diagnosis?
   A. Malignant hypertension
   B. Trachoma
   C. Vitamin A deficiency
   D. Intraocular melanoma
   E. Retinoblastoma

3. A 62-year-old man is suffering from chronic medical conditions such as hypertension, diabetes mellitus. His blood pressure is 140/90 and HbA1c of 9.8%. Fundus examination is shown below. What is the diagnosis?

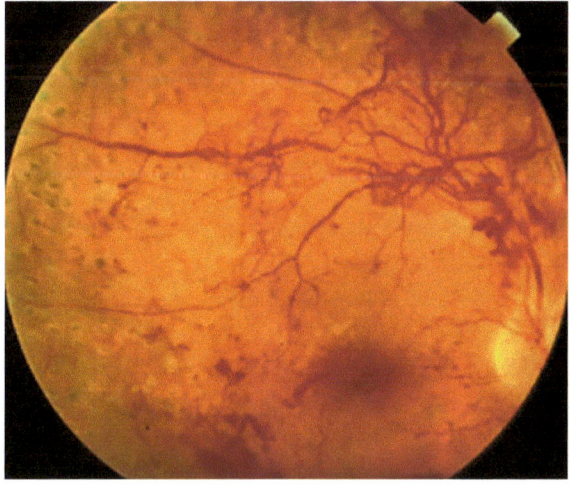

A. Malignant hypertension
B. Glaucoma
C. Macular degeneration
D. Diabetes mellitus
E. Optic neuritis

4. Which of the following tumors are most likely to metastasize to the eye?
   A. Breast carcinoma
   B. Ovarian carcinoma
   C. Lung carcinoma
   D. Renal cell carcinoma
   E. Gastrointestinal carcinoma

5. A middle aged patient with blood pressure of 170/110 is brought to the emergency department. His blood pressure is poorly controlled. Fundus examination is done. The picture is shown below. What are the findings?

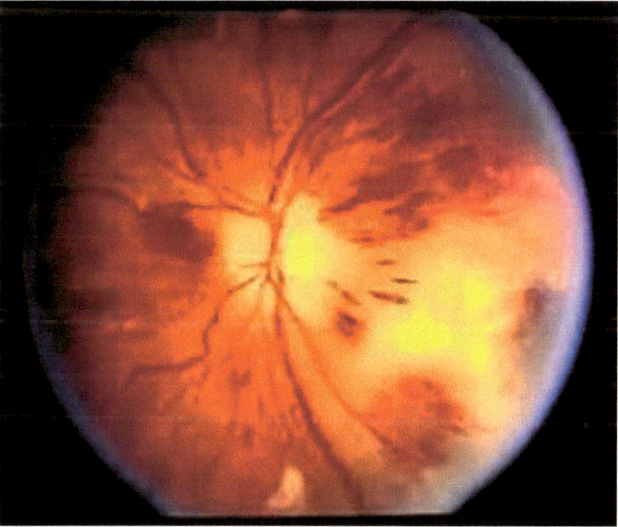

A. Flame shaped hemorrhages
B. Copper wiring of arteriolar walls
C. Silver wiring of arteriolar walls
D. Cotton-wool spots
E. Cherry red spot

V. K. Kohli et al., *Comprehensive Multiple-Choice Questions in Pathology*, https://doi.org/10.1007/978-3-031-08767-7_23

6. What type of secondary malignancy is most likely to occur in the hereditary form of retinoblastoma?
   A. Squamous cell carcinoma
   B. Basal cell carcinoma
   C. Osteosarcoma
   D. Nasal cavity cancers
   E. Lymphoma

7. Trachoma is a major cause of blindness worldwide. Which of the following infectious agent is the cause of trachoma?
   A. Chlamydia trachomatis
   B. Staphylococcus aureus
   C. Neisseria gonorrhoeae
   D. Streptococcus pyogenes
   E. Cytomegalovirus

8. A 10-year-old child comes to pediatrician office with symptoms which include eyelid redness and swelling as well as eye skin swelling. There is also purulent nasal discharge. What is the diagnosis?
   A. Cellulitis
   B. Ocular herpes
   C. Uveitis
   D. Blepharitis
   E. Endophthalmitis

9. A 35-year-old man is receiving long-term high dose glucocorticoid therapy for a chronic medical condition. What ocular complication can develop because of long-term high dose glucocorticoid therapy?
   A. Macular degeneration
   B. Cataract
   C. Nuclear sclerosis of the lens
   D. Open-angle glaucoma
   E. Sympathetic ophthalmia

10. The Kayser Fleischer ring is an ophthalmologic finding. It is strongly associated with which of the following chronic medical condition?
    A. Wilson's disease
    B. Biliary obstruction
    C. Alcoholic cirrhosis
    D. Cryptogenic cirrhosis
    E. Viral induced hepatitis

11. Diagram of a 62-year-old man is shown below. What is the diagnosis?

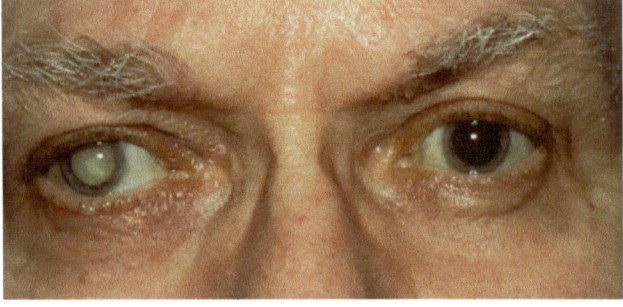

   A. Diabetic cataract
   B. Radiation therapy-induced cataract
   C. Traumatic cataract
   D. Uveitis cataract
   E. Age related cataract

12. What is the diagnosis of the eye lesion shown below:

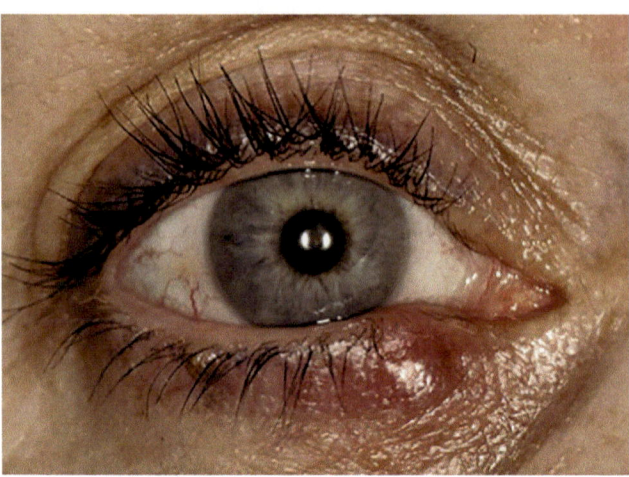

   A. Hordeolum
   B. Chalazion
   C. Basal cell carcinoma
   D. Sebaceous gland carcinoma
   E. Squamous cell carcinoma

13. Which part of the eye is commonly involved in ocular tuberculosis?
    A. Uveal tract
    B. Sclera
    C. Cornea
    D. Lens
    E. Retina

14. Which of the following eye conditions will give rise to cherry red spot at the macula?
    A. Acute angle-closure glaucoma
    B. Anterior ischemic optic neuropathy
    C. Retinal detachment
    D. Central retinal artery occlusion
    E. Vitreous hemorrhage

15. Cupping of the optic disc without hemorrhage is seen in which of the following eye conditions?
    A. Iritis
    B. Closed-angle glaucoma
    C. Episcleritis
    D. Subconjunctival hemorrhage
    E. Infectious keratitis

16. Which of the following eye conditions give rise to night blindness as the earliest symptom?
    A. Traumatic retinopathy
    B. Retinal inflammatory diseases
    C. Autoimmune paraneoplastic retinopathy

D. Drug toxicity

E. Retinitis pigmentosa

17. A 2-year-old male child is brought to the pediatrician office by his mother. Funduscopic examination is done. It shows pale retina with prominent red macular changes. Which of the following eye condition is responsible for this child's eye problems?

A. Sandhoff disease

B. Leigh syndrome

C. Neuronal ceroid lipofuscinoses

D. Tay-Sachs disease

E. GM1 gangliosidosis

18. Which of the following medical conditions give rise to intraretinal hemorrhages?

A. Hereditary spherocytosis

B. Uveitis

C. Keratoconus

D. Keratomalacia

E. Sickle cell anemia

19. Which of the following eye conditions lead to progressive thinning and cone-shaped protrusion of the cornea leading to visual impairment?

A. Keratoconus

B. Pterygium

C. Corneal ectasia

D. Interstitial keratitis

E. Pellucid marginal degeneration

20. Which of the following eye conditions have plaques and nodule composed of lipid laden histiocytes in the skin especially the eyelids?

A. Diabetes mellitus

B. Xanthelasma

C. Necrobiotic xanthogranuloma

D. Tuberous xanthomas

E. Orbital lipogranulomas

21. A 61-year-old female presents with painless proptosis of the left eye and diplopia. Imaging studies show a well-defined soft tissue mass within the left eye. Excision of the soft tissue mass is done. Microscopic picture shows large cystically dilated vascular channels with fibrous septae. What is the diagnosis?

A. Fibrous histiocytoma

B. Cavernous hemangioma

C. Hemangiopericytoma

D. Solitary fibrous tumor

E. Intraocular melanoma

22. A 42-year-old female presents for an evaluation of an eyelid lesion. Biopsy of the lesion shows volcanic-craters. What is the diagnosis?

A. Basal cell carcinoma

B. Squamous cell carcinoma

C. Molluscum contagiosum

D. Melanoma

E. Pyogenic granuloma

23. A 51-year-old male presents with bilateral blood vision and floaters. There is also bilateral intermediate uveitis. Which of the following entities would be consistent with this diagnosis?

A. Sarcoidosis

B. Non-Hodgkin lymphoma

C. Tuberculosis

D. Tularemia

E. Bartonella henselae

Answers and Explanations

1. Answer: D. Herpes simplex virus

The most frequent form of ocular HSV infection is epithelial keratitis. Prominent lesions are dendritic lesions or geographic ulcerations of the cornea. Dendrite is the characteristic form of herpetic keratitis. Epithelial lesions form vesicles. Vesicles coalesce into a linear branching dendritic lesion. Typically, bulbous thickenings are found at the ends of the branches of dendrite.

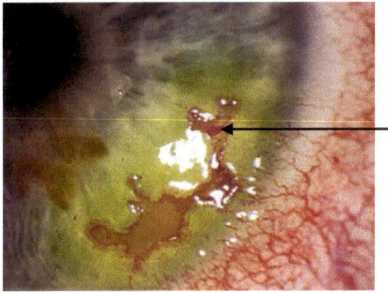

Corneal ulceration of HSV keratitis (Stained with fluorescein and Rose Bengal)

2. Answer: D. Intraocular melanoma

Uveal melanoma is the most common primary intraocular malignant tumor after cutaneous melanoma. Common locations of uveal melanomas are iris, ciliary body, and choroid. Common visual symptoms are blurring, distortion, flashes, floaters, or visual field defects. Choroidal melanomas typically are dome-shaped. Histologically, uveal melanomas are divided into spindle and epithelioid cell types. Spindle cell melanomas involve iris and are associated with better prognosis.

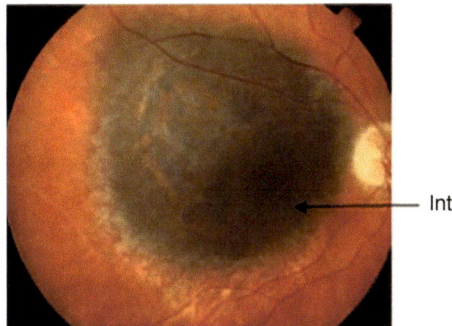

Intraocular melanoma

3. Answer: D. Diabetes mellitus

In nonproliferative type of diabetic retinopathy, findings consist of hard exudates, cotton wool spots (nerve fiber layer infarcts). Microaneurysms and dot blot hemorrhages are also found due to the rupture of microaneurysms. Visual loss is due to macular edema. In proliferative diabetic retinopathy, there is a presence of neovascularization. New vessels are fragile. Traction retinal detachment can also occur.

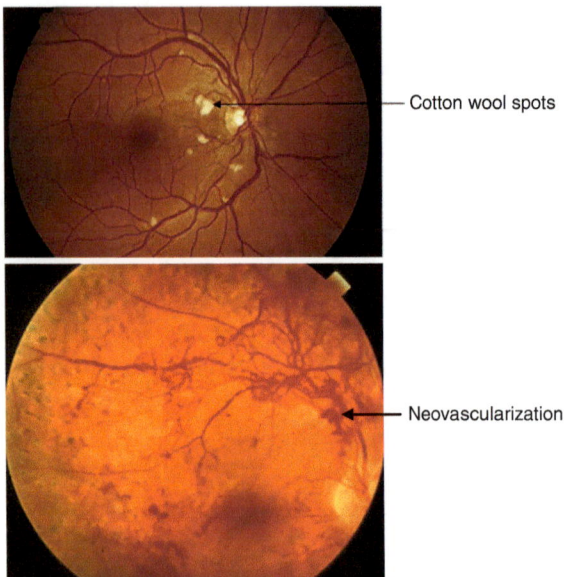
— Cotton wool spots

— Neovascularization

4. Answer: A. Breast carcinoma

Most common tumor with metastasis to the eye is breast carcinoma. Breast carcinoma accounts for approximately 47% of metastasis to the eye. Other organs which cause metastasis to the eye are lung (21%), gastrointestinal tract (4%), and renal (2%).

5. Answer: A. Flame shaped hemorrhages

Severe hypertension causes the damage of the retinal vessels. The signs are arteriovenous nicking, focal arteriolar narrowing, thickening of the arteriolar walls (copper or silver wiring), microaneurysms, cotton wool spots, retinal hemorrhages (dot blot and flame shaped).

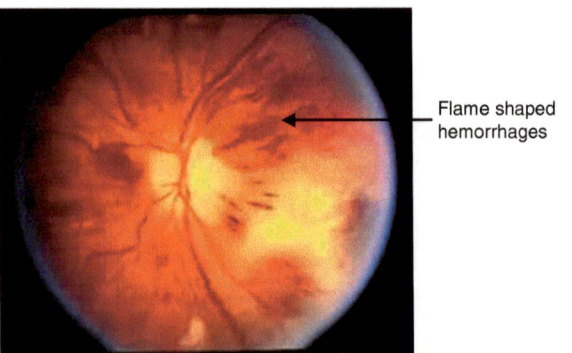
Flame shaped hemorrhages

6. Answer: C. Osteosarcoma

Retinoblastoma is the most common intraocular malignancy of childhood. Almost all cases are diagnosed before 5 years. The common clinical finding is a white eye reflex (leukocoria). Other symptoms may include strabismus, nystagmus, and red eye. Children with congenital or acquired cataract, vitreous hemorrhage may also present with leukocoria. Histologically, Flexner–Wintersteiner rosettes are highly specific of retinoblastoma. Flexner–Wintersteiner rosettes consists of primitive photoreceptor cells which resemble rods and cones, representing retinal differentiation. Individuals who have mutations in the RB1 gene are at high risk of developing secondary tumors in the future. Osteosarcoma is the most common secondary malignancy associated with retinoblastoma.

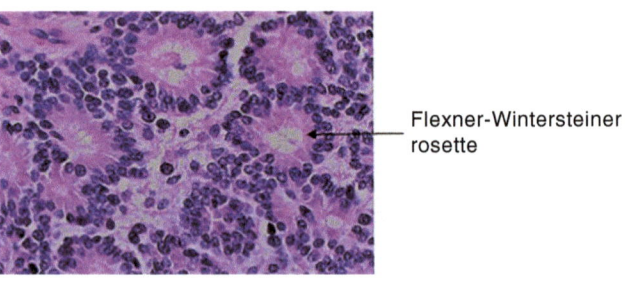
Flexner-Wintersteiner rosette

7. Answer: A. Chlamydia trachomatis

Chlamydia trachomatis is an obligate intraocular bacteria. It causes trachoma which is the leading cause of blindness worldwide.

8. Answer: A. Cellulitis

Infection of the soft tissues within the eye socket is defined as cellulitis. It is common in children. *Staphylococcus aureus* and streptococci are common pathogens which cause orbital cellulitis.

9. Answer: B. Cataract

Cataract and glaucoma are the side effects of systemic glucocorticoids (GC) therapy. Postsubcapsular cataracts (PSCs) in particular are a subtype of cataracts that occur more commonly in patients exposed to GC.

10. Answer: A. Wilson's disease

Wilson's disease is an autosomal recessive disease. It causes the disorder of copper metabolism. Copper is deposited in various organs including the eyes, liver, kidneys, and brain (leading to basal ganglia atrophy). Eye examination demonstrates Kayser Fleischer ring due to the deposition of gold-brown pigment copper within descemet's membrane in the cornea. The rings are best seen on slit-lamp examination.

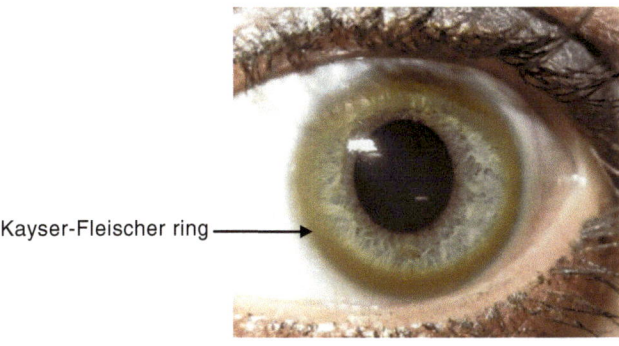

Kayser-Fleischer ring

11. Answer: E. Age related cataract

Gradual clouding and thickening of the lens of the eye is defined as a cataract. It is age related and can be treated by surgery.

12. Answer: A. Hordeolum

Localized painful and erythematous swelling of the eyelid is defined as hordeolum (Stye). It can be external or internal. Glands in the eyelash follicle cause external hordeolum. Internal hordeolum is caused by inflammation of the meibomian gland. Staphylococcus aureus is a common pathogen found in most of the cases. Acute plugging of a meibomian gland and inflammation results in a tender, red bump seen in the medial lower eyelid.

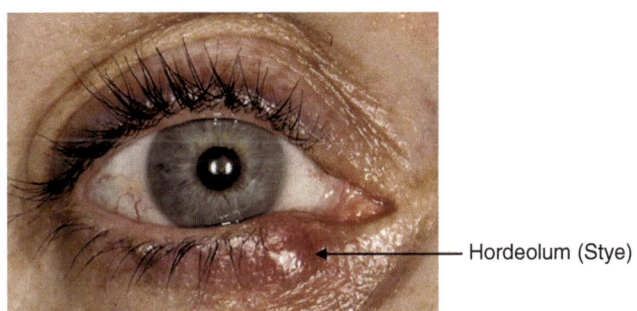

Hordeolum (Stye)

13. Answer: A. Uveal tract

Ocular tuberculosis (TB) can affect any part of the eye and may occur with or without evidence of pulmonary or extrapulmonary TB disease. Intraocular tuberculosis most commonly affects the uveal tract, which includes the iris and ciliary body (anteriorly) and the choroid (posteriorly).

14. Answer: D. Central retinal artery occlusion

In central retinal artery occlusion, there is acute monocular vision loss. On fundus examination, fovea appears as a cherry red spot and the inner layer of the retina appears milky white.

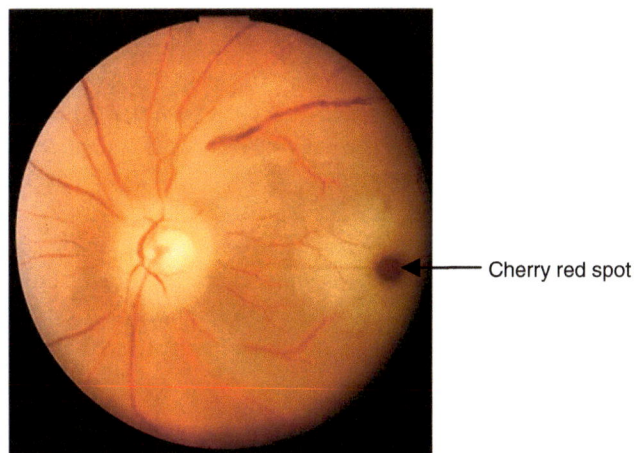

Cherry red spot

15. Answer: B. Closed-angle glaucoma

Increased pressure within the eyeball is called as glaucoma. Impaired aqueous humor drainage causes increased intraocular pressure in closed-angle glaucoma. Symptoms are acute headache, eye pain, and vision loss. Fundus examination shows cupping of the optic disc.

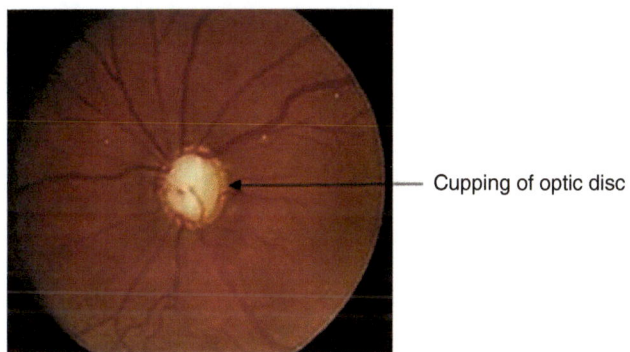

Cupping of optic disc

16. Answer: E. Retinitis pigmentosa

Night blindness (nyctalopia) is one of the earliest symptoms of retinitis pigmentosa. The classic triad of attenuated arterioles, waxy pallor of the optic disc, and intraretinal pigmentation as bone-spicules is seen on fundus examination.

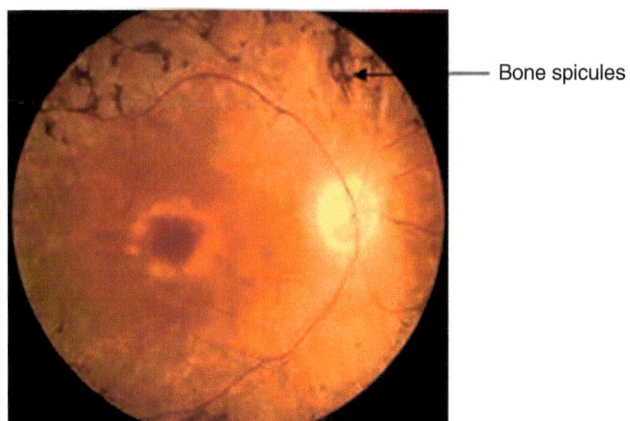

Bone spicules

17. Answer: D. Tay-Sachs disease

Excess storage of Gm2 gangliosides due to deficiency in beta-Hexosaminidase A is found in Tay-Sachs disease. It is an autosomal recessive disorder. Macular cherry red spots are seen on fundoscopic examination in Tay-Sachs disease.

18. Answer: E. Sickle cell anemia

Superficial intraretinal hemorrhages (salmon-patch hemorrhage) are ocular manifestations of sickle cell disease. Ocular manifestations are due to vascular occlusion, which may occur in the conjunctiva, iris, retina, and choroid.

19. Answer: A. Keratoconus

Keratoconus is a disorder of the cornea. It leads to thinning and cone-shaped protrusion of the cornea which causes blurred vision and sensitivity to light and glare. Keratoconus usually affects both eyes and generally affect people aged between 10 and 25 years old.

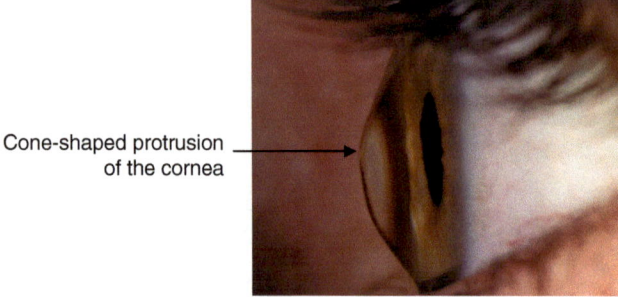

Cone-shaped protrusion of the cornea

20. Answer: B. Xanthelasma

Most eyelid lesions are benign such as hordeolum (stye), chalazion and xanthelasma. Xanthelasma appear as yellow plaques on the medial aspects of the eyelids in adults with hypercholesterolemia.

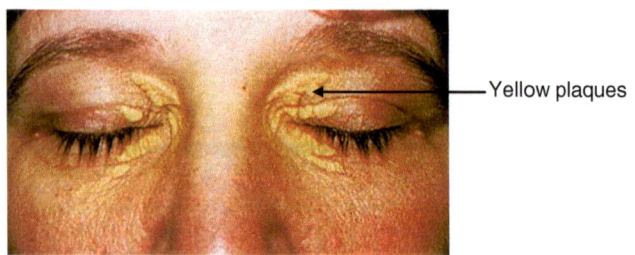

Yellow plaques

21. Answer: B. Cavernous hemangioma

Patients of cavernous hemangioma present with painless proptosis of the eye with diplopia. Histologically, cavernous hemangioma lesions appear with large cystically dilated vascular channels with fibrous septae. Imaging studies help in the diagnosis.

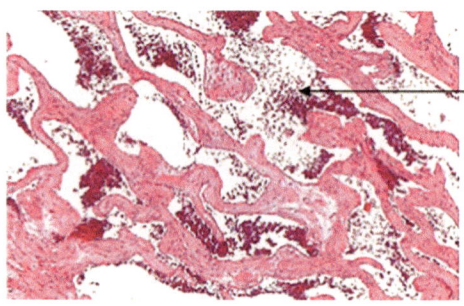

Dilated vascular channels

22. Answer: C. Molluscum contagiosum

Molluscum contagiosum presents with a raised domes polypoid lesion with an umbilicated center. This lesion is a classical form molluscum contagiosum. Histologically, volcanic micro-craters are seen separated by normal areas of skin. Micro-craters are eosinophilic inclusion bodies pathognomonic for molluscum contagiosum, referred to as Henderson–Patterson bodies.

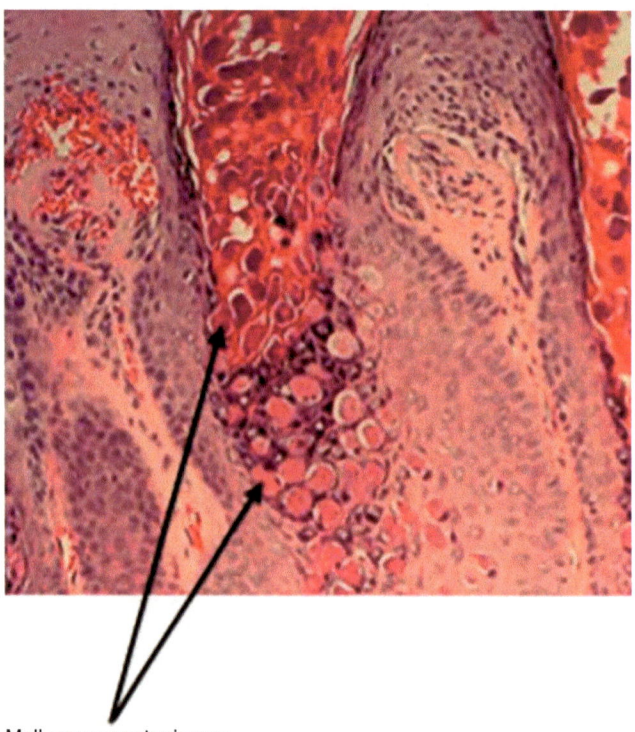

Molluscum contagiosum

23. Answer: A. Sarcoidosis

Sarcoidosis occurs in the eye in approximately 15–50% of the patients who present with systemic disease. Common ocular presentation is uveitis. Inflammatory nodules on the conjunctiva and pupillary margin are commonly seen in sarcoidosis. Histologically, sarcoidosis shows non-caseating, non-necrotizing granulomas with Langerhans giant cells, epithelioid cells along with lymphocytic aggregates.

Bibliography

1. Wang JC, Dahl AA. Herpes simplex virus (HSV) keratitis; 2018.
2. Harbour JW, et al. Initial management of uveal and conjunctival melanomas. Waltham: UptoDate; 2019.
3. McCulloch K, et al. Overview of medical care in adults with diabetes mellitus. Waltham: UptoDate; 2019.
4. Manjandavida FP, Chahar S. The art of retinoblastoma management—curable yet challenging. Kerala J Ophthalmol. 2018;30(1):17–27.
5. Modi P, Arsiwalla T. Hypertensive retinopathy. Treasure Island: StatPearls; 2019.
6. Kaufman PL, Kim J, Berry JL. Approach to the child with leukocoria. Waltham: UptoDate; 2019.
7. Satpathy G, Behera HS, Ahmed NH. Chlamydial eye infections: current perspectives. Indian J Ophthalmol. 2017;65(2):97.
8. Eske J, Griff AM. What is orbital cellulitis? Treasure Island: StatPearls Publishing; 2019.
9. Rachel J, et al. The association between systemic glucocorticoid use and the risk of cataract and glaucoma in patients with rheumatoid arthritis: a systematic review and meta-analysis. PLoS One. 2016;11(11):e0166468.
10. Joshi G, Dhingra D, Tekchandani U, Kaushik S. Kayser–Fleischer ring in Wilson's disease. QJM Int J Med. 2019;112(8):629.
11. Ocampo VVD, Dahl AA. Senile cataract (age-related cataract). New York: Medscape; 2018.
12. Duh EJ, Sun JK, Stitt AW. Diabetic retinopathy: current understanding, mechanisms, and treatment strategies. JCI Insight. 2017;2(14):e93751.
13. Rathinam SR. Tuberculosis and the eye. Waltham: Uptodate; 2019.
14. Hedges TR, et al. Central and branch retinal artery occlusion. Waltham: UptoDate; 2019.
15. Weizer SJ. Angle-closure glaucoma. Waltham: UptoDate; 2019.
16. Givre S, et al. Retinitis pigmentosa: clinical presentation and diagnosis. Waltham: UptoDate; 2019.
17. Roman AS. Preconception and prenatal carrier screening for genetic disease more common in the Ashkenazi Jewish population and others with a family history of these disorders. Waltham: UptoDate; 2019.
18. Ventocilla M. Ophthalmologic manifestations of sickle cell disease. Waltham: UptoDate; 2018.
19. Wayman LL. Keratoconus. Baltimore: Wolters Kluwer; 2019.
20. Ghosh C, Ghoshs T. Eyelid lesions. Baltimore: Wolters Kluwer; 2019.

Index

A

Abdominal aortic aneurysm (AAA), 39, 41
Acalculous cholecystitis, 99
Acanthamoeba encephalitis, 176, 181
Acanthosis nigricans, 149, 152
Acetaminophen, 93, 97
Achalasia, 87, 91
Achondroplasia, 9, 12
Actinic keratosis, 149, 152
Actinomyces israelii, 33, 36
Acute cholecystitis, 95, 99
Acute erythroid leukemia, 58, 66
Acute lymphoblastic leukemia, 56, 64
Acute monocytic leukemia, 56, 63
Acute myeloblastic leukemia without maturation (AML-M1), 58, 66
Acute myeloid leukemia, 53, 59
Acute promyelocytic leukemia, 53
Acute respiratory distress syndrome (ARDS), 69, 71
Addison's disease, 143, 145
Adenocarcinoma of gallbladder, 95, 100
Adenoid cystic carcinoma (ACC), 79, 83, 136, 139
Adenomyosis, 129, 132
Alcoholic fatty liver, 94, 98
Alcoholic hepatitis, 96, 97, 101, 103
Alcoholism, 57
Alpha-1 antitrypsin (AAT) deficiency, 93, 97
Alport syndrome, 114, 119
Alveolar soft part sarcoma (ASPS), 159, 165
Alzheimer disease, 176, 182
Amylin, 108
Amyloidosis, 62, 118
Amyotrophic lateral sclerosis, 169, 171
Anaplastic large cell lymphoma, 25, 28
Anaplastic lymphoma kinase (ALK) fusion oncogene, 70, 73
Anemia, 58
Anemia of chronic disease (ACD), 66
Anencephaly, 177, 184
Angiogenesis, 2, 5
Angionimmunoblastic T-cell lymphoma, 25, 28
Angiosarcoma, 95, 100
Anitschkow cells, 47
Ankylosing spondylitis (AS), 18, 21
Ankyrin, 56, 63
Anorexia nervosa (AN), 145, 148
Antineutrophil cytoplasmic antibodies (ANCA), 116
Antiplatelet antibodies, 53, 58
Aplastic anemia, 54, 59
Apoptosis, 1, 4, 102
Apoptotic bodies, 4
Arachidonic acid, 6
Arachidonic acid metabolites, 2, 5
Aschoff body, 45, 47

Aspergillosis, 31, 34
Asplenia, 53, 59
Astrocytoma, 178, 186
Ataxia telangiectasia, 11, 14
Atherosclerosis, 39, 41, 117
Atrophy, 2, 5
Atypical (walking) pneumonia, 34
Atypical ductal hyperplasia, 135, 137
Auspitz sign, 152
Autoimmune adrenalitis, 143, 145
Axillary lymph node status, 136, 138

B

Bacterial pneumonia, 70, 73
Balanitis, 121, 123
Balanoposthitis, 123
Barrett esophagus, 86, 88, 90
Basal cell adenoma, 79, 83
Basal cell carcinoma, 150, 153
Basophilic stippling, 60
Becker muscular dystrophy (BMD), 169, 171
Beckwith-Wiedemann syndrome, 96, 102, 116
Bell's palsy, 184
Benign prostatic hyperplasia, 122, 124
Benign salivary gland tumors, 80
Benign tumor, 25
Berger's disease, 113, 118
Beta-cell tumors, 105, 107
β Thalassemia, 54, 59
Birbeck granule, 149, 151
Bite cells, 61
Bloom syndrome, 9, 12
Bones, joints, and soft tissue disorders
    ASPS, 159, 165
    avascular necrosis, 158, 164
    chondroblastoma, 162, 166
    chondrosarcoma, 158, 164
    desmoid tumor, 161, 166
    DFSP, 159, 165
    Ewing sarcoma, 158, 164
    fibrous dysplasia, 161, 166
    giant cell tumor, 157, 163
    gout, 157, 163
    hibernoma, 160, 165
    lipoma, 159, 165
    liposarcoma, 160, 165
    multiple myeloma, 160, 165
    nodular fasciitis, 161, 166
    onion peel appearance, 158, 163
    osteoarthritis, 162, 167
    osteoblastoma, 157, 163